Best Care in Early Psychosis Intervention

Best Care in Early Psychosis Intervention

Global Perspectives

Edited by

Tom Ehmann PhD
Consultant Psychologist
Early Psychosis Intervention (EPI) Program
White Rock, BC; and Provincial Liaison,
British Columbia Schizophrenia Society,
Vancouver, BC
Canada

G William MacEwan MD
Director, Schizophrenia Program
Department of Psychiatry
Division of Clinical Neuroscience
University of British Columbia
St Vincent's Hospital
Vancouver, BC
Canada

William G Honer MD
Jack Bell Chair of Schizophrenia Research
Department of Psychiatry
University of British Columbia
Vancouver, BC
Canada

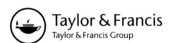

Taylor & Francis
Taylor & Francis Group

LONDON AND NEW YORK

A MARTIN DUNITZ BOOK

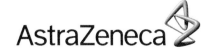

The AstraZeneca logotype is a trademark of the AstraZeneca group of companies

Made possible by an unrestricted educational grant from AstraZeneca

© 2004 Taylor & Francis, an imprint of the Taylor & Francis Group

First published in the United Kingdom in 2004
by Taylor & Francis, an imprint of the Taylor & Francis Group, 2 Park Square,
Milton Park, Abingdon, Oxon OX14 4RN

Tel.:   +44 (0) 1235 828 600
Fax.:   +44 (0) 1235 829 000
E-mail: info@dunitz.co.uk
Website: http://www.dunitz.co.uk

Although every effort has been made to ensure that all owners of copyright material have been acknowledged in this publication, we would be glad to acknowledge
in subsequent reprints or editions any omissions brought to our attention.

Although every effort has been made to ensure that drug doses and other information are presented accurately in this publication, the ultimate responsibility rests
with the prescribing physician. Neither the publishers, nor the authors, nor
AstraZeneca can be held responsible for errors or for any consequences arising
from the use of information contained herein.

A CIP record for this book is available from the British Library.

Library of Congress Cataloging-in-Publication Data
Data available on application

ISBN 1 84184 403 9

Composition by Wearset Ltd, Boldon, Tyne and Wear, UK

Printed and bound in Spain by Grafos SA Arte Sobre Papel

Contents

Section III State-of-the-Art Applications

Contributors

Donald Addington MD
Professor and Head
Department of Psychiatry and Psychosis Research
Unit, University of Calgary
Early Psychosis Program
Calgary Health Region
Calgary, Alberta
Canada T2N 2T9

Jean Addington PhD
Associate Professor
Department of Psychiatry
University of Toronto
Center for Addiction and Mental Health
250 College Street
Toronto, Ontario
Canada M5T 1R8

G Paul Amminger MD
Associate Professor
Department of Child and Adolescent Psychiatry
PACE Clinic Vienna
Medical University of Vienna
Währinger Gürtel 18–20
Vienna
Austria A-1090

Sawagata Bapat
ORYGEN Youth Health
Locked Bag 10
Parkville
Vic 3052
Australia

Richard P Bentall PhD
Professor of Experimental Clinical Psychology
Department of Psychology
University of Manchester
Coupland 1 Building
Oxford Road
Manchester M13 9PL
UK

Max J Birchwood
Director, Birmingham Early Intervention Service
Birmingham and Solihull Mental Health Trust
Professor, Department of Psychology
University of Birmingham
Edgbaston
Birmingham
B15 2TT
UK

Warrick Brewer PhD
Senior Lecturer
ORYGEN Research Centre
Department of Psychiatry
University of Melbourne
Locked Bag 10
Parkville, Vic 3052
Australia

Jenny L Bywaters MA BM
Director of Professional Liaison and Public
Health
National Institute for Mental Health in England
Blenheim House, West One
Duncombe Street
Leeds LS1 4PL
UK

Eric Chen
Department of Psychiatry
The University of Hong Kong
Queen Mary Hospital
Hong Kong, China

Philippe Conus
Privat Docent University Lausanne, Switzerland;
and Senior Lecturer, University of Melbourne,
Australia
Clinique de Cery
10098 Prilly
Switzerland

Eric Davis
Director
Gloucester Early Intervention Service

Jane Edwards
Associate Professor
Director, Clinical Services
ORYGEN Youth Health
Locked Bag 10
Parkville, Vic 3052
Australia

Tom Ehmann PhD
Consultant Psychologist
Early Psychosis Intervention (EPI) Program
White Rock, BC; and Provincial Liaison, British
Columbia
Schizophrenia Society
Vancouver, BC
Canada

Peter Falkai MD
Professor and Head of the Department of
Psychiatry and Psychotherapy
University of Saarland
Kirrberger Strasse, 66421 Homburg/Saar
Germany

Robin Friedlander MD
Psychiatrist; Clinical Associate Professor, UBC;
Clinical Director, West Coast and Fraser Valley
MHSTs
BC Childrens Hospital
Neuropsychiatry Clinic
4480 Oak Street
Vancouver,
BC, Canada V6H 3V4

Wolfgang Gaebel MD
Professor and Speaker of the Network
Schizophrenia
Head of the Department of Psychiatry at the
Heinrich-Heine-University
Rheinische Kliniken Düsseldorf, University of
Düsseldorf
Bergische Landstrasse 2, 40649 Düsseldorf
Germany

John Gleeson
Associate Professor
Department of Psychology
ORYGEN Youth Health
University of Melbourne
Locked Bag 10
Parkville, Vic 3052
Australia

Kimberley P Good PhD
Department of Psychiatry
Dalhousie University
9216-5909 Veteran's Memorial Lane
Halifax, NS B3H 2E2
Canada

Steve Haines
Formerly EPPIC Statewide Services
ORYGEN Youth Health
University of Melbourne
Locked Bag 10
Parkville, Vic 3052
Australia

Laura Hanson PhD
Project Manager
Early Psychosis Intervention (EPI) Program
15521 Russell Avenue
White Rock, BC V4B 2R4
Canada

Meredith Harris
Research Fellow
ORYGEN Research Centre
Department of Psychiatry
University of Melbourne
Locked Bag 10
Parkville, Vic 3052
Australia

William G Honer MD
Jack Bell Chair of Schizophrenia Research
Department of Psychiatry
University of British Columbia
Vancouver, BC
Canada

Irfan Khanbhai MD
Department of Psychiatry
St. Paul's Hospital
Vancouver, BC, Canada

Claudia Klier MD
PACE Clinic Vienna
Medical University of Vienna
Währinger Gürtel 18–20
A-1090 Vienna
Austria

Lili Kopala MD FRCPC
Clinical Professor of Psychiatry
Center for Complex Disorders
University of British Columbia
Vancouver
Canada

Helen Krstev
Northwestern Mental Health Program
ORYGEN Youth Health
University of Melbourne
Locked Bag 10
Parkville, Vic 3052
Australia

Tania Lecomte
Assistant Professor of Psychiatry
University of British Columbia
828 West 10th Avenue, Room 214
Vancouver, BC V52 1L8
Canada

Jeffrey A Lieberman MD
Professor of Psychiatry, Pharmacology and
Radiology
Vice-Chair, Department of Psychiatry
Director of the Mental Health Research Center
CB# 7160
University of North Carolina
Chapel Hill, NC 27599-7160
USA

G William MacEwan MD
Director, Schizophrenia Program
Department of Psychiatry
Division of Clinical Neuroscience
University of British Columbia
St Vincent's Hospital
Vancouver, BC
Canada

Eric MacNaughton MA
Canadian Mental Health Association
Vancouver, Canada

William R McFarlane MD
Department of Psychiatry
Maine Medical Center
University of Vermont
Columbia University, College
of Physicians and Surgeons
22 Bramhall Street
Portland, ME 04102
USA

Patrick D McGorry MBBS PhD FRANZCP
Professor and Executive Director
Department of Psychiatry
ORYGEN Youth Health
University of Melbourne
Locked Bag 10
Parkville, Vic 3052
Australia

Kathryn Mckay
Department of Psychiatry
University of British Columbia
Vancouver, BC
Canada

Ross Norman PhD
Department of Psychiatry
London Health Sciences Centre
University of Western Ontario
392 South Street
London, Ontario N6A 4G5
Canada

Ruth Ohlsen
Clinical Research Nurse
Section of Neurochemical Imaging and Psychiatry
PO Box 54
Institute of Psychiatry
De Crespigny Park
London SE5 8AF
UK

Kerryn Pennell
Department of Psychiatry
ORYGEN Youth Health
University of Melbourne
Locked Bag 10
Parkville, Vic 3052
Australia

Diana O Perkins MD MPH
Associate Professor of Psychiatry
University of North Carolina School of Medicine
Department of Psychiatry CB# 7160
Chapel Hill, NC 27599-7160
USA

Lyn S Pilowsky MRCPsych PhD
Reader and Head of Section of Neurochemical
Imaging and Psychiatry
Box 54
Institute of Psychiatry
De Crespigny Park, Denmark Hill
London SE5 8AF
UK

Deepika Ratnaike BA
Evaluation and Quality Coordinator
ORYGEN Research Centre
Department of Psychiatry
University of Melbourne
Locked Bag 10
Parkville, Vic 3052
Australia

Karen Tee PhD
Program Manager
Early Psychosis Intervention Program
15521 Russell Avenue
White Rock, BC
V4B 2R4
Canada

Laurel A Townsend PhD
Saanich Child and Youth Mental Health Services
Ministry of Children and Family Development
PO Box 9753 Stn Prov Govt
Victoria, BC V8W 953
Canada

David Shiers
Primary Mental Health Care Lead
West Midlands Regional Development Centre
(NIMHE) and Carer.

Geoffrey N Smith
Department of Psychiatry
British Columbia
Vancouver, BC
Canada

Jo Smith
Director
Worcester Early Intervention Service

Darryl Wade MA
Clinical Psychologist
ORYGEN Youth Health
Locked Bag 10
Parkville, Vic 3052
Australia

Thomas Wobrock MD
Department of Psychiatry and Psychotherapy,
University of Saarland
Kirrberger Strasse
66421 Homburg/Saar
Germany

Lisa Wong GradDipEdPsych
Senior Research Assistant
ORYGEN Research Centre
Department of Psychiatry
University of Melbourne
Locked Bag 10
Parkville, Vic 3052
Australia

Annemarie Wright
ORYGEN Youth Health
University of Melbourne
Locked Bag 10
Parkville, Vic 3052
Australia

Foreword

In recent years early diagnosis and phase-specific treatment of psychotic disorders has been pioneered and progressively translated to countless clinical settings and communities around the world. Canada has played a unique leadership role in this international reform process and early psychosis programs span the nation from coast to coast. It is therefore not a surprise that the editors of this volume are Canadian, based in Vancouver, the host city for the 4th International Early Psychosis Conference (2004). They have done a remarkable job in assembling a unique resource for this growing clinical field.

The ultimate aim of early intervention in psychotic disorders is to bring about maximum and sustained recovery from these potentially fatal and disabling illnesses with minimum disruption and collateral damage to the lives of those affected and their families. To achieve these goals requires serious endeavour on a number of fronts. Firstly, the logic and conceptual basis for early intervention must be clearly understood by all concerned and it must be seen as a realistic possibility. This is an educational task, almost a form of 'deprogramming' for many, since the therapeutic nihilism surrounding schizophrenia in particular remains tenacious. The case for early detection and diagnosis, and the value of

phase-specific interventions, which differ qualitatively from those appropriate to later stages of disorder, must be made. Secondly, the need for service reform and restructuring must be embraced, and strategies, tactics and models to engineer this described with the aid of multiple examples of successful approaches from a variety of settings. Thirdly, the building blocks of clinical interventions in early psychosis need to be created and described in detail and training in this new skill set developed. A related aspect is the fundamental requirement for expertise in quality assurance and the measurement of health outcomes. Fourthly, the central place of clinical research in such an innovative field should be celebrated and endorsed as a vital strategy to ensure that reform and clinical care is supported as far as possible by a solid evidence base. Evidence-based medicine is best seen as a genuine guide, even an insurance policy for sustainable reform. It should not be misused, as some have advocated, as a constraint or reason to stand still. Truly evidence-based health care remains an ideal at this stage. Yet the highest ideal remains quality of life and better outcomes for patients and families.

This wonderful book covers all of these central tasks, providing state-of-the-art knowledge from a superb array of international pioneers and contributors from North America, Asia, Europe and Australia. It will prove an essential resource for years to come in countless settings across the globe.

Patrick McGorry MD PhD FRCP FRANZCP
Director, ORYGEN Youth Health (incorporating EPPIC) and ORYGEN Research Centre; Professor, University of Melbourne Department of Psychiatry, Australia

Preface

Early intervention in psychotic disorders represents a paradigm shift in our conceptualization and treatment of psychosis. This development has generated worldwide excitement among professionals, patients, and their families. The creation and effective delivery of appropriate clinical services in early psychosis promises to have the most significant impact upon outcomes for serious mental illness since the introduction of the antipsychotic medications in the 1950s.

There has long been understanding that psychotic disorders, such as schizophrenia, schizo-affective disorder and related psychotic disorders, are severe illnesses with high morbidity and mortality. The World Health Organization (WHO) ranked active psychosis as the third most disabling medical condition with the main psychotic disorders decreasing lifespan by about 10 years. According to the WHO, about 2% of all disability-adjusted life years (i.e. years of 'healthy living' lost) are accounted for by schizophrenia and bipolar disorder alone.[1] Unfortunately, improvements in the treatment of psychosis have failed to improve outcomes significantly. Antipsychotic medications have helped to relieve some of the suffering of psychosis and allowed more patients to live in the community, but fully two thirds of patients still have an unsatisfactory response. Similarly, deinstitutionalization has not achieved its goals of improving psychiatric and social functioning while integrating persons into the community. Finally, therapeutic pessimism has impeded the advance of fresh approaches to psychotic illnesses.

The early psychosis movement fostered new ways to view the treatment and outcome of psychosis. Early intervention in psychosis, which started as a research approach to understanding schizophrenia, generated debate regarding its validity and utility. We wholeheartedly endorse the view stated by Edwards and McGorry that 'to argue against early detection and optimal treatment seems to defend the indefensible'.[2] Max Birchwood, more playfully, noted that it is quite incredible that arguments could be forwarded advocating for late, rather than early intervention and that nowhere else in medicine would such a concept be seriously considered. We believe the more sober debate now revolves around the question of defining 'early' in early intervention. Our experience is that many professionals and the public confuse intervention shortly after the onset of psychosis with the idea that psychosis onset itself can be averted via intervention with someone who may be experiencing an onset prodrome. The field needs clarity in communicating the difference between these issues as the latter carries many ethical and practice issues that merit the considerable research and debate it is receiving.

The early psychosis clinical treatment movement, typified by the Early Psychosis Prevention and Intervention Center (EPPIC) in Melbourne, spearheaded the concepts that appropriate comprehensive care of persons with psychosis begin quickly but not so aggressively that long-term engagement is jeopardized. Durations of untreated psychosis dropped from averages of two years prior to interventions to less than six months. The concept gained such strength that in countries like Denmark and Britain national early psychosis intervention (EPI) programs were developed. Positive research findings from projects such as OPUS in Scandinavia,[3] Canada,[4] and elsewhere showed that early intervention programs were effective. Earlier, carefully conducted research showed that full symptomatic recovery was possible in 80% within one year for first episode patients with schizophrenia and other psychoses.[5]

These developments began to change the view of the psychosis landscape. Schizophrenia went from being 'chronic and debilitating' to potentially curable. Patients were seen rapidly and often. Interventions were expected to have outcomes in weeks rather than months. If no positive results occurred early, treatment teams asked why and moved onto different interventions rather than wait and wait. Treatment moved from high dose antipsychotics only to combination therapies. For example, low dose atypical antipsychotic medications combined with psychoeducational and other group treatments are now the expected form of therapy in all programs. Other treatments, such as cognitive behavioral therapy and substance abuse programs, were included. Families became an integral part of the treatment process, as a source of collateral information and support.

Early psychosis intervention (EPI) became a medical and social phenomenon. Early psychosis programs proliferated from a few in Australia and Scandinavia to all regions of the globe. These programs embraced the new age of information technologies in contrast to other areas in psychiatry. Early psychosis websites, such as www.psychosissucks.ca in Canada, and public awareness campaigns, such as the TIPS project in Norway, brought issues of burden of disease for psychosis, and its potential treatments, to the forefront in both medical and public arenas.

As EPI matured, many clinical groups realized that to say you were treating psychosis early could mean many things. Treatment protocols and monitoring of outcomes have become ways to address the potential variance in the treatment of patients with early psychosis and how well they recovered over time. Delivering optimal practices in EPI is now an expectation.

Our book intends to capture the excitement and energy of the early days of EPI and help funnel it towards implementing current best practices. We hope to supplement the dialogue that is already occurring both informally between treatment teams worldwide and more formally through organizations such as the International Early Psychosis Association (IEPA).

This book is divided into three sections. The Guide to Clinical Care, authored by Drs Tom Ehmann and Laura Hanson, aims to assist clinicians and administrators. This guide is intended both as a stimulus for EPI and as a fairly comprehensive reference source. It represents a synthesis of the latest and most significant research and practices in delivering comprehensive care. Topics include the rationale for early intervention, assessment, pharmacologic, psychotherapeutic, and psychosocial treatments and discussions of special populations, such as those with intellectual disability or substance abuse. The guide also examines service delivery systems and outcome measurement, and provides a compendium of early psychosis resources. In sum, it lays out a framework for EPI best care practices and constitutes a good primer in other specialized areas.

In the book's second section, clinicians and researchers from around the world describe how EPI principles are translated into the development of service programs. This section is meant to highlight how different programs have identified barriers to EPI and then describe the solutions they have achieved. Topics range from Dr Eric Chen's review of the ethnocultural issues his program faced in Hong Kong to the complexity of the national initiative in the UK. Specific programs in various stages of development are presented from Vancouver, London, Lausanne, and rural Australia.

The third section of the book offers commentary by leading practitioners and researchers in specific areas, including pharmacotherapy, cognitive therapy, prodromal intervention, family and other psychosocial interventions, the utility of neurocognitive assessment and maintaining treatment integrity. It also contains chapters that illustrate the relevance of basic research and epidemiology to early intervention. These chapters are not intended to be an extensive review of these topics but rather more focused perspectives from experts in the area.

This book seeks to guide readers on current optimal practices, provide diverse perspectives on service delivery efforts, and update some interesting clinical and research developments. Our greatest hope is that the discussions presented will resonate with your own interests and experiences and energize you further to advance the global early intervention movement.

Acknowledgment

We would like to thank AstraZeneca Canada Inc. for fully funding the development of this book through an unrestricted educational grant. The selection of editors, authors and the content of the book were strictly independent of the grant.

Tom Ehmann
White Rock, British Columbia, Canada
GW MacEwan
Vancouver, British Columbia, Canada
WG Honer
Vancouver, British Columbia, Canada

References

1. World Health Organization. *World Health Report 2001. Mental Health: New Understanding, New Hope.* Geneva: World Health Organization; 2001.

2. Edwards JM, McGorry PD. Implementing Early Intervention in Psychosis: A Guide to Establishing Early Psychosis Services. London: Martin Dunitz; 2002.

3. Jorgensen P, Nordentoft M, Abel MB, et al. Early detection and assertive community treatment of young psychotics: the Opus Study Rationale and design of the trial. Soc Psychiatry Psychiatr Epidemiol 2000; **35**(7):283–7.

4. Malla A, Norman R, McLean T, et al. A Canadian programme for early intervention in non-affective psychotic disorders. Aust N Z J Psychiatry 2003; **37**(4):407–13.

5. Lieberman J, Jody D, Geisler S, et al. Time course and biologic correlates of treatment response in first-episode schizophrenia. Arch Gen Psychiatry 1993; **50**(5):369–76.

Section I Guide to Clinical Care for Early Psychosis

Senior authors

Tom Ehmann PhD
Laura Hanson PhD

Assistant authors for selected materials

Robin Friedlander MD (Developmental disabilities)
Irfan Khanbhai MD (Acute inpatient presentations)
Eric MacNaughton MA (Psychoeducation, Community functioning)

Acknowledgments

This *Guide to Clinical Care* was created with the support of the BC Schizophrenia Society aided by an unrestricted development grant from Eli-Lilly Canada. An earlier version was written in support of the British Columbia Early Psychosis Initiative, an inter-ministerial project funded by the Ministry of Health and the Ministry of Children and Family Development and administered by the Mental Health Evaluation and Community Consultation Unit of the University of British Columbia.

Emmanuel Stip MD, Donald Addington MD and Philippe Conus MD kindly provided comments on this document.

We also wish to thank the following individuals for their comments and contributions to earlier drafts of the manuscript. These contributors included researchers, clinicians, administrators and consumer representatives: Jean Addington PhD, Miriam Cohen RN, Jane Duval, Dave Erickson PhD, Sean Flynn MD, John Gray PhD, Jim Harris BSc Pharm, Ruth Hess-Dolgin MSW, William Honer MD, Josephine Hua BSc, Peter Liddle MD, Otto Lim MSW, GW MacEwan MD, Fred Ott BSc OT, LauraLynn Rheinhardt MSc and Karen Tee PhD.

1

Introduction

Tom Ehmann and Laura Hanson

This guide summarizes current knowledge of early psychosis intervention and intends to:

- Increase understanding of the rationale behind early intervention and the guiding principles of care and support for persons in the early phase of psychotic disorders
- Guide clinicians in specific aspects of management
- Reduce unwanted variations in clinical practice by encouraging the use of appropriate procedures and services
- Act as a planning vehicle to improve service delivery systems and guide policymakers in implementing changes to mental health systems and policies.

The emphasis of this guide is on service delivery for adolescent and young adult populations presenting with early psychosis. Research related to etiology, pathophysiology, or epidemiology of early psychosis is not within the scope of this review. The goal of attempting to prevent onset of a psychotic disorder is also not addressed with the exception of Chapter 21, concerning the onset prodrome.

An evidence-based approach was employed. Information and advice are based on a thorough review of published research evidence plus comprehensive published reviews, existing clinical practice guidelines, and meta-analyses. Emphasis was placed on controlled studies, with uncontrolled trials and quasi-experimental designs used where they provided information unavailable through controlled trials. Priority was given to literature specific to early psychosis. When such evidence was not available, studies from the general literature on schizophrenia, bipolar disorder, and other psychoses were utilized. Finally, published expert opinion formed an important third source upon which discussions are based. Many of the practices being undertaken to support the principles of early intervention are quite new and the body of research available on those practices is often limited.

Information in this guide is not intended to apply to psychotic conditions that have become chronic. However, many individuals who have experienced several psychotic episodes would likely benefit from the interventions discussed. The term 'early psychosis' is loosely defined as approximately five years after onset of psychotic symptoms. In the text, readers will find references to both 'first episode' and 'early psychosis'. The terms are not necessarily interchangeable and the authors strove to indicate when a study was restricted to first episode cases by retaining that term.

The assessment and treatment discussions are applicable to individuals presenting with various psychotic disorders. However, most knowledge is derived from studies of schizophrenia and, to a lesser extent, bipolar disorder. Whenever possible, evidence directly pertaining to other psychotic disorders has been incorporated.

This guide covers fundamental clinical care issues. It is not a critique of all possible approaches nor is it a 'how-to-cook' book outlining specific techniques in detail. It is not exhaustive and does not rule out numerous approaches that may be merited in particular cases. It is not a standard of care and does not stipulate a single correct approach for all clinical situations. Decisions regarding specific procedures for specific individuals with psychosis remain the responsibility of the attending professionals.

The following principles pertaining to psychosis and early intervention were adhered to in writing the guide:

- The stress-vulnerability model accounts for the development of psychosis.
  - This model asserts that predisposing factors such as genetic make-up can render an individual susceptible to developing a psychotic disorder. The disorder becomes manifest given sufficient triggering factors. This process can pertain to both initial onset and subsequent episodes of psychosis.

- Interventions should be phase- and age-specific.
  - There are phases to a psychotic disorder: vulnerability (high risk), prodromal, acute, recovery, remission, and relapse. Each phase carries implications for assessment, treat-

ment, and support. The types of care offered should be age-appropriate.

- Optimal care consists of integrated biopsychosocial approaches tailored to each individual.
  - Psychotic disorders produce pervasive changes in individuals and social networks. Care needs to encompass the entire spectrum of areas important to an individual's well-being rather than focus solely on the signs and symptoms of psychosis. Psychosocial treatments have both direct effects and interactive effects when combined with pharmacologic interventions targeting psychosis and associated secondary problems.

- Empirically validated interventions lead to better outcomes.
  - Validated interventions undertaken by trained caregivers produce better outcomes. This guide can help educate professionals as to those practices currently believed to be optimal. Practitioners should strive to stay within their competencies, advocate for and receive training where needed, and seek others' expertise through referral and consultation.

- Care should be provided in the least restrictive setting possible.
  - The least restrictive setting is one that affords the individual the greatest possible number of personal rights and choices, yet still provides necessary services and safety.

2

Rationale for Early Intervention

Tom Ehmann and Laura Hanson

The costs of psychosis

Psychotic conditions constitute a major public health issue. A person in the midst of a psychotic episode experiences tremendous distress and may engage in actions that are dangerous to themself or others. The burden resulting from psychosis is substantial. Onset in late adolescence causes major disruptions in the ability of individuals to meet developmental tasks. Social, sexual, academic, and vocational challenges may be threatened as are consolidation of personal independence, identity, and values. Family relationships are often severely stressed, and individuals experiencing psychosis are prone to other psychopathologies, victimization, poverty, and increased medical problems.

Together with the horrific personal costs to individuals and families come immense economic and societal costs. The World Health Organization (WHO) ranked active psychosis as the third most disabling condition—higher than paraplegia and blindness. According to the WHO, about 2% of all disability-adjusted life years (i.e. years of 'healthy living' lost) are accounted for by schizophrenia and bipolar disorder, and lifespan is decreased by about 10 years.[1] About 40% of males and 25% of females in western nations show persistent moderate-to-severe disability.[2]

The introduction of the atypical antipsychotics in the last 15 years has been coupled with a renewed interest in social and psychological processes, such as neuropsychological functioning, and psychotherapeutics, such as cognitive therapy. These developments, together with the emphases on community care and research into the causes and course determinants of the major psychotic disorders, produced both a new optimism and increased interest in the onset and early stages of psychotic disorders. Research pointed out that young persons with psychoses often experienced significant delays before assessment and treatments were started. Also, these procedures were often traumatizing, alienating, and poorly applied over time.[3] Together, these events led to the creation and refinement of service delivery systems around the world, such as the Early Psychosis Prevention and Intervention Centre (EPPIC) program in Melbourne and the spawning of the International Early Psychosis Association. Despite the research efforts of these programs to use data to refine clinical practice, there remain many areas of clinical care that do not enjoy quality research support. The pioneering innovations made by many groups in response to perceived clinical need are now being improved and subjected to empirical validation. Thus, the challenge of caring for persons early remains a work in progress. The rationale for intervening early, rather than late, in the course of illness retains a logic that is very difficult to criticize. Before examining the rationale and goals of early intervention in greater detail, a review of the course and outcomes of psychotic disorders is warranted.

Course and outcomes in psychotic disorders

The most common diagnoses associated with psychosis are schizophrenia, schizophreniform disorder, schizoaffective disorder, bipolar disorder, and major depression with psychotic features. The use of substances that can induce psychosis has increased significantly and clinicians are encountering such psychotic presentations in many settings around the world.

Most psychotic disorders tend to follow a relapsing course wherein periods of acute psychosis are preceded by periods of disruption (a 'prodrome') and followed by recovery, deterioration, and subsequent re-emergence of florid psychosis. Conceptualizing the disorder as consisting of these phases suggests that different strategies become appropriate for assessment and treatment at each stage.[4]

With respect to outcome, when all psychotic disorders are considered, about half of patients were considered to have a good outcome after 15 years (schizophrenia 38% vs other psychoses 55%).[5] However, if more stringent criteria are used that exclude patients who had an episode of treatment in the previous two years, showed no symptoms, and enjoyed a reasonably high level of functioning, the proportion of recovered patients falls to 16% for those with schizophrenia and 36% for those with other psychoses.[5]

Schizophrenia

For schizophrenia, males generally have an onset of psychosis during adolescence or early twenties. Females tend to have an onset when they are several years older. About 39% of males and 23% of females have onset of schizophrenia before age 19.[6] Onset of bipolar disorder is slightly later with about 25% occurring before age 20.[7]

Numerous studies of first episode patients with schizophrenia have reported on long-term outcomes. Typically, about 20–30% of first episode patients recover with no persisting symptoms.[8] Poor symptomatic outcomes are found in 20–42% of cases. Moderate-to-severe functional and/or social impairment is found in at least half of patients after five years.[9] One five-year prospective study found that 30% of patients were considered to have a good outcome with 14% doing poorly and 56% having an intermediate outcome.[10] About 27% had competitive employment and good social networks and almost 40% showed no or minimal symptoms. About half of the 20% not on medication at five years had good outcomes. However, other studies have reported worse outcomes with about 50% doing poorly and less than 20% being in remission after five years.[11] A recent epidemiological outcome study reported that three quarters of first episode patients with schizophrenia and almost half of those with non-affective psychoses were receiving work disability benefits after five years. Nine percent of the schizophrenia patients and 39% of the non-schizophrenia patients were rated as not being in need of treatment.[12] In contrast to these overall general response rates, data from studies with high medication adherence rates present a more favorable picture of recovery. For example, one study employing injectible medication reported that about 85% of first episode patients were considered symptomatically recovered by one year,[13] while another early psychosis program reported that less than 10% of patients showed positive symptoms at one year.[14]

Persons with schizophrenia who are male, with cognitive impairment, less education, and lower premorbid functioning levels tend to have poorer outcomes.[15] Additional predictors of poorer long-term outcomes include onsets associated with younger age, history of drug abuse, lack of close friends, and negative symptoms.[5] Schizophrenia is associated with poorer functional outcomes and slower recoveries from episodes than other psychotic disorders.[5,16]

Bipolar disorder

Bipolar disorder is a prototypical relapsing-remitting psychiatric disorder. Lifetime prevalence is about 1.6%.[17] Patients who have ever been hospitalized are expected to spend about 20% of their lifetime in episodes (starting from the onset of their disorder).[18] One half of bipolar episodes last between two and seven months (median three months), with inter-episode intervals shortening over time, 10–15% of persons will have at least 10 lifetime episodes,[19] and about 90% of youths with mania will continue to have adult recurrences.[20]

A 15 year follow-up of bipolar patients found that 17% showed a poor overall long-term outcome. Full compliance with medication, younger age at onset, and male sex predicted good outcome. Younger age at onset as well as male sex, but not full compliance, also predicted a favorable psychosocial outcome.[21] These results are not all duplicated as others reported that time to syndromal recovery and functional recovery was associated with older age at onset and shorter hospitalization.[22] In that study, syndromal recovery was attained by 84% and 97% of subjects at six and 24 months, respectively, but functional recovery was attained by only 30% at six months and 38% at 24 months. Another one year follow-up of first episode cases found that 56% achieved syndromal recovery but only 35% achieved symptomatic or functional recovery.[23] The finding that better socioeconomic status portends better outcomes may suggest that early intervention and relapse prevention might be protective by allowing socioeconomic development to be well established.[24] Finally, major depression accompanied by psychosis leads to poorer five and 10 year symptomatic and functional outcomes compared to non-psychotic depressions.[25]

Premises and goals

From reviewing the data on course and outcomes in psychotic disorders, it is apparent that determination of prognosis is multifactorial. However, for all psychotic disorders, the better the short-term course, the better the long-term outcome with the percentage of time spent with psychotic symptoms in the first few years being the best predictor.[5]

Many studies found long delays before treatment began in first episode psychosis including bipolar disorder.[26] Long durations of untreated psychosis (DUP) have been associated with slower and less complete recovery, more biological abnormalities, more relapses, and poorer long-term outcomes.[27–29] A newer concept, delay in intensive psychosocial treatment (DIPT), may also be related to outcome and associated with negative symptoms.[30]

The early phase of psychosis, the period when most deterioration occurs, may represent a 'critical period' for determining long-term outcome.[31] This period may present an important treatment opportunity because course-influencing bio-psychosocial variables, including patient and family reactions, develop and show maximum ability to change positively during this time.[32] The relationship of the duration of untreated psychosis to outcomes is complex. Research findings are not unanimous in showing that longer duration signals poorer outcome.[33] Although the relationship between duration of untreated psychosis and outcomes awaits further clarification, truncating the time to effective treatment is one of several ways that improvement in long-term outcomes may be produced.

In recent years, interest has grown in treating psychotic disorders as early as possible in order to reduce immediate suffering and danger and to improve both short- and long-term prognoses[34,35] (see Box 2.1).

Onset of psychosis typically occurs in late adolescence or early adulthood, thereby causing a major disruption in the ability of individuals with the disorder to meet developmental challenges. Family relationships suffer and parents and

---

Box 2.1 Goals of early intervention

- Better short- and long-term prognoses
- Increased speed of recovery
- Lower use of hospitalization
- Decreased risk of damaging socioeconomic consequences to the individual
- Reduced secondary psychiatric problems (e.g. depression, substance abuse, etc.)
- Minimization of family disruption
- Optimization of personal assets, psychosocial skills, role functions, and social/environmental supports
- Reduced relapse risk.

---

siblings experience significant distress.[36] Individuals experiencing psychosis are more prone to suicide, depression, aggression, substance abuse, cognitive impairment, and anxiety disorders.

Effective early intervention seeks to address these problems by:

- Providing age-appropriate support to minimize disruption in the lives of these individuals and enable them more successfully to meet their developmental challenges
- Limiting the suffering and possible negative repercussions of psychotic behavior
- Assisting families
- Remaining sensitive to factors that may hinder successful ongoing treatment, such as
  - negative effects generated by aversive procedures
  - medication side effects
  - stigma and other impediments to collaborative relationships.
- Providing treatment for associated problems, such as suicidal tendencies, depression, aggression, substance abuse, cognitive impairment, and anxiety disorders, rather than simply assuming that these features are secondary phenomena.

Evidence regarding the effectiveness of early intervention is accumulating. Participation in early psychosis programs has been reported to decrease DUP,[29,37] decrease hospitalization,[37–39] decrease police involvement in admissions,[37] lower medication use,[38,39] improve functional outcome,[28] lower relapse rates,[40] improve treatment adherence,[41] and lead to greater patient satisfaction.[39] These programs also appear to be cost effective.[42,43]

Despite these achievements, the answers to many other questions await the development and empirical validation of appropriate interventions and service systems. For example, research is needed to determine how long intensive intervention should last and whether these interventions improve long-term outcome or delay deterioration. Even if early intervention simply delays deterioration, it may raise the recovery bar since the developmental tasks the patient faces are further developed.

References

1. World Health Organization. *World Health Report 2001. Mental Health: New Understanding, New Hope.* Geneva: World Health Organization; 2001.
2. Barbato A. *Schizophrenia and Public Health.* Geneva. World Health Organization; 1998.
3. Edwards J, McGorry P. *Implementing Early Intervention in Psychosis: A Guide to Establishing Early Psychosis Services.* London: Martin Dunitz; 2002.
4. Birchwood M, McGorry P, Jackson H. Early intervention in schizophrenia. Br J Psychiatry 1997; **170**:2–5.
5. Harrison G, Hopper K, Craig T, et al. Recovery from psychotic illness: a 15- and 25-year international follow-up study. Br J Psychiatry 2001; **178**:506–17.
6. Loranger AW. Sex difference in age at onset of schizophrenia. Arch Gen Psychiatry 1984; **41**(2):157–61.
7. Faedda GL, Baldessarini RJ, Suppes T, et al. Pediatric-onset bipolar disorder: a neglected clinical and public health problem. Harv Rev Psychiatry 1995; **3**(4):171–95.
8. Ram R, Bromet EJ, Eaton WW, et al. The natural course of schizophrenia: a review of first-admission studies. Schizophr Bull 1992; **18**(2):185–207.

9. Wing JK. Five-year outcome in early schizophrenia. Proc R Soc Med 1966; **59**(1):17–18.

10. Wieselgren IM, Lindstrom LH. A prospective 1–5 year outcome study in first-admitted and readmitted schizophrenic patients; relationship to heredity, premorbid adjustment, duration of disease and education level at index admission and neuroleptic treatment. Acta Psychiatr Scand 1996; **93**(1): 9–19.

11. Carone BJ, Harrow M, Westermeyer JF. Posthospital course and outcome in schizophrenia. Arch Gen Psychiatry 1991; **48**(3):247–53.

12. Svedberg B, Mesterton A, Cullberg J. First-episode non-affective psychosis in a total urban population: a 5-year follow-up. Soc Psychiatry Psychiatr Epidemiol 2001; **36**(7):332–7.

13. Robinson DG, Woerner MG, Alvir JM, et al. Predictors of treatment response from a first episode of schizophrenia or schizoaffective disorder [see comments]. Am J Psychiatry 1999; **156**(4):544–9.

14. Edwards J, McGorry PD, Waddell FM, Harrigan SM. Enduring negative symptoms in first-episode psychosis: comparison of six methods using follow-up data. Schizophr Res 1999; **40**(2):147–58.

15. Green MF. What are the functional consequences of neurocognitive deficits in schizophrenia? [see comments]. Am J Psychiatry 1996; **153**(3):321–30.

16. Harrow M, Sands JR, Silverstein ML, Goldberg JF. Course and outcome for schizophrenia versus other psychotic patients: a longitudinal study. Schizophr Bull 1997; **23**(2):287–303.

17. Kessler RC, McGonagle KA, Zhao S, et al. Lifetime and 12–month prevalence of DSM-III-R psychiatric disorders in the United States. Results from the National Comorbidity Survey. Arch Gen Psychiatry 1994; **51**(1):8–19.

18. Angst J, Sellaro R. Historical perspectives and natural history of bipolar disorder. Biol Psychiatry 2000; **48**(6):445–57.

19. Goodwin GM, Jamison KR. *Manic Depressive Illness*. Oxford University Press; 1990.

20. Kessler RC, Avenevoli S, Ries Merikangas K. Mood disorders in children and adolescents: an epidemiologic perspective. Biol Psychiatry 2001; **49**(12): 1002–14.

21. Tsai SM, Chen C, Kuo C, et al. 15-year outcome of treated bipolar disorder. J Affect Disord 2001; **63**(1–3):215–20.

22. Tohen M, Hennen J, Zarate CM, Jr, et al. Two-year syndromal and functional recovery in 219 cases of first-episode major affective disorder with psychotic features. Am J Psychiatry 2000; **157**(2): 220–8.

23. Strakowski SM, Keck PE, Jr, McElroy SL, et al. Twelve-month outcome after a first hospitalization for affective psychosis. Arch Gen Psychiatry 1998; **55**(1):49–55.

24. Conus P, McGorry PD. First-episode mania: a neglected priority for early intervention. Aust N Z J Psychiatry 2002; **36**(2):158–72.

25. Coryell W, Leon A, Winokur G, et al. Importance of psychotic features to long-term course in major depressive disorder. Am J Psychiatry 1996; **153**(4):483–9.

26. Lish JD, Dime-Meenan S, Whybrow PC, et al. The National Depressive and Manic-depressive Association (DMDA) survey of bipolar members. J Affect Disord 1994; **31**(4):281–94.

27. McGlashan TH. Early detection and intervention of schizophrenia: rationale and research. Br J Psychiatry Suppl 1998; **172**(33):3–6.

28. Harrigan SM, McGorry PD, Krstev H. Does treatment delay in first-episode psychosis really matter? Psychol Med 2003; **33**(1):97–110.

29. Malla A, Norman R, McLean T, et al. A Canadian programme for early intervention in non-affective psychotic disorders. Aust N Z J Psychiatry 2003; **37**(4):407–13.

30. de Haan L, Linszen DH, Lenior ME, et al. Duration of untreated psychosis and outcome of schizophrenia: delay in intensive psychosocial treatment versus delay in treatment with antipsychotic medication. Schizophr Bull 2003; **29**(2):341–8.

31. Birchwood M, Todd P, Jackson C. Early intervention in psychosis. The critical period hypothesis. Br J Psychiatry Suppl 1998; **172**(33):53–9.

32. Birchwood M. Early intervention and sustaining the management of vulnerability. Aust N Z J Psychiatry 2000; **34**(Suppl):S181–4.

33. Norman RM, Malla AK. Duration of untreated psychosis: a critical examination of the concept and its importance. Psychol Med 2001; **31**(3):381–400.

34. Wyatt RJ, Henter ID. The effects of early and sustained intervention on the long-term morbidity of schizophrenia. J Psychiatr Res 1998; **32**(3–4): 169–77.

35. Wyatt RJ, Green MF, Tuma AH. Long-term morbidity associated with delayed treatment of first

admission schizophrenic patients: a re-analysis of the Camarillo State Hospital data. Psychol Med 1997; **27**(2):261–8.

36. Addington J, Coldham EL, Jones B, et al. The first episode of psychosis: the experience of relatives. Acta Psychiatr Scand 2003; **108**(4):285–9.

37. Yung AR, Harris BA. Management of early psychosis in a generic adult mental health service. Aust N Z J Psychiatry 2003; **37**(4):429–36.

38. Carbone S, Harrigan S, McGorry PD, et al. Duration of untreated psychosis and 12–month outcome in first-episode psychosis: the impact of treatment approach [see comments]. Acta Psychiatr Scand 1999; **100**(2):96–104.

39. Cullberg J, Levander S, Holmqvist R, et al. One-year outcome in first episode psychosis patients in the Swedish Parachute project. Acta Psychiatr Scand 2002; **106**(4):276–85.

40. Linszen D, Dingemans P, Lenior M. Early intervention and a five year follow up in young adults with a short duration of untreated psychosis: ethical implications. Schizophr Res 2001; **51**(1): 55–61.

41. Jorgensen P, Nordentoft M, Abel MB, et al. Early detection and assertive community treatment of young psychotics: the Opus Study Rationale and design of the trial. Soc Psychiatry Psychiatr Epidemiol 2000; **35**(7):283–7.

42. Moscarelli M, Capri S, Neri L. Cost evaluation of chronic schizophrenic patients during the first 3 years after the first contact. Schizophr Bull 1991; **17**(3):421–6.

43. Mihalopoulos C, McGorry PD, Carter RC. Is phase-specific, community-oriented treatment of early psychosis an economically viable method of improving outcome? Acta Psychiatr Scand 1999; **100**(1):47–55.

3

Early Psychosis Services

Tom Ehmann and Laura Hanson

Fundamental components of early psychosis services

Effective early psychosis intervention consists of multiple components that progress from recognition and referral, through assessment and treatment, and ultimately, to evaluation. In clinical practice, the focus of early intervention is on the early phases of psychosis. Treatment specific for psychosis should only be initiated upon the emergence of signs and symptoms of acute psychosis. Treatment for individuals who appear to be at very high risk for psychosis should be limited to interventions for presenting complaints, stress management, and close monitoring. High risk individuals may also be candidates for quality research studies examining interventions.

International interest in early psychosis is burgeoning. There are many well developed services throughout the world and new programs are forming. The rapid growth in interest produces the risk of uneven or inadequate practices being provided because of a limited conceptualization of the pertinent issues. The implementation of well intentioned but piecemeal interventions in the absence of adherence to sound theoretical or evidentiary bases is unlikely to produce the desired results. The evolving research on early psychosis intervention suggests that the whole is

potentially much greater than the sum of its parts. Therefore, it is important both for the integrity of the field and for persons with early psychosis that early intervention is applied comprehensively and in accordance with the identified clinical needs.

Several documents, such as the draft consensus statement, outline fundamental principles and practices of care in early psychosis.[1] These principles of care and best practices are overarching and apply to all the components of early psychosis intervention. It is recognized that fundamental components can be incorporated into a variety of models that all retain fidelity to the primary goals and practices. The recommendations presented in this chapter are consistent with the draft consensus statement on principles and practice in early psychosis from the International Early Psychosis Association,[1] and were partly derived from the *Australian Clinical Guidelines for Early Psychosis*.[2] Figure 3.1 outlines the fundamental components to early psychosis intervention.

Recognition: increasing recognition of emerging psychosis

Public and professional education should be properly planned, resourced and recognized as a priority. The following educational strategies should help enhance early psychosis recognition.

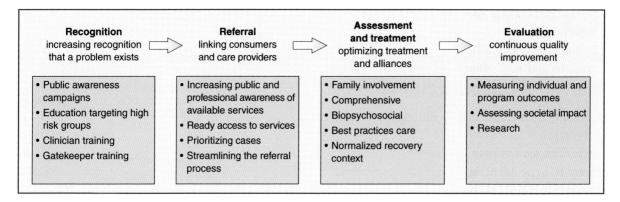

Figure 3.1 Fundamental components of early psychosis services

Increase public awareness

The first step toward enhancing early intervention is to increase public awareness about psychosis. The recognition of psychotic symptoms and awareness of the need for treatment are low in the general public.[3] Education helps to dispel myths and misconceptions that result in stigma and counter the false belief that little can be done to treat psychoses effectively. Awareness campaigns should aim to educate the public about the nature of early psychosis, the signs and symptoms of psychosis, and the importance of timely treatment. Public education should provide accurate information about psychosis and aim to dispel misconceptions.

Target education to high risk groups

Education should target persons at increased risk for developing psychosis. Education on psychosis should be incorporated into school settings and school curricula. Early intervention services may consider partnering with local community consumer groups to provide this education more broadly. Efforts must be made to ensure that educational material and information is age-appropriate and focused on early psychosis. Meeting a young person with a diagnosis of schizophrenia has been demonstrated to lead to a significant reduction in the negative stereotypes held by students.[4] Where this is not possible or practical, videos showing young people describing their experiences with psychosis and treatment may prove helpful in reducing the stigma associated with psychotic disorders.

Train gatekeepers to recognize psychosis

Professionals positioned to interact with individuals who may be experiencing incipient psychosis and who are poised for liaison with specialized early psychosis services should be trained to recognize symptoms of psychosis and understand the importance of early intervention. This gatekeeper training should include groups such as teachers, school counselors, and forensic personnel. This training may be introduced as part of their educational curriculum or provided in the workplace.

Train health clinicians in early psychosis evaluation

Education should be provided to general practitioners, mental health clinicians, hospital staff, and emergency room personnel to raise the 'index of suspicion' that a psychotic process may be occurring. Education should correct negative misconceptions regarding prognosis and course still held by many clinicians. By providing a greater awareness of new developments in the treatment of early psychosis, education will produce realistic optimism rather than a defeatist perspective. This would further serve to promote prompt action rather than a passive 'wait and see' approach.

Referral: linking consumers and care providers

By improving the efficiency of the pathway into care the harmful effects of delayed care can be minimized. The following strategies should help remove obstacles that sometimes impede referral to mental health services.

Increase awareness of services

Even if a problem is recognized, patients and families may not be familiar with existing services. Public awareness of available services and ease of accessing information about these services facilitate first contact. Health professionals and other service providers should inform patients and families of the range of services available. Special efforts must be made to educate teachers, physicians, counselors, and other service providers about early intervention services and how to access them. Increasingly, the internet is employed as a first step in persons' search for information. The development of websites can serve to provide education and specific information on local services. Gatekeepers, high risk groups, and the general public should be informed of the available and appropriate resources if early psychosis is suspected. Information should be provided on how to gain access to these services.

Make access to services quick and simple

Individuals should find access to services simple and convenient rather than stressful, confusing, and complicated. Psychotic symptoms and cognitive deficits can significantly impair an individual's ability to access services. Entry can be facilitated by accepting referrals from a wide variety of sources and situating services in discrete, accessible settings. Services should be easily accessible and include self- and family-referral. Both the number of steps needed for a person to receive appropriate care and the time spent seeking treatment should be minimized.

Respond to referrals rapidly

Response to referrals should be rapid and appropriate. After a referral is made, individuals should not have to wait for extended periods before being seen. If the interval is long, ambivalence the individual may have about entering treatment could result in a failure to follow through. Fewer than 40% of persons with severe mental disorders receive ongoing treatment.[5] Young adults and those living in urban areas are especially likely to have unmet needs for treatment. The majority of those who did not receive treatment felt that they did not have an emotional problem requiring treatment. Among those who did recognize a need for treatment, 52% reported situational barriers, 46% reported financial barriers, and 45% reported perceived lack of effectiveness as reasons for not seeking treatment. The most commonly reported reason both for failing to seek treatment and for treatment dropout was a desire to solve the problem without treatment.[5] If an individual believes there is a need for treatment yet is denied prompt access to services, there is a risk that the individual's distress will be exacerbated and that psychotic symptomatology will worsen. What was a situation that could be handled in the community may deteriorate into one needing hospitalization. Services should be organized so that clinicians can respond quickly, efficiently, and humanely. Creative alternatives to traditional office visits may facilitate early treatment. For example, a first meeting could occur at a school and include someone such as a teacher or friend, if the patient wishes it. Clinical services need to have a system for prioritizing, streamlining, and advertising the referral process.

Assessment and treatment: optimizing treatment and alliances

Optimal care consists of integrated biopsychosocial approaches (i.e. medication, psychosocial interventions, and patient and family education) tailored to the unique characteristics of each individual and the phases of their illness. Care that is culturally and age-appropriate must be provided in a context that normalizes recovery. Early psychosis services should be guided by the following principles to help ensure that optimal care is provided.

Comprehensive services

Services must be comprehensive and involve multiple sectors. The housing, educational, vocational, and general healthcare requirements of individuals with early psychosis need to be addressed. Such social determinants of health are predictive of:

- The onset of illness
- Access, adequacy, and compliance with diagnosis and treatment
- Likelihood and severity of relapse.

Communities need to ensure there are broad mechanisms to assist individuals through acceptance and support. This includes peer support, family support networks, and appropriate community resources. Given the high incidence of comorbid conditions in early psychosis, services must have a means of both assessing and treating these conditions that remains integrated with interventions provided for psychosis.

Prompt initiation of care

Services must ensure that assessment and treatment delays are avoided in order to reduce the length of time young people remain untreated. Assessment must be comprehensive and performed by a skilled professional. The emphases of treatment should be on managing symptoms and role fulfilment rather than diagnosis.

Continuity of care

Services have an obligation to ensure that care is continuous over time and across involved systems. Care needs to be user-centered and seamlessly available for those with early psychosis across all ages. The challenge for early psychosis services is heightened when the responsibility for service delivery shifts from one authority to another solely due to the chronological age of the individual. All too often this results in disruption, dis-

continuity, treatment dropout, and the risk of 'falling between the cracks'. Collaboration between governmental systems and agencies beyond healthcare is necessary for effective identification and treatment of illness. Services need to effectively integrate child, adolescent, and adult mental health services and work in partnership with primary care, education, social services, youth, and other relevant services.

Focus on the individual and family

Services should be youth-friendly and flexible in their approach. Assessment should be performed in the most comfortable environment possible (e.g. home visits and outreach). Family and other supports should be actively engaged from the outset. Care should address the 'whole person', including their ethnic and cultural background, rather than solely the signs and symptoms of psychosis. The person and the family should be engaged as active collaborators in care.

Best practices care

Clinicians must have the time, knowledge, and skills to provide best practices. A clear distinction is made between the clinical skills needed for working with individuals with early psychosis compared to those with persistent and chronic psychotic disorders. Care should be intensive and comprehensive. Rather than await symptom remission, recovery is actively promoted during the early phase of illness with emphases on normal social roles and developmental needs (e.g. attaining educational, employment, and social goals). The person and the family should be engaged for extended periods (e.g. perhaps several years or longer). At the end of the treatment period, care needs to be transferred thoughtfully and effectively facilitated.

Evaluation: continuous quality improvement

Evaluation and research must be recognized as a priority in order to ensure consistent adherence to best practices, continuously improve care and expand knowledge. Early psychosis services should consider inclusion of a variety of evaluative methods to help guide refinements in services and care.

Evaluation strategy

The use of shared strategies and indicators across services will strengthen evaluation efforts. The development of indicators should include measures of outcome as well as those related to process and implementation. These indicators should be reviewed for their pertinence and effort should be made to ensure that they are collected in a reliable and valid fashion. Information systems need to be built into programs as part of their basic operation. Evaluation should directly assess the routine use of clinical guidelines and inform the teaching of best practices to professionals. Publication of evaluation methodologies,[1,6] and results,[7] will allow for greater sharing of evaluation strategies and provide comparative data.

Outcome evaluation

Outcome evaluation is the process of identifying benefits to individuals receiving the services. Intake assessment, which is obviously important to formulate problems, plan interventions, and administer systems of care, can provide the baseline for outcome data to be compared against. Outcome measurement is useful for clinical, administrative, and research purposes. The study of outcomes complements the measurement of structural features (organizational design, staffing attributes, facility properties) and care processes (the services rendered to a patient).[8]

Measurement not only assists administration but also directly influences clinical activity. Consequently, clinical outcome data for individual patients needs to be approached with care and respect for the data collection process. All too often decisions regarding treatments and services are made without the benefit of good data. Unfortunately, busy clinicians are often unable to find time to collect measurements. Many clinicians tend to see data collection as a misplaced attempt to enforce accountability or as being irrelevant to their jobs.

These factors can produce perfunctory data collection that leads to a 'garbage in–garbage out' situation wherein useful results cannot be derived from the data. Although many clinicians do not see themselves as data collectors, information gathering is an essential and ongoing process that all clinicians routinely undertake. The use of rating scales, forms or other psychometric instruments merely formalizes the processes clinicians already do every day.

Outcome evaluation should incorporate measures of symptomatology, functioning, and quality of life. Standardized rating scales will help ensure reliability of data collected. Data should be collected routinely from a variety of perspectives including clinician, patient, and family (see Chapter 9 on measuring care for examples of assessment instruments).

Process evaluation

Process evaluation should be performed to assure quality service delivery. Process evaluation includes indicators that reflect how the services are implemented and whether they were implemented in a manner that is consistent with the program description and early psychosis best practices. Case reviews or audits can identify recurring problematic areas. This information will prove particularly useful in guiding future service refinements. Process data should be collected routinely from a variety of perspectives. Obtaining multiple perspectives can identify differences between the priorities of patients and family members and the treating clinicians.[9] Knowing and changing aspects of care that cause patient and family dissatisfaction can help ensure better engagement with services.

Societal impact

Evaluation needs to include parameters that reach beyond clinical service provision. This may consist of many parameters including epidemiological research, medicoeconomic evaluation, cross-field applicability of service delivery models, and assessment of training programs for new providers.

Research

The field of early psychosis is filled with unanswered questions pertaining to risk, mechanisms of psychosis, assessment, treatment, service systems, and outcome. Although many clinicians believe that doing research is alien to their daily work, this is not true. Research can be experimental, quasi-experimental, or uncontrolled, yet all can be extremely useful. Clinicians can provide valuable contributions when they keep good records and judiciously employ standardized and non-standardized measures. Such data can be used for local research projects and for external research in a variety of ways. Research should be an integral part of early intervention services that serves continuously to improve knowledge and treatments of psychosis.

Models of care for early psychosis services

In an integrated approach, community services are not isolated from inpatient units. Whereas many early psychosis programs begin at inpatient units and gradually add outreach components, others start in the community and then integrate hospital services into their programs. An empirical comparison of these approaches to early intervention has not been conducted. Perhaps a more critical issue concerns the skills available to the team members and the support they receive from management and policymakers in being able to utilize those skills.

Edwards and McGorry in *Implementing Early Intervention in Psychosis: A Guide to Establishing Early Psychosis Services* (2002) have described various models for care delivery, ranging from the establishment of centers of excellence to 'spoke and hub models' where regionalized services are linked to a common center. They also provide detailed information on the steps involved in setting up early psychosis services. Readers are recommended to refer to this book for a fuller treatment of these service-related topics. The following discussion is limited to highlighting the key aspects of delivering care in inpatient settings, community settings, and to individuals with comorbid substance abuse.

Inpatient services

Although early intervention hopes to avoid hospitalization through early identification and avoid re-hospitalization by decreasing relapse, the fact remains that 50% of first episode cases will be hospitalized within a week of first making contact with psychiatric services and 80% within three years.[10]

Ideally, specialized inpatient units catering to the unique needs of young persons with early psychosis should be available. Such facilities would have the capability of providing early-psychosis-specific interventions in the context of a homogenous patient population. Staff would have available early-psychosis-specific resources and be well trained in their utilization. Patients of a similar age and stage of illness could benefit each other, as they are undergoing a similar experience. They would also be shielded from the apprehension that can be produced by being grouped with more chronically ill patients. Sufficient numbers of patients would allow age-appropriate and stage-appropriate group interventions to be offered. Also, recreational activities and general ward atmosphere could be tailored to reflect youth culture, thereby helping to normalize the experience and provide continuity with their normal pursuits.

Unfortunately, the development of such units would be restricted to large urban areas. The vast majority of early psychosis cases will present to general inpatient units. Ward managers should be sensitive to optimal early psychosis practices and strive to incorporate them into daily practice. One initial strategy would be to provide staff training in these issues and assign staff with the greatest interest and expertise to first episode admissions.

Avoiding hospitalization when possible may decrease system costs and represent a less trying experience for the patient and family. Alternatives to hospitalization include home care, outpatient services, or specialized halfway houses. These settings must have adequate supportive capacities and are not usually suitable for individuals at risk for harm to self or others.

Inpatient–outpatient liaison

If outpatient services are ongoing before a first admission is needed, the outpatient mental health worker should be involved in the intake procedures, throughout the period of hospitalization, and in discharge planning. This may mean having the mental health worker accompany the person to hospital.

Conversely, if first contact is hospitalization, early engagement of community services should be established. This will help ensure smooth transition and reduce the likelihood of the patient becoming lost to the system after discharge from hospital. It is particularly important in early psychosis cases to initiate discharge planning as soon as possible after admission since the patient is unlikely to have any familiarity with community resources and housing options.

Community services

Case management is at the center of comprehensive community treatment of psychosis. It provides a continuing relationship between service providers, the patient, and his or her family. The goals of case management are to:

- Engage and maintain contact with the patient
- Ensure continuity of care
- Provide comprehensive treatment
- Increase accountability of service providers.

At a minimum, a case manager should be:

- Knowledgeable about theories of psychosis, presentation and course, and the range of treatments appropriate for early psychosis
- Skilful at assessing psychosis, early warning signs, other potential comorbid conditions, level of functioning, and medication side effects

- Proficient at providing suitable psychoeducation
- Aware of other appropriate available services.

Additional training in a variety of psychosocial treatments allows the case manager to offer more comprehensive care without having to refer to another professional. Case managers should only provide treatments consistent with their level of expertise.

Forms of case management

The many different forms of case management are often categorized into three main models.

1. Brokerage
   The case manager's role is to refer the patient to services and coordinate care. The case manager does not usually provide direct care to the patient.
2. Clinical case management
   Within this model, the approaches differ in emphasis (i.e. rehabilitation, personal strengths) and intensity (i.e. intensive case management, which includes frequent contact and proactive outreach). An individual case manager directly provides the majority of services/treatments. Referrals are made to other services on an as-needed basis.
3. Assertive community treatment
   Intensive support and rehabilitation are provided where the patient resides. Support and treatment responsibilities for a case are shared by a team of mental health workers rather than by one individual case manager.

Clinical case management has been shown to increase contact with mental health services and treatment adherence.[11] There is less evidence that it results in improvements in mental state or social functioning when compared to standard care. Within the general model of clinical case management, intensive case management is associated with better short-term outcomes and lower rates of hospital admission.[12,13]

Compared to clinical case management, there is more evidence demonstrating the effectiveness of assertive community treatment.[14] In addition to increasing contact with services and improving treatment adherence, assertive community treatment is associated with a lower rate of hospital admission, improved accommodation and employment status, and higher levels of patient satisfaction.[12,15,16] Patient-focused case management (in which the patient is seen as an equal partner in treatment) is also associated with greater patient satisfaction with services.[17]

Case management for early psychosis

The vast majority of studies examining clinical case management and assertive community treatment have focused on patients with significant social disability and chronic psychotic illnesses. Most early psychosis programs utilize a model of intensive clinical case management. In one study, at three month follow-up, there were greater improvements in treatment alliance and adherence with assertive community treatment than with standard clinical case management.[18]

> Either assertive community treatment teams or intensive case management with team back-up appear to be the most desirable case management approaches to providing community care for individuals with early psychosis.

Case management tasks and phase of psychosis

Case management tasks have been subdivided according to phase of disorder.[19]

1. Acute phase
   Priorities in this phase are to establish engagement, provide symptomatic relief, perform a comprehensive assessment, and provide information about psychosis and treatments.

Although there is considerable variability across individuals, the acute phase typically lasts several weeks. Patients and families are usually seen several times per week.

2. Early recovery phase
   As the psychosis begins to respond to treatment, the case manager starts to address secondary problems (e.g. depression, anxiety, substance abuse), provides psychoeducation, encourages adherence, monitors for side effects, explores the patient's explanatory model, teaches coping strategies, and gradually begins the reintegration process. This phase frequently lasts several months and visits occur about one to two times per week.

3. Later recovery phase
   Later in recovery, the case manager continues to treat secondary problems, works on relapse prevention, assists with problem solving, and monitors for return of symptoms. Visits are about once per week, moving to once per month as recovery progresses.

The case manager should become actively involved with the patient and family as soon as possible—at the initial assessment or as soon as possible after hospital admission.[19,20] The case manager typically carries the bulk of responsibility for providing direct service to the patient and family. The case manager must be accessible to the patient and family should a crisis arise, flexible to meet the individual needs of patient and family, as well as being optimistic and encouraging in the promotion of recovery.

The transition from adolescent to adult services may be particularly awkward. If such a transition is unavoidable or associated with possible benefits to the patient (i.e. access to other services not available in adolescent services), case managers are advised to gradually transfer therapeutic contact until engagement with the new case manager is established.

Group interventions

Case managers often act as leaders in therapeutic and educational groups. Groups can be a useful and cost-effective method for providing education, support and treatment to people with psychosis and their families. Group work may cover a wide variety of topics including psychoeducation, health education, lifestyle issues, stress management, social skills training, occupational preparation, academic upgrading, and recreational pursuits. Specific benefits of the group approach include:

- A sense of belonging for those whose social circles have diminished
- An opportunity to develop interpersonal skills
- A rich source of ideas for problem-solving regarding specific situations.[21,22]

Group approaches need to include individuals who are at a similar stage in terms of phase of illness and need. Efforts should be made to create a climate that is safe for disclosure, allows discussion of individual views of the illness, and allows equal participation. Group membership should be kept as consistent as possible. Skilled facilitation must be available to minimize the possible deterioration into 'gripe sessions'.[23,24] When case managers facilitate the sessions, clinical issues that arise can be handled in the context of continuity of care. Ideally, there should be two facilitators, and the group should run in parallel with individual psychoeducational interventions, including home-based interventions.[23,25]

Experience from early psychosis patient-group programs shows that they may be less desirable for individuals who are further along in their recovery, and less convenient for people who continue to attend school or work.[26]

> Group-based education and interventions should be considered as an adjunct (not an alternative) to individually based work.

Models of care for comorbid substance abuse

In initializing early psychosis services, consideration should be given to the model of care to be utilized for those patients presenting with comorbid substance abuse. This comorbidity is common in early psychosis,[27,28] and can complicate both assessment and treatment. The inherent difficulties in providing services to patients with psychosis and comorbid substance abuse are exacerbated by the separation of treatment programs for mental illness from those for substance abuse. The problems resulting from such a division of service are further compounded by the frequent exclusion of patients with substance abuse from entry into mental health programs and vice versa. Ultimately, few treatment options are left open to this population. The separation of these services appears to be associated with poor outcomes for people with mental illness and comorbid substance abuse.[29]

Three outpatient service delivery models have been used for treating comorbidity:[30]

1. Sequential or serial
   This model involves treating one disorder until it is under control, and then referring the patient to another agency to treat the other comorbid disorder. Both agencies often prefer to be second in line.
2. Parallel
   In this model, two agencies work with the patient at the same time, each treating one disorder.
3. Integrated
   This model incorporates substance abuse and mental health interventions in one clinical program.

The following problems are associated with the sequential and parallel models:[29,31–33]

1. Lack of comprehensiveness in assessment and treatment
   Clinicians do not gain an understanding of how problems interact and maintain one another. These interactions and maintenance factors are not addressed in treatment.

2. Poor continuity of care

Interventions can be incompatible with the goals of the other service (e.g. confrontative treatment for substance abuse). Engagement is threatened by requiring patients to attend two different services and have significantly more professionals involved in their care. There is often inadequate information exchange or little collaboration between treating professionals.

3. An association with poor patient outcome

Attrition rates are high. Generally, these models are less effective at reducing abuse severity and psychiatric symptoms compared to integrated approaches.

Integration of treatments may be necessary to address both the lack of effectiveness and the other problems apparent with these methods of service provision.[29,30,34] The National Institute of Mental Health in the United States funded 13 community demonstration projects to determine if integrated treatment was feasible and effective. The evaluation concluded that integrated services can be developed successfully in a number of different clinical settings and appear to improve patient outcome (i.e. reductions in substance use and hospitalization rates).[35] More information on integrated treatment for comorbid substance abuse can be found in Chapter 8.

References

1. Edwards J, McGorry P. *Implementing Early Intervention in Psychosis: A Guide to Establishing Early Psychosis Services.* London: Martin Dunitz; 2002.
2. *Australian Clinical Guidelines for Early Psychosis.* Melbourne: National early psychosis project, University of Melbourne; 1998.
3. Jorm AF, Korten AE, Jacomb PA, et al. Helpfulness of interventions for mental disorders: beliefs of health professionals compared with the general public. Br J Psychiatry 1997; **171**(11):233–7.
4. Schulze B, Richter-Werling M, Matschinger H, et al. Crazy? So what! Effects of a school project on students' attitudes towards people with schizophrenia. Acta Psychiatr Scand 2003; **107**(2):142–50.
5. Kessler RC, Berglund PA, Bruce ML, et al. The prevalence and correlates of untreated serious mental illness. Health Serv Res 2001; **36**(6 Pt 1): 987–1007.
6. Turner M. *Evaluation of Early Intervention for Early Psychosis Services in New Zealand. What Works?* Auckland: Health Research Council of New Zealand; 2002.
7. Preston NJ, Stirling ML, Perera K, et al. A statewide evaluation system for early psychosis. Aust N Z J Psychiatry 2003; **37**(4):421–8.
8. Sederer L, Dickey B, Hermann R. The imperative of outcomes assessment in psychiatry. In: Sederer L, Dickey B (eds). *Outcomes Assessment in Clinical Practice.* Baltimore: Williams & Wilkens; 1996.
9. de Haan L, Kramer L, van Raay B, et al. Priorities and satisfaction on the help needed and provided in a first episode of psychosis. A survey in five European Family Associations. Eur Psychiatry 2002; **17**(8):425–33.
10. Sipos A, Harrison G, Gunnell D, et al. Patterns and predictors of hospitalisation in first-episode psychosis. Prospective cohort study. Br J Psychiatry 2001; **178**:518–23.
11. Marshall M, Gray A, Lockwood A, Green R. Case management for people with severe mental disorders. Cochrane Database Syst Rev 2000; 2.
12. Mueser KT, Bond GR, Drake RE, Resnick SG. Models of community care for severe mental illness: a review of research on case management. Schizophr Bull 1998; **24**(1):37–74.
13. Aberg-Wistedt A, Cressell T, Lidberg Y, et al. Two-year outcome of team-based intensive case management for patients with schizophrenia. Psychiatr Serv 1995; **46**(12):1263–6.
14. Marshall M, Lockwood A. Assertive community treatment for people with severe mental disorders. Cochrane Database Syst Rev 2000;2.
15. Bond GR, Witheridge TF, Dincin J, et al. Assertive community treatment for frequent users of psychiatric hospitals in a large city: a controlled study. Am J Community Psychol 1990; **18**(6):865–91.
16. McGrew JH, Bond GR, Dietzen L, et al. A multisite study of client outcomes in assertive community treatment. Psychiatr Serv 1995; **46**(7):696–701.
17. O'Donnell M, Parker G, Proberts M, et al. A study of client-focused case management and consumer

advocacy: the Community and Consumer Service Project. Aust N Z J Psychiatry 1999; **33**(5):684–93.

18. Jorgensen P, Nordentoft M, Abel MB, et al. Early detection and assertive community treatment of young psychotics: the Opus Study Rationale and design of the trial. Soc Psychiatry Psychiatr Epidemiol 2000; **35**(7):283–7.

19. Edwards J, Cocks J, Bott J. Preventive case management in first-episode psychosis. In: McGorry PD, Jackson HJ (eds). *The Recognition and Managment of Early Psychosis*. Cambridge University Press; 1999.

20. Falloon IR, Fadden G. *Integrated Mental Health Care*. Cambridge University Press; 1993.

21. Atkinson JM, Coia DA, Gilmour WH, Harper JP. The impact of education groups for people with schizophrenia on social functioning and quality of life. Br J Psychiatry 1996; **168**(2):199–204.

22. Kansas N. Group therapy and schizophrenia: An integrative model. In: Martindale B, Bateman A, Crowe M, Margison F (eds). *Psychosis: Psychological Approaches and their Effectiveness*. London: Gaskell; 2000.

23. North CS, Pollio DE, Sachar B, et al. The family as caregiver: a group psychoeducation model for schizophrenia. Am J Orthopsychiatry 1998; **68**(1):39–46.

24. McFarlane WR, Dunne E, Lukens E, et al. From research to clinical practice: dissemination of New York State's family psychoeducation project. Hosp Community Psychiatry 1993; **44**(3):265–70.

25. Leff J, Berkowitz R, Shavit N, et al. A trial of family therapy v. a relatives group for schizophrenia [see comments]. Br J Psychiatry 1989; **154**:58–66.

26. Francey S. The role of day programmes in recovery in early psychosis. In: McGorry PD, Jackson HJ, (eds). *The Recognition and Management of Early Psychosis*. Cambridge University Press; 1999.

27. Rabinowitz J, Bromet EJ, Lavelle J, et al. Prevalence and severity of substance use disorders and onset of psychosis in first-admission psychotic patients. Psychol Med 1998; **28**(6):1411–19.

28. Cantwell R, Brewin J, Glazebrook C, et al. Prevalence of substance misuse in first-episode psychosis. Br J Psychiatry 1999; **174**:150–3.

29. Ridgely MS, Goldman HH, Willenbring M. Barriers to the care of persons with dual diagnoses: organizational and financing issues. Schizophr Bull 1990; **16**(1):123–32.

30. Drake RE, Mercer-McFadden C, Mueser KT, et al. Review of integrated mental health and substance abuse treatment for patients with dual disorders. Schizophr Bull 1998; **24**(4):589–608.

31. Ridgely MS, Goldman HH, Talbott JA. Treatment of chronic mentally ill young adults with substance abuse problems: emerging national trends. Adolesc Psychiatry 1989; **16**:288–313.

32. Hellerstein DJ, Rosenthal RN, Miner CR. Integrating services for schizophrenia and substance abuse. Psychiatr Q 2001; **72**(4):291–306.

33. Barrowclough C, Haddock G, Tarrier N, et al. Randomized controlled trial of motivational interviewing, cognitive behavior therapy, and family intervention for patients with comorbid schizophrenia and substance use disorders. Am J Psychiatry 2001; **158**(10):1706–13.

34. McLellan AT, Luborsky L, Woody GE, et al. Predicting response to alcohol and drug abuse treatments. Role of psychiatric severity. Arch Gen Psychiatry 1983; **40**(6):620–5.

35. Mercer-McFadden C, Drake RE. *A Review of 13 NIMH Demonstration Projects for Young Adults with Severe Mental Illness and Substance Abuse Problems*. Rockville, MD: Community Support Program, Center for Mental Health Services, US Department of Health and Human Services; 1995.

4

Assessment

Tom Ehmann and Laura Hanson

Introduction

Assessment and treatment constitute the core of early intervention. Ongoing accurate assessment guides treatment decisions, monitors changes over time, reveals additional areas in need of attention, and allows for program evaluation and research. Assessment domains and procedures are examined here in sufficient detail to allow clinicians meaningfully to review their own practices.

Goals of assessment

Assessment provides sufficient information for diagnosis, guides treatment planning, and helps development of a therapeutic alliance. Assessment must be ongoing in order to ascertain change, uncover new problem areas, and evaluate service delivery. The quality and breadth of any assessment session will be affected by time constraints, degree of rapport, the assessor's skill, and the patient's insight and ability to cooperate. A mental status exam should ascertain the presence, severity, and duration of signs and symptoms. A thorough assessment ensures collection of collateral information from family, friends, social worker, school, police, or others. Many of the following assessment recommendations were derived from existing clinical practice guidelines.[1,2–6]

Focus of assessment

Signs and symptoms

Regardless of the stage of illness, assessments of symptoms and functioning are essential. The assessor not only focuses on the referral symptoms suggestive of psychosis, but also conducts a comprehensive assessment of symptoms to allow for the diagnosis of comorbid conditions, such as depression and substance abuse.

> Particular attention should be paid to any risk indicators for suicide, violence, or victimization.

Functioning

The status and rate of change in the following should be established:

- Social relationships
- School and/or work performance
- Recreational pursuits
- Finances and ability to manage money
- Self-care
- Religious activities
- Domestic roles
- Housing and clothing
- Community involvement.

History

From interview and collateral information, the following histories should be taken:

- Birth and development
- Medical—including any neurological problems such as head injury, loss of consciousness, or difficulties with walking, coordination, or speech
- Psychiatric
- Forensic
- Academic/occupational
- Recreational
- Social
- Trauma
- Family history including queries regarding past and present psychiatric conditions, adjustment issues, interaction, and environment
- Past involvement with services, previous treatments, and the outcomes of those treatments.

Cognition

The assessment of intellectual and cognitive function can foster understanding of current functioning and has ramifications for occupational and educational possibilities, rehabilitation training, and the provision of services and financial support.[7,8] A preliminary estimate of cognitive and intellectual functioning can be derived from the mental status exam. Neuropsychological assessment may detect unusual patterns of deficit that could have diagnostic implications. Also, cognitive assessment can help a patient understand personal limits and the fact that their illness is a brain disorder. Conversely, areas of relative strength can be identified.

Stress, coping, and personality

Enquires should be made about:

- Significant life events and social stressors
- Instrumental needs
- Chronic and daily hassles
- Family conflicts
- Developmental adjustment issues, such as sexual difficulties, school/work problems, identity formation, and separation-individuation.

- Assessment of self-concept, personality, and coping styles may assist diagnosis and treatment.
- In addition to taking histories and conducting interviews, the assessor can use one or more of the many standardized instruments available.
- The assessment of strengths and intact functions benefits intervention targeting, retention of self-efficacy, and the relationship between patient and provider.

The patient's explanatory model

Understanding the patient's explanation of his or her condition should help promote a collaborative alliance. Emotional and behavioral responses to the psychosis can be explored along with the strategies employed to relieve distress.

Patient and family attitudes to mental health services, medications, and alternative therapies may be related to the degree of convergence between their explanatory models and what they believe to be the conceptual models underlying various services.

Physical assessment

The presence of physical disorders in patients with psychiatric disorders is high. Problems with eyesight, dentition, and high blood pressure become especially common as the illness progresses.[9] A greater number of current medical problems appear to contribute to more severe psychosis, depression, and greater likelihood of suicide attempts.[9]

- Every patient should receive basic neurological and general physical examinations.
- The presence of movement abnormalities prior to initiating antipsychotic drug treatment should be carefully noted.
- Basic laboratory tests can help identify the presence of psychosis-inducing medical illnesses and provide baseline information

that may have implications for the treatment plan. Include: complete blood count; electrolyte and glucose measurements; tests for hepatic, renal and thyroid function; and tests to determine HIV and STD status.

- A toxicology screen should be ordered.
- Urine and blood analysis can also help detect systemic infections.
- Heart function (perhaps including electrocardiogram) should be ascertained since antipsychotic medications may have adverse cardiac effects.

The patient should be weighed before beginning treatment and body mass index (BMI) calculated.

Imaging

The use of brain scans (i.e. computed tomography scans) of individuals with recent onset psychosis is justified in order to rule out neurological diagnoses that may mimic schizophrenia in their early stages. A scan also serves to reassure patient, family, and physician that diagnostic possibilities with visible cerebral insult have been considered. Certain brain abnormalities frequently found in schizophrenia are not diagnostically specific and, therefore, neuroimaging is not necessarily indicated if the neurological exam and history are normal.[4]

Initial interview considerations

Good rapport produces better information and greater adherence to treatment. Initial contact should focus on engaging the patient while obtaining critical clinical information on risk and symptoms. Both patient and interviewer must feel safe.

Inform the patient about:

- Who made the referral and why
- What the assessment will consist of
- What the interviewer's role will be
- Who else will have access to the assessment information

- The provisions for explaining the results of the assessment.

The limited experience of most young persons with government agencies or mental health professionals might increase their level of stress. Attempts to minimize distress or reluctance around a first visit may include conducting the initial assessment in an environment comfortable for the patient (e.g. the home), avoiding a long period in the waiting room, and encouraging someone the person trusts to attend the session. A fairly short interview, concern for the person's physical space, and encouragement of participation and input into the pace and content of the visit can all facilitate a successful initial visit.

Some patients may have a history of violence, be under the influence of drugs or alcohol, or present as physically intimidating. Interviewers can minimize the risk of being assaulted by conducting an interview in close proximity to other staff, maintaining non-threatening verbal and non-verbal communications and paying attention to escape routes. If the patient picks up on the interviewer's discomfort, anxiety, or fear he or she may not engage well with the process. For further information on addressing potentially threatening situations refer to the section below on acute inpatient presentations.

Paranoia and distrust, substance abuse, preoccupation with psychotic experiences, difficulty identifying feelings or finding words to express their experiences, and lack of knowledge about the abnormality of certain experiences can all hamper assessment. The quality of information may be affected by the patient's intelligence, language, and cultural heritage. The family or other persons close to the patient can usually help the assessor determine whether certain beliefs or behaviors are abnormal.

Family members, friends, school personnel such as teachers and counsellors, and others who know the patient well can all be sources of collateral information The impact of the patient's condition on them should be explored and acknowledged. When a patient is hesitant to allow family involvement in the assessment, the clinician should be patient, continue to develop rapport, and explore the reasons behind the patient's hesitation.

Semi-structured interviews increase diagnostic reliability and may help elicit features overlooked in unstructured clinical interviews. Standardized clinical rating scales also help ensure consistent coverage, quantify symptom severity, and permit later comparisons.[10]

Discordance between a patient's perceived needs and those of a service provider frequently occur. A recently published instrument may reveal these discrepancies and facilitate communication.[11]

Assessment feedback and diagnosis

Assessment feedback that is informative and positive is usually effective and helps to initiate therapy. Discussing the diagnostic possibilities with the patient and the family provides an opportunity to provide realistic hope and understanding about effective treatment. It is best not to be overly speculative about diagnoses. The patient and others involved in the process need to understand that accurate diagnosis often requires observation of symptoms over a period of many months. In these instances it is better to retain a focus on effectively treating the presenting problems while acknowledging the uncertainty. Given that psychotic experiences appear to form a continuum and are frequently reported in non-clinical populations, attempts to help normalize the experience of psychosis might be abetted by carefully providing this information.[12] It is important for the assessor to be sensitive to the rate and amount of information that others can absorb. Feedback that addresses personal strengths and resources should be provided in addition to information about identified problem areas.

Diagnosis

Diagnosis provides important information on possible treatments and outcomes. A diagnostic formulation should be completed, including all five DSM-IV axes and possible rule-out diagnoses. In early psychosis cases, a specific diagnosis may be ambiguous, even though the need for treatment is clearly present. Presenting symptoms prioritized by a provisional diagnosis (e.g. psychotic symptoms) should form the main focus of initial treatment.

Changes in the diagnosis are frequent in first-episode psychosis. The temporal criteria in DSM-IV necessitate some diagnostic changes (e.g. schizophreniform to schizophrenia). Other changes in diagnosis over the early course could result from a reluctance to label illness early, a shift in symptoms over time, and neglect of the importance of affective features. This diagnostic instability may be particularly evident in adolescents where almost 50% of initial diagnoses are subsequently changed.[13] In adolescents, diagnoses of schizophrenia and affective disorder demonstrate good stability compared to other diagnoses.[14,15] With earlier identification, this stability may be lessened, since longitudinal course-related variables will not yet be manifest.

Diagnostic reassessment several times a year is recommended. Use of diagnostic criteria checklists or direct consultation of DSM-IV is likely to result in greater diagnostic precision. Failure to re-diagnose can result in problems, such as the possible application of inappropriate treatments in the future, provision of inappropriate educational information, or the development of misleading expectations on the part of both patient and treatment professionals.

References

1. *Australian Clinical Guidelines for Early Psychosis.* Melbourne: National early psychosis project, University of Melbourne; 1998.
2. Practice guideline for the treatment of patients with bipolar disorder. American Psychiatric Association. Am J Psychiatry 1994; **151**(12 Suppl):1–36.

3. Treatment of schizophrenia. The Expert Consensus Panel for Schizophrenia. J Clin Psychiatry 1996; **57**(Suppl 12B):3–58.

4. Practice guideline for the treatment of patients with schizophrenia. American Psychiatric Association [see comments]. Am J Psychiatry 1997; **154**(4 Suppl):1–63.

5. Canadian clinical practice guidelines for the treatment of schizophrenia. The Canadian Psychiatric Association [see comments]. Can J Psychiatry 1998; **43**(Suppl 2):25S-40S.

6. AACAP official action. Summary of the practice parameters for the assessment and treatment of children and adolescents with schizophrenia. American Academy of Child and Adolescent Psychiatry. J Am Acad Child Adolesc Psychiatry 2000; **39**(12):1580–2.

7. Velligan DI, Bow-Thomas CC, Huntzinger C, et al. Randomized controlled trial of the use of compensatory strategies to enhance adaptive functioning in outpatients with schizophrenia. Am J Psychiatry 2000; **157**(8):1317–23.

8. Green MF, Kern RS, Braff DL, Mintz J. Neurocognitive deficits and functional outcome in schizophrenia: are we measuring the 'right stuff'? Schizophr Bull 2000; **26**(1):119–36.

9. Dixon L, Postrado L, Delahanty J, et al. The association of medical comorbidity in schizophrenia with poor physical and mental health. J Nerv Ment Dis 1999; **187**(8):496–502.

10. Kay SR, Opler LA, Spitzer RL, et al. SCID-PANSS: two-tier diagnostic system for psychotic disorders. Compr Psychiatry 1991; **32**(4):355–61.

11. van Os J, Altamura AC, Bobes J, et al. 2–COM: an instrument to facilitate patient-professional communication in routine clinical practice. Acta Psychiatr Scand 2002; **106**(6):446–52.

12. Verdoux H, van Os J. Psychotic symptoms in non-clinical populations and the continuum of psychosis. Schizophr Res 2002; **54**(1–2):59–65.

13. Menezes NM, Milovan E. First-episode psychosis: a comparative review of diagnostic evolution and predictive variables in adolescents versus adults. Can J Psychiatry 2000; **45**(8):710–16.

14. Hollis C. Adult outcomes of child- and adolescent-onset schizophrenia: diagnostic stability and predictive validity. Am J Psychiatry 2000; **157**(10): 1652–9.

15. Jarbin H, von Knorring AL. Diagnostic stability in adolescent onset psychotic disorders. Eur Child Adolesc Psychiatry 2003; **12**(1):15–22.

5

General Treatment Considerations

Tom Ehmann and Laura Hanson

Introduction

Treatment in early psychosis demands a wide spectrum of pharmacological, psychological, psychosocial, and educational interventions. The information provided in this section is intended to generalize to many forms of service delivery. For example, a family physician working alone may use this guide as a framework for a general approach, a prompt to seek out other appropriate resources, or as a source for specific medication information. Those working within multidisciplinary teams may compare the style and content of the services they provide to the approaches discussed here. More specialized interventions are not provided in exhaustive detail. Rather, evidence for their effectiveness is presented, along with references that the reader can consult for more information on specific procedures.

General treatment targets

Psychotic symptoms

Historically, the primary target symptoms for a person presenting with psychosis for the first time were positive symptoms of psychosis (e.g. delusions, hallucinations, thought disorder, and disorganization) and/or manic symptoms. Later, the importance of treating negative symptoms became apparent. These defining features of psychosis, along with acute distress, remain the primary targets of initial treatment efforts.

Psychosocial functioning

Social relationships, academic and vocational pursuits, and role functioning all contribute to an individual's quality of life and should form a vital focus of treatment. Preservation of opportunities, environmental supports, and social relationships should be followed by psychosocial rehabilitation if necessary.

Comorbid psychiatric conditions

The rate of comorbid psychiatric conditions in those with psychosis appears to be over 50%,[1] even in first episode cases.[2] Associated psychiatric features of psychosis include suicide, depression, aggression, substance abuse, and anxiety disorders, such as post-traumatic stress disorder.[3–6] About 45% of drug-free patients with schizophrenia were found to have significant depressive symptoms.[7] Psychosis, regardless of type, carries an increased risk of suicide—half of the persons with schizophrenia who commit suicide do so in the first five years of illness.[8] The rate of completed suicide in patients with schizophrenia is usually estimated to be about 10%, a rate 25 times greater than in the general population.[9] Annual rates in treated psychotic patients of attempted and completed suicides are about 5% and 1%, respectively.[10] In first episode schizophrenia spectrum cases, 11% attempted suicide within one year.[11]

A recent study of first episode admissions found a 68% rate of lifetime exposure to trauma and that 14% of cases met criteria for post-traumatic stress disorder.[12] The presence of symptoms suggesting comorbid conditions must therefore be carefully assessed. Only after this assessment is done can a judgment be made regarding whether the symptoms can be considered integral to the primary or provisional diagnoses. This may be difficult. For example, although panic attacks may be an associated feature of schizophrenia, the treating team must evaluate the presence of certain cognitions about the attacks that, if present, would merit making a diagnosis and treating the panic disorder. Similar arguments could be made for other conditions including obsessive-compulsive disorder, post-traumatic stress disorder, and major depression.

Cognitive deficits

More recently, it has been recognized that cognitive deficits are associated with psychotic disorders but do not necessarily vary with positive psychotic symptoms.[13] Cognitive deficits may both mediate functional performance and form the substrate of many psychotic experiences. Patients with a first episode of schizophrenia frequently show a large generalized neuropsychological deficit along with more selective deficits in attention, learning, memory, speeded visuomotor, and executive functions.[14–16] Similar cognitive impairments are also present in other psychotic disorders.[17,18] Poorer long-term social functioning has been related to impaired cognitive functioning and more severe negative symptoms.[19–21] Cognition is increasingly being targeted through both pharmacological[22,23] and psychosocial approaches.[24–26]

General treatment principles

A strong working alliance facilitates successful ongoing treatment

Development of the therapeutic relationship may take precedence over treatment initiation in order to increase the probability of long-term success. All too frequently, alliance is forsaken because of demands on staff time or because its importance is not recognized.

The patient's initial discomfort should be minimized

Professional caregivers now recognize there are many opportunities for the person with psychosis to become distressed or traumatized. These can include:

- The nature of the symptoms (hallucinations, passivity experiences, delusions, etc.)
- Insight that something is terribly wrong
- Coercive or confusing admission procedures
- Fear, loss of independence, and heavy-handed interventions in an inpatient unit
- Poor interviewing styles
- Bothersome or dangerous side effects from treatment.

Minimization of distress and trauma is therapeutically beneficial over both short and longer terms.

Treatment should target a broad range of treatment goals

Treatment should be comprehensive, individually tailored, and adhere to best practices. General goals for treatment include:

- Amelioration of psychotic symptoms
- Amelioration of non-psychotic symptoms
- Well-timed effective re-entry into the person's normal roles and environments
- Prevention of secondary morbidity
- Minimization of relapse risk
- Retention of a positive self-concept
- Enhancement of self-efficacy
- Maximization of quality of life.

Diagnostic classifications frequently demand temporal criteria, yet the individual is clearly suffering before a diagnosis can be definitively assigned. Therefore, the patient should be treated initially for manifest psychopathology. Although merely treating symptoms is at odds with the principle of treating syndromes, it is consistent with the fact that antipsychotic medications basically treat psychosis and are not antischizophrenia medications.

Professional involvement should be ongoing and intensive

The levels and types of interventions will vary according to individual readiness. The concept of a critical period, wherein early course predicts later course, suggests that ongoing intensive involvement should occur for at least several years after the resolution of the initial episode.[27] Evidence to confidently inform the duration and intensity of interventions is generally lacking. Further, discontinuities in care can confuse and upset a patient and result in uneven treatment applications. These disruptions pose potential threats to engagement and may lead to relapse either directly or via non-adherence to treatment. In many jurisdictions the transition from youth to adult services is especially awkward.

Practices should be age- and stage-appropriate

Specific interventions are appropriate to different stages of a disorder. Both pharmacological and psychosocial interventions are affected by this principle. Similarly, the content and process of interventions should be consistent with the developmental stage of the individual.

The pace and timing of reintegration should be carefully considered

Successful rapid reintegration back into social, occupational/scholastic, and other roles is a primary goal of early intervention. The pace and extent of return to each area calls for sensitive handling. Confidence and self-esteem can easily be damaged if the individual experiences failures rather than successes. Careful assessment and planning are needed to avoid problems such as academic failure that can occur when the individual is expected to assume a full course load from where he or she left off. Intellectual declines and cognitive deficits may persist, even though symptomatic remission has been attained.

Family involvement should be early, intensive, and sustained

Families need support both for themselves and to assist the ill family member. Recognizing the enormous implications for a family when a member develops a psychotic disorder, the alleviation of family disruption should be fostered along with engagement of the family as a therapeutic partner. Despite significant evidence that family involvement leads to lowered relapse rates, improved patient functioning, and enhanced family well-being,[28–33] delivery of mental health services to persons with psychosis often bypasses the family.[34]

Collaboration between care providers and families should begin immediately, with consideration given to the pace and extent to which a family can participate. Regardless of the patient's age, family involvement should be part of a specific treatment plan rather than informal and as needed. Work with the family should include supportive counselling, psychoeducation, relapse prevention, stress management, and enhancement of coping skills.

Acute inpatient presentations

Special concerns regarding hospitalization

The experience of the early psychosis patient is markedly different from the experience of someone who has been hospitalized repeatedly. First episode patients may find their initial hospital experience to be traumatizing.[3] Inpatient staff should promptly allay any unfounded fears that first episode patients may have, or concerns that they will inevitably come to resemble some of the more chronic patients seen in inpatient settings. Instructions regarding how to maintain personal safety may be of benefit if there are potentially aggressive patients on the ward. Inpatient staff should attempt to include family or close friends in as many intake procedures and interviews as possible. It is important that proceedings are explained to the patient and family, and that realistic reassurance regarding shorter-term outcomes be given. Early psychosis patients should be assigned priority for private rooms.

Handling emergency department presentations

A patient in crisis presenting at hospital emergency may show significant behavioral difficulties. An expert consensus panel has published its recommendations on appropriate procedures to manage behavioral emergencies.[35] In such situations, staff must be aware of the factors that can jeopardize or enhance their own safety. Measures that minimize risk include an open demeanor, room logistics (e.g. a safe escape route, a location for conducting assessments in clear view of other staff), and the ability to access security personnel quickly. One of the most important forms of psychological management is to approach an anxious or agitated patient openly and genuinely to contain the situation verbally. This includes communicating a reasonable summary of the situation along with your psychiatric concerns in a clear, easy-to-understand manner. Tone of voice should be soft and non-threatening. Clinicians should describe the treatment plan and sequence of upcoming events as a set of short-term and longer-term goals. If verbal containment is not adequate to complete the assessment or allay agitation, pharmacological methods may need to be employed as described in Chapter 6 on pharmacotherapy.

Seclusion and restraint

Seclusion and restraint are measures of last resort used when there exists a threat of imminent physical harm to patient and staff or, more rarely, when significant property damage is occurring. These procedures should be used for the minimal time necessary and should be preceded by a clear explanation of the reason for their implementation. When the seclusion or restraint procedures are terminated, it is important to discuss with the patient the expectations for his or her behavior and restate the treatment plan. The use of seclusion and restraint in early psychosis cases is especially worrisome since it can seriously damage the relationship between the patient and mental health services.[36] One study found that patients reported a preference for medication over physical restraint in psychiatric emergencies.[37] Further discussions of some of the medical and ethical questions involved in the use of restraint can be found elsewhere.[35,38]

References

1. Cassano GB, Pini S, Saettoni M, et al. Occurrence and clinical correlates of psychiatric comorbidity in patients with psychotic disorders. J Clin Psychiatry 1998; **59**(2):60–8.
2. Strakowski SM, Tohen M, Stoll AL, et al. Comorbidity in psychosis at first hospitalization. Am J Psychiatry 1993; **150**(5):752–7.
3. McGorry PD, Chanen A, McCarthy E, et al. Posttraumatic stress disorder following recent-onset psychosis. An unrecognized postpsychotic syndrome [see comments]. J Nerv Ment Dis 1991; **179**(5):253–8.
4. Westermeyer JF, Harrow M, Marengo JT. Risk for suicide in schizophrenia and other psychotic and nonpsychotic disorders. J Nerv Ment Dis 1991; **179**(5):259–66.
5. Aguilar EJ, Haas G, Manzanera FJ, et al. Hopelessness and first-episode psychosis: a longitudinal study. Acta Psychiatr Scand 1997; **96**(1):25–30.
6. Humphreys MS, Johnstone EC, MacMillan JF, Taylor PJ. Dangerous behaviour preceding first admissions for schizophrenia [see comments]. Br J Psychiatry 1992; **161**:501–5.

7. Leff J, Tress K, Edwards B. The clinical course of depressive symptoms in schizophrenia. Schizophr Res 1988; **1**(1):25–30.

8. Wieselgren IM, Lindstrom E, Lindstrom LH. Symptoms at index admission as predictor for 1–5 year outcome in schizophrenia. Acta Psychiatr Scand 1996; **94**(5):311–19.

9. Meltzer HY. Suicide and schizophrenia: clozapine and the InterSePT study. International Clozaril/ Leponex Suicide Prevention Trial. J Clin Psychiatry 1999; **60**(Suppl 12):47–50.

10. Khan A, Khan SR, Leventhal RM, Brown WA. Symptom reduction and suicide risk among patients treated with placebo in antipsychotic clinical trials: an analysis of the Food and Drug Administration database. Am J Psychiatry 2001; **158**(9): 1449–54.

11. Nordentoft M, Jeppesen P, Abel M, et al. OPUS study: suicidal behaviour, suicidal ideation and hopelessness among patients with first-episode psychosis. One-year follow-up of a randomised controlled trial. Br J Psychiatry Suppl 2002; **43**:S98–S106.

12. Neria Y, Bromet EJ, Sievers S, et al. Trauma exposure and posttraumatic stress disorder in psychosis: findings from a first-admission cohort. J Consult Clin Psychol 2002; **70**(1):246–51.

13. Green MF, Nuechterlein KH. Should schizophrenia be treated as a neurocognitive disorder? Schizophr Bull 1999; **25**(2):309–19.

14. Bilder RM, Goldman RS, Robinson D, et al. Neuropsychology of first-episode schizophrenia: initial characterization and clinical correlates. Am J Psychiatry 2000; **157**(4):549–59.

15. Albus M, Hubmann W, Wahlheim C, et al. Contrasts in neuropsychological test profile between patients with first-episode schizophrenia and first-episode affective disorders. Acta Psychiatr Scand 1996; **94**(2):87–93.

16. Saykin AJ, Shtasel DL, Gur RE, et al. Neuropsychological deficits in neuroleptic naive patients with first-episode schizophrenia. Arch Gen Psychiatry 1994; **51**(2):124–31.

17. Martinez-Aran A, Penades R, Vieta E, et al. Executive function in patients with remitted bipolar disorder and schizophrenia and its relationship with functional outcome. Psychother Psychosom 2002; **71**(1):39–46.

18. Zarate CA, Jr, Tohen M, Land M, Cavanagh S. Functional impairment and cognition in bipolar disorder. Psychiatr Q 2000; **71**(4):309–29.

19. Bellack AS, Sayers M, Mueser KT, Bennett M. Evaluation of social problem solving in schizophrenia. J Abnorm Psychol 1994; **103**(2):371–8.

20. Dickerson F, Boronow JJ, Ringel N, Parente F. Social functioning and neurocognitive deficits in outpatients with schizophrenia: a 2–year follow-up. Schizophr Res 1999; **37**(1):13–20.

21. Addington J, Addington D. Neurocognitive and social functioning in schizophrenia: a 2.5 year follow-up study. Schizophr Res 2000; **44**(1):47–56.

22. Meltzer HY, McGurk SR. The effects of clozapine, risperidone, and olanzapine on cognitive function in schizophrenia. Schizophr Bull 1999; **25**(2): 233–55.

23. Harvey PD, Green MF, McGurk SR, Meltzer HY. Changes in cognitive functioning with risperidone and olanzapine treatment: a large-scale, double-blind, randomized study. Psychopharmacology (Berl) 2003; **169**(3–4):404–11.

24. Hogarty GE, Flesher S. Practice principles of cognitive enhancement therapy for schizophrenia. Schizophr Bull 1999; **25**(4):693–708.

25. Brenner HD, Hodel B, Roder V, Corrigan P. Treatment of cognitive dysfunctions and behavioral deficits in schizophrenia. Schizophr Bull 1992; **18**(1):21–6.

26. Roder V, Zorn P, Muller D, Brenner HD. Improving recreational, residential, and vocational outcomes for patients with schizophrenia. Psychiatr Serv 2001; **52**(11):1439–41.

27. Birchwood M. Early intervention and sustaining the management of vulnerability. Aust N Z J Psychiatry 2000; **34**(Suppl):S181–S184.

28. Barbato A, D'Avanzo B. Family interventions in schizophrenia and related disorders: a critical review of clinical trials. Acta Psychiatr Scand 2000; **102**(2):81–97.

29. Pharoah FM, Mari JJ, Streiner D. Family intervention for schizophrenia. Cochrane Database Syst Rev 2000; 2.

30. Dyck DG, Short RA, Hendryx MS, et al. Management of negative symptoms among patients with schizophrenia attending multiple-family groups. Psychiatr Serv 2000; **51**(4):513–19.

31. Falloon IR, Boyd JL, McGill CW, et al. Family management in the prevention of morbidity of schizophrenia. Clinical outcome of a two-year

longitudinal study. Arch Gen Psychiatry 1985; **42**(9):887–96.

32. Falloon IR, Pederson J. Family management in the prevention of morbidity of schizophrenia: the adjustment of the family unit. Br J Psychiatry 1985; **147**:156–63.

33. Falloon IR, McGill CW, Boyd JL, Pederson J. Family management in the prevention of morbidity of schizophrenia: social outcome of a two-year longitudinal study. Psychol Med 1987; **17**(1):59–66.

34. Lehman AF, Steinwachs DM. Translating research into practice: the Schizophrenia Patient Outcomes Research Team (PORT) treatment recommendations. Schizophr Bull 1998; **24**(1):1–10.

35. Allen MH, Currier GW, Hughes DH, et al. The Expert Consensus Guideline Series. Treatment of behavioral emergencies. Postgrad Med 2001(Spec No):1–88; quiz 89–90.

36. Macnaughton E. *The BC Early Intervention Study: Report of findings*. Vancouver: Canadian Mental Health Association, BC Division; 1999.

37. Sheline Y, Nelson T. Patient choice: deciding between psychotropic medication and physical restraints in an emergency. Bull Am Acad Psychiatry Law 1993; **21**(3):321–9.

38. Hem E, Steen O, Opjordsmoen S. Thrombosis associated with physical restraints. Acta Psychiatr Scand 2001; **103**(1):73–5; discussion 75–6.

6

Pharmacotherapy

Tom Ehmann and Laura Hanson

Status of antipsychotic medications in early psychosis

Typical antipsychotics

Older antipsychotic medications ('typicals') have been successfully used for almost 50 years. Although effective at reducing psychotic symptoms, they are often associated with various acute and chronic side effects, including significant motor effects.[1,2] These motor effects include acute dystonia, parkinsonism, akathisia, tardive dyskinesias, dystonia, and tremor.[3]

Typical antipsychotics appear equivalent to each other in the treatment of psychotic symptoms.[4] This may result from their shared ability to antagonize the dopamine subtype-2 receptor (D_2).[5] There appears to be a narrow window of D_2 blockade between antipsychotic efficacy and the development of adverse side effects. It has been reported that while less than 70% D_2 blockade does not usually ameliorate psychosis, prolactin starts rising at 72% blockade and extrapyramidal symptoms emerge at close to 80% D_2 occupancy.[6] However, optimal subjective experience for first episode patients may occur at 60–70% D_2 occupancy.[7] Given their therapeutic similarity, the choice of typical antipsychotic has often been made on the basis of type and degree of side effects, patient preference, availability, and the presence of other psychiatric disturbances.

Atypical antipsychotics

'Atypical' antipsychotics developed over the past two decades are much less likely to produce the types of side effects often found with the typical antipsychotics.[8] Atypical antipsychotics (e.g. clozapine, risperidone, olanzapine, quetiapine, amisulpride, arapiprizole, zotepine, and ziprasidone) have all been shown to decrease positive and negative psychotic symptoms.[9–14] Numerous reviews have noted that all antipsychotics reduce negative symptoms significantly more reliably than placebo, with some data showing that risperidone, olanzapine, and amisulpride do so slightly better than typicals.[10,12,15,16] Compared to typical antipsychotics, the effect sizes for overall symptomatic improvement appear superior for clozapine, amisulpride, olanzapine, and risperidone.[17]

Within the atypicals, overall efficacy appears to be similar,[10,17–20] although the data are not unequivocal.[21]

Atypicals are associated with fewer extrapyramidal side effects and reduced need for anticholinergic medication.[10,22–25] They also carry more benign side effect profiles in a number of other areas.[26] However, some atypicals are associated with significant weight gain and endocrine/sexual effects.

The atypical antipsychotics can roughly be grouped into those resembling clozapine (e.g.

olanzapine and quetiapine) and those that do not, but have similar receptor profiles (e.g. risperidone and ziprasidone).[27] Clozapine has high affinity for many receptors including $5\text{-}HT_{2A}$, M_1, H_1, and D_4, while olanzapine is similar but has higher D_2 and D_1 affinities. The other group of atypicals has high affinities for D_2 and $5\text{-}HT_{2A}$ receptors along with their adrenergic α_1 blocking characteristics. Perhaps the most 'atypical' atypical is amisulpride, which selectively antagonizes D_2 and D_3 receptors.[28] Most atypicals, including olanzapine, risperidone, quetiapine, zotepine, ziprasidone, and clozapine, have a high $5\text{-}HT_{2A}$ to D_2 receptor ratio. It is believed that $5\text{-}HT_{2A}$ blockage in the striatum increases dopamine transmission and therefore lessens the tendency to cause extrapyramidal side effects (which are due to reduced dopamine transmission in the striatum). However, it has also been suggested that the atypicals' shared tendency to dissociate from the D_2 receptor more quickly than typicals may result in decreased motor and cognitive dysfunction.[29] In turn, the atypicals vary in their D_2 dissociation rates.[30]

Response in first episode psychosis to antipsychotics

The vast majority of patients with schizophrenia or schizoaffective disorders will show a good symptomatic response to antipsychotic medication.[31] Most improvement tends to occur within the first six months of treatment.[32] Trials lasting shorter periods reported response rates of around 60–70% on atypicals,[33,34] and about 50% on typical antipsychotics.[35,36]

Olanzapine, risperidone, and clozapine are the only atypicals for which there exist reported data from controlled clinical trials showing efficacy in early psychosis. The efficacy of risperidone[22,37] and olanzapine[36,38] in first episode cases has been established. Clozapine has been shown to be effective for treatment-resistant first episodes.[39] A recently published trial found clozapine was equal to chlorpromazine in the number of patients con-

sidered remitted after one year.[40] Clozapine is generally reserved for refractory cases, because its associated risk of agranulocytosis necessitates rigorous monitoring procedures. Also, a recent prospective naturalistic study that showed comparable proportions of first episode and multi-episode patients were responders to clozapine suggests there may be no loss of clozapine efficacy if treatment refractory patients are first given trials of less onerous agents.[41]

Controlled trials examining quetiapine, zotepine, amisulpride, aripiprazole, and ziprasidone in first episode cases have not been conducted. Several open trials of quetiapine in first episodes involving a variety of diagnoses found a significant reduction in psychotic and manic symptoms using doses around 500 mg/day.[42,43] No trials specific to first episodes were found to date for the other atypicals.

Male sex, a history of obstetrics complications, more severe symptoms, younger age of onset, and the development of parkinsonian symptoms predict poorer initial response to medication.[31,44–47] Poor premorbid adjustment has been related to lesser remission of positive symptoms,[48] insidious onset, poorer social course, and persistent negative symptoms.[44,49] Longer duration of untreated psychosis has been associated with poorer response in first episode patients.[40]

Side effects of antipsychotic medications

Motor side effects

Antipsychotics with high affinities for cholinergic receptors are less likely than those without such affinities to generate extrapyramidal side effects, and most atypicals tend to have anticholinergic activity. The exception is risperidone, which, if given in higher doses, may induce more extrapyramidal side effects than other atypicals.[10] The atypicals present a more favorable side effect profile than the typicals. Neuroleptic-naïve patients are more susceptible to develop extrapyramidal side effects than chronically treated patients.[50,51] In neuroleptic-naïve patients with schizophrenia, risperidone produced fewer extrapyramidal side effects than haloperidol.[52] Patients with mania may also be more vulnerable to developing acute dystonia than patients with schizophrenia.[53] In general, extrapyramidal side effect rates are lower for all atypicals compared to typicals.[15]

Approximately 4% of patients receiving typical antipsychotic medications will develop tardive dyskinesia (TD) each year.[54,55] The one year incidence in first episode psychosis treated with low dose haloperidol was 12%.[56] In comparison, the one year TD risks are 0.52% for olanzapine,[57] and 0.3% for risperidone.[26] Data were not located for TD risks from other atypicals.

Elevated prolactin and sexual side effects

One study found that over 50% of males reported sexual difficulties while treated with typical antipsychotics and over 90% of women reported menstrual changes.[58] These changes were associated with elevated prolactin levels.

The atypicals, with the exception of risperidone,[59] are much more prolactin sparing than the typical antipsychotics.[60,61] In women, hyperprolactinemia may cause amenorrhea, galactorrhea, vaginal dryness, hirsutism, reduced bone density, and decreased libido. In men, it can result in erectile dysfunction, ejaculatory dysfunction, gynecomastia, hyperspermatogenesis, and decreased libido. Younger women may be especially prone to these side effects because their higher estrogen levels (e.g. on birth control pills) may potentiate the prolactin-elevating properties of typical antipsychotics.[62,63]

Although the atypicals (with the exception of risperidone) are more prolactin sparing than the typicals, they do not appear to be associated with a low incidence of sexual side effects during longer-term treatment.[64]

Among bipolar patients, over 50% reported sexual dysfunction when treated with benzodiazepines and lithium (compared to 17% treated with lithium and any other drug).[65] Treatment

with bromocriptine or amantadine[66] may be effective but the risk of exacerbating psychotic symptoms must be considered.[67] Dose reduction has been the treatment of choice to date.

Weight gain

All antipsychotic medications can cause weight gain.[1] A sample of 114 patients treated with atypicals were found to show an average weight gain of 12% in one year and the percentage of patients considered obese rose from 36% to 60%.[68] Among atypical antipsychotics, clozapine appears to cause the most weight gain followed by olanzapine, quetiapine, and then risperidone. For example, quetiapine, one of the two drugs least likely to cause weight gain, is associated with greater than 7% increase over baseline in about 25% of patients with the gains continuing over the first year of treatment.[69] Weight gain on olanzapine appears to be associated with younger age.[70] Ziprasidone appears less likely to cause weight gain.[69] Lithium and valproate are considered more likely to cause weight gain than carbamazepine.[71]

Weight is best monitored by taking a baseline measurement of body mass index (BMI: weight in kg/height in meters[2]). The Canadian Practice Guidelines recommend monitoring lipids and glucose if the BMI increases by 10%.[72] The BMI should be calculated monthly for the first six months, or weekly if rapid weight gain is occurring. Significant weight gain could be a risk factor for non-adherence, especially in young females. It also poses increased risk for other obesity related disorders, such as diabetes and heart disease.

Dietary strategies and exercise remain the principal treatments for weight gain. Support groups may be helpful to some individuals. Atypicals have also been implicated in the exacerbation or precipitation of diabetes regardless of the amount of weight gain.[73] Risperidone has not been implicated in reports of impaired glucose regulation. Caregivers in both community and inpatient settings should take baseline glucose measures and continue monitoring over time. The use of pharmacological agents to control weight gain is generally not recommended,[74] although some experts do see a role for them in some patients.[75]

Other side effects

Most sedation from atypicals is transitory.[76] Low potency medications, such as clozapine and chlorpromazine, appear to pose a greater risk of sedation than most high potency typicals. However, the atypicals olanzapine, quetiapine and risperidone all appear more sedating than haloperidol.[71]

Jaundice is an infrequent occurrence with antipsychotic medications but has been found in 1–5/1000 patients on chlorpromazine.[54] Leukopenia has been found in almost 10% of patients on chlorpromazine with 0.3% developing agranulocytosis. Extensive blood monitoring must be undertaken with clozapine use because of the 1% rate of agranulocytosis.[77] Clozapine also has a dose-dependent risk for seizures with an overall rate of 2.8%.[54]

Overdose of antipsychotic medications rarely causes death unless accompanied by alcohol/ drug ingestion or pre-existing medical conditions.[54] Treatment of overdose is symptomatic and supportive. Neuroleptic malignant syndrome has been associated with virtually all antipsychotic medications including atypicals.[78,79] Antipsychotic medications should be discontinued immediately and symptomatic treatment instituted.

The rate of sudden death among those on antipsychotic medications is no higher than that for the general population.[54] Nevertheless, the risk for heart arrhythmias may be lessened by using low doses of medications, ensuring patients are well hydrated, monitoring vitals, and, finally, minimizing use of restraints, since cardiovascular and autonomic instabilities could result from the interaction of agitation/stress and medication effects.[54] Failure to understand the patient's subjective experience of both mental and physical side effects can lead to treatment failure because the patient may develop a negative attitude to the medication and cease to take it.[80]

Therapeutic use of side effects associated with medication

In some instances, the side effect associated with a medication is useful therapeutically. For example, sedation may be desirable in a patient who is agitated, anxious, or unable to sleep. The sedating potential of a drug can be reasonably predicted by its ability to antagonize H_1 receptors. Thus, a clinician using a typical antipsychotic might choose one from the low potency group (e.g. chlorpromazine) since low potency typicals have a high affinity for histamine subtype 1 receptors (H_1) in addition to cholinergic receptors. The rank order of H_1 blockade for selected antipsychotics starting with the highest is: clozapine, olanzapine, chlorpromazine, quetiapine, fluphenazine, risperidone, and haloperidol.[15,22,34,39,81,82]

Table 6.1 Receptor profiles and medication side effects

Receptor	Side effects
Dopamine (D_2)	Extrapyramidal, elevated prolactin
Acetylcholine (Muscarinic: M1)	Blurred vision, dry mouth, urinary hesitation, cognitive impairment, constipation
Histamine (H_1)	Sedation, weight gain
Serotonin (5-HT_{2A})	Increased appetite, sexual performance difficulties
Adrenergic (α_1)	Hypotension, nasal congestion, ejaculatory dysfunction

Table 6.1 provides a simple overview of some of the main effects associated with some transmitters.

Of course, all predictions of effects based on receptor profiles must consider dosage. A drug with a low affinity for a specific receptor may still create a side effect associated with that receptor if the dose is increased sufficiently. However, the increased dose would also affect other receptors and produce consequent effects associated with those transmitters.

Treatment of side effects

When very low doses of typicals or risperidone are used, the rates of extrapyramidal side effects are low, and anticholinergic medications are not needed. If extrapyramidal side effects develop during treatment with an atypical, the dose should be lowered. Anticholinergic medications, such as benztropine, are effective for treating extrapyramidal symptoms. They may also be used prophylactically. Because of the very high rates of extrapyramidal side effects in neuroleptic-naïve and young patients, anticholinergics should be used if the initial medication is a typical antipsychotic given in more than very low doses (which itself is generally not recommended). Nevertheless, prophylactic use of biperiden lowered the rate of dystonia in first episode cases from 60% to 7%.[51]

Drug interactions

Cytochrome P450 enzymes, predominantly found in the liver, metabolize many psychiatric drugs. Understanding the effects involving cytochrome P450 enzymes has implications for avoiding unwanted drug interactions and for developing rational dosing strategies.[83,84] Ethnic differences exist in hepatic enzyme activity. In general, younger age, female sex, and tobacco smoking lead to faster drug metabolism. In some cases (e.g. risperidone), this has little practical effect since the metabolite is equipotent to the parent compound.[85] Although the following interactions are far from exhaustive, they do represent several of the more common situations that may be encountered.[86,87]

- All antipsychotics decrease the effects of dopamine agonists.
- Carbamazepine increases clearance of most atypicals.
- Quetiapine clearance is increased by phenytoin and decreased by cimetidine.
- Quetiapine increases clearance of lorazepam.
- Tobacco can lower blood levels of some antipsychotics by up to 50%.
- Large amounts of grapefruit juice increase olanzapine and clozapine levels.
- Clozapine, ziprasidone, and quetiapine levels can be increased by protease inhibitors, antifungals, and some antibiotics.
- Selective serotonin receptor inhibitors (SSRIs) can increase plasma levels of the atypicals.
- Benzodiazepines and clozapine can induce respiratory depression.

Targets for antipsychotic medications

In addition to the positive, negative, and disorganized symptoms of psychosis, the atypicals also target broader areas of psychopathology.

Cognition

Cognitive performances appear to improve on all atypicals (albeit in slightly different domains), whereas typicals generally do not lead to cognitive improvement.[88–93] Clinicians should be aware that anticholinergic effects impair several cognitive abilities.[93]

Depression and suicide

Some research suggests that antipsychotics lower the risk of suicide,[94] with evidence being strongest for clozapine.[95,96] The use of lithium has also been shown to lower suicide.[97] Significant reductions in depression have been reported for risperidone, olanzapine, quetiapine, amisulpride, and ziprasidone.[98–105]

Agitation and aggression

Many antipsychotics have been used to control agitation. Some evidence suggests that clozapine use, in particular, may be associated with decreased aggression over extended periods.[101]

Substance abuse

Typical antipsychotics may be less effective in controlling psychotic symptoms in individuals with schizophrenia and a history of psychotogenic substance abuse,[104] and higher doses may be required to achieve stabilization in alcohol abusers.[105] Additionally, typical antipsychotic medications do not appear helpful in decreasing substance abuse, and there is some evidence that they might even be associated with increased use.[106,107] A number of case studies and non-controlled studies suggest that clozapine is effective in reducing both psychotic symptoms and substance abuse.[108–111] Theoretical development that implicates enhanced reward-related circuitry in the corticolimbic system might contribute to further investigation of the atypicals' use in treating substance abuse.[112] There are only preliminary data for the other atypicals,[113–115] and the only direct comparison between atypicals was a small retrospective study that favored clozapine over risperidone.[116]

Quality of life

Life satisfaction may be mediated by psychosocial factors and symptom reduction more than side effects.[117] Better studies are needed,[118] but preliminary data are encouraging in that improved quality of life is associated with atypical antipsychotics.[119]

Pharmacotherapy of non-affective psychosis

If a non-affective psychotic disorder is suspected, pharmacological treatment should centre on the use of antipsychotic medication. The target symptoms should be broad in scope. Advances in assessment and delineation of various components of psychotic symptomatology have led to an emphasis on treatment of negative, as well as positive, symptoms of psychosis.[120] Mood symptoms, anxiety, aggression, and other symptoms are commonly found along with psychosis and cognitive deficits.

Targets should vary according to individual presentations. Although pharmacological treatments should ultimately target all of the above symptoms, wholesale polypharmacy is neither recommended nor proven to be beneficial.[121]

> It is recommended that treatment begin with one antipsychotic, preferably an atypical.

Response to treatment should be defined multidimensionally, with consideration given to psychotic symptoms, mood, social and occupational functioning, acute and chronic side effects, cognition, subjective response, and quality of life (see Table 6.2).

Starting medication treatment

Treatment should be initiated as soon as possible. An antipsychotic-free period for a few days may be useful if there are any possible diagnostic concerns (such as substance involvement). If necessary, antipsychotic treatment can be delayed for weeks without adversely affecting outcome.[122]

Table 6.2 Rationale for use of atypicals in early psychosis

- Effective at treating psychotic symptoms
- Less likely to cause adverse side effects that produce non-adherence
- Appear to have beneficial effects on cognition
- Appear effectively to treat some non-psychotic symptoms
- May be associated with less hospitalization
- May be more cost effective
- May be associated with better quality of life.

Perhaps because young people are usually more sensitive to both beneficial and negative effects of antipsychotic medications,[123] there is increasing evidence that much lower doses are needed.[52,124] The dictum 'start low and go slow' is indicated.

Doses of less than 3 mg risperidone,[125] and about 2 mg of haloperidol have been shown to be optimal in first episode cases (Table 6.3).[124,126] In a study with 106 patients of which 32 were neuroleptic-naïve patients, 73% attained remission after five weeks on an average of 3.4 mg (± 2.3 mg) of haloperidol.[127]

Oral doses of atypical antipsychotics usually reach peak plasma concentrations after 2–4 hours, are metabolized in the liver, and have half-lives of 20–40 hours. Most atypicals reach steady state plasma levels in five half-lives. The use of polypharmacy is generally discouraged. However, in many cases, several medications may need to be concurrently administered.

Assessment of response

Psychotic and other psychiatric symptoms, side effects, daily functioning, and subjective response should all be assessed repeatedly. Assessments should occur on multiple occasions in the first week and at least biweekly for the first month. Response is best assessed in the context of the types of target symptoms identified. For example,

agitation should respond within days, while negative symptoms may take much longer to respond. Clinicians should not solely rate improvement according to positive symptoms. The use of rating scales allows objective progress—especially over time—and is suitable for routine clinical use. Several measures are listed in Chapter 9 on measuring the effectiveness of care.

Increasing doses

An initial period of about one to two weeks should allow the clinician to determine if the patient is tolerating the medication and deriving benefit. Positive symptoms, along with general symptoms, such as anxiety and agitation, often show discernible improvement within one week. A recent first episode study that restricted haloperidol doses to 1 mg for the first four weeks found that 55% of patients remained stabilized on that dose.[212] Further, 83% remained on haloperidol after a 12 week trial at an average dose of 1.78 mg per day. The concept of a 'neuroleptic threshold' (dosing to the threshold of motor side effects) has been used successfully in several first episode studies using typicals to keep doses and side effects low while attaining excellent clinical responses.[124,127]

Several guides that list the approximate lowest doses expected to be effective were used to devise Table 6.4.[27,128] The list is derived either from

Table 6.3 Suggested initial dosage for first-episode cases

Medication	Starting daily dose
Haloperidol	1 mg
Amisulpride	50–100 mg ?
Aripiprazole	5–10 mg ?
Risperidone	0.5–1 mg
Olanzapine	2.5–5 mg
Quetiapine	50–100 mg
Ziprasidone	40 mg ?
Zotepine	25 mg ?

?=insufficient data from controlled trials to be more exact

Table 6.4 Expected lowest effective doses

Medication	Dose/day
Haloperidol	1–2 mg
Amisulpride	300 mg
Aripiprazole	15 mg
Risperidone	1–2 mg
Olanzapine	5 mg
Quetiapine	300–400 mg
Ziprasidone	80 mg
Zotepine	100 mg

studies using the drugs in early psychosis, or by calculating chlorpromazine equivalents. Of course, many patients will require significantly higher doses and it must be reiterated that controlled studies using most of these medications in first episodes have yet to be completed.

Up to 30% of first episode cases of schizophrenia will not respond within six weeks of treatment. Since non-responders taking reasonable doses do show adequate binding to D_2 receptors, it is unlikely that dose increases will be effective.[27] Instead, switching to another medication should be considered.

Utility of antipsychotic plasma levels

About 75% of first episode responders to low dose haloperidol had blood plasma levels well below those commonly believed to be associated with response.[124] Therefore, plasma monitoring is not recommended as a good predictor of response but may be undertaken to assess non-adherence, to identify unusual drug metabolism when a seemingly adequate dose fails to produce an adequate clinical response, and to help distinguish psychopathology from side effects.[121] Plasma levels are of more importance with clozapine.[129,130]

Use of other medications

Little is known about the use of adjunctive agents, such as antidepressants, benzodiazepines, and mood stabilizers in first episode cases of schizophrenia. This is because most studies utilized refractory chronic patients.[121] The use of two antipsychotics in first episodes is generally unwarranted.

Mood stabilizers

Lithium used alone for schizophrenia is likely to be ineffective or even to worsen symptoms, but it may enhance the effects of antipsychotics when given adjunctively.[54] Lithium should not be employed before an adequate trial of an antipsychotic alone. The lithium add-on should show a beneficial response in most patients within four weeks. Clinicians must closely monitor for lithium toxicity, since lithium-antipsychotic combinations place patients at greater risk for side effects, including neuroleptic malignant syndrome.[54] Valproate and carbamazepine are not effective antipsychotics, but may have a role in patients with persistent agitation, aggression, or electroencephalogram (EEG) irregularities.[54]

Benzodiazepines

The benzodiazepines are helpful in managing sleep disturbances, agitation, and anxiety very early in the treatment process.[131] Benzodiazepines also appear to possess some antipsychotic activity, albeit considerably less than antipsychotic medications.[132] Their use can foster greater diagnostic clarity and improve engagement. Benzodiazepines may be beneficial adjuncts to antipsychotics in reducing positive symptoms, anxiety, agitation, and overall psychopathology,[121] although these effects may be limited in duration.[54] If a benzodiazepine is used with an antipsychotic, the dose of antipsychotic should be lowered. When lithium or carbamazepine is employed in acute mania, benzodiazepines may be effectively combined with them,[133] especially to help treat behavioral disturbance.[134,135] Given that benzodiazepines can cause disinhibition, abuse, and rebound withdrawal symptoms, their use for more than brief periods demands caution.

Antidepressants

The covariation of mood symptoms with psychotic symptoms in many patients with schizophrenia suggests that depression is integral to the illness and that monotherapy with an antipsychotic is viable.[136] Others argue that neuroleptics themselves produce depressive symptoms that are distinguishable from akinesia.[137]

Although antidepressants, electroconvulsive therapy (ECT), and mood stabilizers are all effective treatments for depression in bipolar patients,[138] their place in treating schizophrenia is less clear. Antidepressants may not be particularly helpful once the illness is established.[139–141] Nevertheless, the use of antidepressants is justified if antipsychotic monotherapy or in combination with a mood stabilizer, such as lamotrigine, fails adequately to treat depressive syndromes.[121] With respect to early psychosis, initially prescribing antidepressant medications cannot be condoned when reluctance to start antipsychotics is simply due to the lack of a definite diagnosis of schizophrenia.

Switching antipsychotics after a partial or poor response

When a patient fails to show significant improvements within four to six weeks, experiences ongoing distressing side effects, or is dissatisfied with the treatment, the clinician should consider switching to another medication. A poor initial response is not cause for therapeutic pessimism, since about 16% of early unremitting cases will achieve late-phase recovery.[142] As noted previously, the ongoing use of two antipsychotics in early psychosis is generally unwarranted. A discussion should be undertaken regarding the risk of symptom exacerbation and length of time that might be needed to see results. If symptoms worsen or other difficulties arise during a switch, the clinician should consider if the method of switching is leading to dosing effects or rebound phenomena (e.g. anticholinergic).

Three main approaches to switching exist and little research has been done to show overall superiority of one method. In the cross-taper approach, the old and new medications are gradually interchanged over weeks or months. The dose of the existing medication should be slowly reduced at a maximal rate of 30–50% every week or slower. Youth are at higher risk of exacerbations.[143] The second method involves reaching a therapeutic dose of the new medication and only then gradually reducing the dose of the old medication. A study using this technique found that achieving a therapeutic dose of the new medication, before gradual withdrawal of the old agent, resulted in fewer relapses.[144] The final method, an abrupt stop accompanied by a rapid push to

expected effective dose is less likely to be relevant to first episode cases treated with atypicals. Although this approach does not involve the polypharmacy-related risks associated with the other methods, rebound effects may occur.

Criteria for considering clozapine

Clozapine is regarded as the gold standard in treatment-resistant cases.[145,146] The clinician must decide how long to wait before a treatment-resistant patient is prescribed clozapine. The American Psychiatric Association Guidelines for Schizophrenia suggest that an acute episode be treated with either one typical or atypical for six weeks. If response is poor after six weeks, these guidelines recommend consideration of clozapine.[54] A set of expert consensus guidelines suggests use of one typical then a trial of an atypical before switching to clozapine.[147] The Texas algorithms suggest three trials before clozapine,[148] while the PORT group recommended two trials from different classes of either typicals or atypicals.[121] The Canadian Clinical Practice Guidelines for Schizophrenia imply that physicians consider one trial of a typical and at least one, if not two, trials of atypicals before moving to clozapine.[72] The only guidelines specifically written to date for early psychosis advocate two six week trials of atypicals, then either adding lithium to the atypical or going directly to clozapine.[149]

> It is recommended that clozapine should not be prescribed before at least two trials, at least one of which should be either risperidone or olanzapine.
> Each trial should last at least six weeks, unless discontinued earlier due to side effects.

Duration of treatment following a good response

An expert consensus guideline document recommended that a first episode patient with schizophrenia who shows a good initial response to medication and is able to return to work full time should be maintained on the medication for 12–24 months before considering dose reduction and discontinuation.[147] An evidence-based report recommended at least one year of maintenance therapy after an acute episode.[121] Guidelines for children and adolescents also recommended 12–24 months of maintenance.[150] However, the data from at least one study using typical antipsychotics in first episode schizophrenia suggested that patients receive maintenance medication for two to five years after initial recovery because of the increased risk of relapse, especially in those who discontinue medication.[151] The influences of the atypical antipsychotics and specialized early psychosis psychosocial interventions on relapse and course remain unresolved at this time. Therefore, it is recommended that patients with first episode schizophrenia remain on maintenance medication for a minimum of one year unless there are circumstances that might merit the intermittent targeted strategy described below.

Patients frequently discontinue medications when they have recovered from a first episode. Unfortunately, there is no reliable way to predict who belongs to the substantial subgroup of persons with schizophrenia (about 20%) who will not experience a second episode regardless of whether they take maintenance antipsychotic medication. Therefore, some researchers and clinicians have advocated a medication strategy that entails restarting the antipsychotic at the first signs of a relapse. Earlier studies showed that relapse rates using this 'intermittent targeted' approach were higher than when medication was continuously prescribed,[152] that a low dose was almost as effective as a regular dose and that restarting medication before the person is in crisis produces less risk of relapse than starting after a crisis has begun.[153] A recent study that compared first and multi-episode patients with schizophrenia found that multi-episode patients relapsed least over two years under continuous medication but the first episode patients did just

as well in terms of relapse, psychopathology, and social functioning when they received relapse prodrome-based interventions. Also, compliance was better for prodromal intervention.[154] Other evidence supports the approach that symptomatic exacerbations in recent-onset schizophrenia when off medication can be successfully managed in most cases by providing support and restarting medication rather than resorting to hospitalization.[155] Some researchers are examining drugs other than antipsychotics using the intermittent approach. One recent study showed that diazepam significantly outperformed placebo (as did fluphenazine) in preventing progression from early warning signs to full relapse.[156]

Despite the fact that an intermittent dosing strategy may be less than ideal, it will occur in clinical situations quite frequently. If the person has had only one episode, experienced a complete symptomatic recovery, and is willing to be closely followed but is very reluctant to take medication, it appears reasonable to try the intermittent approach. However, for someone with schizophrenia who has relapsed quickly, medication should probably be maintained for at least five years.[54]

In general, a patient in the maintenance phase is well served through:

- Close monitoring
- Engagement of family or others close to the patient
- Timely review of the diagnosis
- Keeping the dose as low as possible
- Facilitation of ongoing psychosocial interventions
- Ensuring easy access to services if a relapse appears possible.

Consequences of stopping treatment

About 60% of patients who recovered from a first episode of psychosis relapsed within a year if they stopped receiving medication, whereas 40% of those on a maintenance dose of an antipsychotic relapsed.[157] Other studies report that 70% of patients with schizophrenia on placebo will relapse within one year compared to 30% on active medication,[158] while estimations of 'real world' one year relapse rates of patients on medication are about 50%. When persons with schizophrenia were taken off typical antipsychotic medication, almost 75% relapsed within two years.[159] A recent analysis of recovered first episode patients with schizophrenia or schizoaffective disorder found that the cumulative first relapse rate after five years was over 80%. Of those who had a second relapse, 86% had a third relapse within four years after recovery from a second relapse. Discontinuing antipsychotic drug therapy increased the risk of relapse by almost five times. Subsequent analyses controlling for antipsychotic drug use showed that patients with poor premorbid adaptation to school and premorbid social withdrawal relapsed earlier.[151]

A recent report highlights the interpretive problems that arise when the definition of relapse varies. When hospitalization was used as a criterion for identifying relapse, only 13% of recent-onset patients with schizophrenia were found to have relapsed within two years after discontinuation of a typical antipsychotic (that had been prescribed for one to two years).[155] When increased symptomatology was employed as the criterion, 96% experienced a 'relapse' within two years. Only six out of 46 patients who suffered symptom exacerbation could not be successfully managed in the community. Therefore, although maintenance medication therapy is associated with lower relapse rates, many patients will either request withdrawal or discontinue on their own. In these cases, clinically supervised discontinuation with rapid reintroduction is preferable to covert non-compliance. A cooperative patient with good insight and a history of excellent response to medication may be a better candidate for supervised withdrawal than one lacking these qualities. For a fuller discussion on non-adherence refer to the section on relapse in Chapter 7.

Pharmacotherapy of affective psychoses

Response rates in affective psychoses are relatively good. A recent study found that 84% of bipolar patients attained syndromal recovery within six months (80% of the sample had psychotic features) compared to 59% syndromal recovery among patients with non-affective psychoses.[160]

Guidelines for the treatment of bipolar disorder and other affective disorders with psychotic features are available.[135,161,162] A recent paper thoroughly reviews the pharmacotherapy of first episode bipolar disorder.[128] Side effects are extensive with medications used to treat bipolar disorder. A review of those effects is beyond the scope of this discussion and the reader should consult one of the many resources available.[162]

Acute phase treatment

If a first episode psychosis patient presents with mania and the clinician suspects bipolar disorder, treatment with an antipsychotic and a mood stabilizer is recommended as both lithium and valproate are effective treatments for acute mania.[163] Lithium's utility in adolescents with mania has been established regardless of the presence of depressive symptoms, substance abuse, or history of attention deficit hyperactive disorder (ADHD).[164]

Although both typical and atypical antipsychotics are effective treatments for acute mania,[165] the literature on antipsychotic medications in first episode mania is sparse. In acute mania, several atypicals and typicals have been shown to be more effective than placebo.[166] Atypicals also appear to hold promise as monotherapy.[167–169] The use of atypicals as monotherapy in acute mania has also been confirmed for risperidone and olanzapine, compared to lithium and valproate, with the atypicals perhaps leading to remission more quickly.[170–172] Case reports suggesting that atypicals can induce mania have not been confirmed by larger group studies.[173]

Risperidone or haloperidol added to either valproate or lithium produced a significant reduction in manic symptoms versus placebo but they did not differ from each other.[174] Also, both olanzapine and risperidone have been shown to be effective adjuncts to mood stabilizers in persons with bipolar or schizoaffective disorders.[175,176] Adolescents with bipolar disorder also responded significantly better when quetiapine versus placebo was added to valproate.[177]

> It is recommended that initial treatment of a patient with psychosis and manic symptoms suggestive of bipolar disorder begins with an atypical antipsychotic to which is added lithium or valproate.

Since stimulants may exacerbate mania, it is recommended that the stimulant be discontinued when ADHD is also present.[178] If the patient presents with psychosis and depression, it is recommended that an atypical antipsychotic be combined with an antidepressant. However, 13% of patients first admitted with a major depressive disorder with psychosis developed manic symptoms within two years.[179]

Maintenance phase treatment

Psychotic disorders, other than schizophrenia, merit shorter maintenance periods with antipsychotics after symptomatic recovery, although close monitoring is essential. For example, with first episode manic patients it is common practice for antipsychotics to be discontinued in about 75% of patients within six months.[160] One study on combined lithium/antipsychotic therapy in bipolar patients found that discontinuation of the antipsychotic one month after a good therapeutic response was not maintained (especially in those with a longer duration of untreated psychosis).[180] In recurrent major depression with psychotic features, some data indicate that treatment with an antipsychotic (and an antidepressant) was not required beyond 4–8 months for about 75% of patients.[181] The relapse rate in persons with bipolar disorder on lithium is about 35–40% compared to about 80% on placebo.[182] Lithium treatment extends the time to relapse into mania but not depression versus placebo.[183,184] Discontinuation of lithium must not be abrupt in order to avoid the risk of relapse.[185] Comprehensive practice guidelines for first episode mania have not been developed but a recent set of evidence-based guidelines for bipolar disorder suggests indefinite maintenance treatment for good responders who have tolerated medication well for several years.[161] Conversely, the effect of maintenance lithium or carbamazepine on the subsequent course was not affected by the duration of illness when starting treatment.[186]

Persons with bipolar disorder are at high risk for developing tardive dyskinesia.[165] Also, the available evidence is currently limited to demonstrating effectiveness in the atypical antipsychotics in the acute phase.[187] Olanzapine appears to be the first medication for which data are accumulating showing efficacy for maintenance. It appears to be at least as effective as divalproex,[172] and very recent data found it to be as effective as lithium.[188]

Lithium remains the most well researched choice for maintenance therapy.[189] Valproate and carbamazepine also appear to be effective maintenance agents.[131,190] Lamotrigine and valproate may be especially useful in preventing relapse into depression.[191,192] Valproate inhibits the metabolism of lamotrigine.

> Maintenance on a mood stabilizer is recommended until further evidence accrues showing the viability of atypicals, other than olanzapine, as monotherapy.

Ongoing depression is a major problem after recovery from the initial acute episode and adjunctive treatment with an antidepressant produces only a modest success rate.[193] In bipolar patients it is well recognized that antidepressants, especially tricylics, can induce mania.[45] However, those patients who discontinued antidepressants within six months of treatment with an antidepressant were more likely to relapse into depression than those who maintained the antidepressant for a year.[194] Therefore, for that small proportion of responders to antidepressants who remain euthymic for months, it is recommended that antidepressant therapy be continued. A recent large trial found that olanzapine was superior to placebo in treating bipolar depression over eight weeks and olanzapine combined with fluoxetine was even better (with no active treatment increasing risk of developing mania).[195] In pediatric bipolar disorder, some evidence suggests that use of selective serotonin reuptake inhibitors (SSRIs) in follow-up both reduces risk of depression and increases risk of mania yet did not interfere with the reduced mania risk of mood stabilizers.[196]

> For a patient initially presenting with mania and psychosis who relapses, exhibiting depression and psychosis, treatment with an antipsychotic, antidepressant, and mood stabilizer is recommended.

Although it may be helpful, the common practice of maintaining a patient on a combination of mood stabilizers is not informed by a large body of evidence from controlled trials. Failure to derive a good response after three weeks may prompt the use of a second mood stabilizer, or a different antipsychotic.[167–169,175,176]

Benzodiazepines can also be considered if severe behavioral disturbance is present.[131,134,135,162] (See Figure 6.1 for a flowchart of pharmacotherapy from the onset of psychosis.)

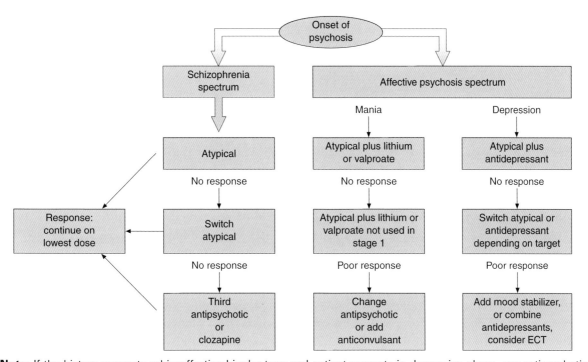

Note: If the history suggests schizoaffective bipolar type and patient presents in depressive phase, use antipsychotic and mood stabilizer, and follow bipolar manic stream.

Figure 6.1 Pharmacotherapy flowchart

Adolescents: pharmacological considerations

The practice parameters for schizophrenia by the American Academy of Child and Adolescent Psychiatry caution that their treatment recommendations are based on the adult literature because of a paucity of research on adolescents with schizophrenia.[150] However, typical antipsychotic medications are effective in youth.[197] It appears that adolescents' response to atypicals is similar to that of adults with the schizophrenia spectrum,[198–204] and bipolar disorder.[177] Dose finding studies in youth are needed since sensitivity to extrapyramidal symptoms and weight gain appear to be increased in younger patients.[106,197] Effects on cognition do not appear to have been examined, and long-term data on dyskinesias and other adverse effects are lacking. However, data are accumulating documenting the effective use of lithium and valproate in younger populations.[164,205]

Emergency room presentations

Pharmacotherapy priorities

Several general pharmacotherapy strategies apply to presentations in hospital emergency departments:[206]

- Determine if any psychiatric medications are currently prescribed. If so, it is advisable to continue with those medications, rather than switch to a new agent.
- Reserve as-needed medications for situations (such as anxiety or mild aggression) in which psychological interventions prove ineffective. If as-needed medication is required, benzodiazepines rather than antipsychotics are recommended. The use of benzodiazepines allows for observation of the presenting symptoms and their course over the initial few days as well as time to investigate possible etiologies of the presenting psychosis. Use of atypical antipsychotics should be considered after the initial period of observation when the psychosis persists and the provisional diagnosis appears more robust.[128]

- The ideal response to the acutely agitated or aggressive state is not necessarily sedation, but a reduction in agitation accompanied by an alert, oriented cooperative state, whereby the patient can be assessed.
- Moderate agitation may be treated with low-to-moderate doses of benzodiazepines (e.g. 1–2 mg lorazepam given orally or sublingually), while severe agitation usually merits higher doses (e.g. 3–4 lorazepam).
- If a patient is combative, a show of numbers may be helpful along with the offer of higher doses of benzodiazepines (e.g. 3–4 mg lorazepam) given orally if possible or intramuscularly, if necessary.

When a combative patient fails to respond to the above interventions, a combination of an intramuscular benzodiazepine and a moderately sedating antipsychotic might be considered. It is important to remember calm, clear communication, and a united attitude when explaining the need for parenteral medication.

A patient may require an injectible benzodiazepine (e.g. 2 mg lorazepam) and antipsychotic (e.g. loxapine 5–25 mg), depending on his or her size, ethnicity, and level of agitation. A new injectible form of olanzapine has been developed that may be useful in this regard. If repeated doses fail to settle a patient, the use of zuclopenthixol represents a viable option, as its effects last for 2–3 days. Dose in first episode patients is 50–100 mg. However, the use of injectible antipsychotics prompts questions about the impact upon patient autonomy and informed consent.[207]

New intramuscular (IM) treatment possibilities include IM olanzapine and IM ziprasidone. However, all trials of these medications were restricted to adult populations. IM ziprasidone controlled agitation in 57% of patients at 10 mg, whereas 90% responded at 20 mg, with little adverse events that include nausea, headache, and dizziness (nearly free of extrapyramidal side effects (EPS) and the magnitude of QTc interval increase was very modest and comparable to oral ziprasidone).[208] IM olanzapine was also efficacious in four randomized, double blind placebo-controlled trials at doses of 5–10 mg (comparable to IM lorazepam and IM haloperidol). It is also generally safe and well tolerated with fewer than 5% of acutely agitated patients experiencing sinus bradycardia with little EPS. The optimally efficacious dose appears to be 10 mg, which is comparable to the 20 mg dose of oral (or dissolving) olanzapine.[209]

Liquid risperidone and the rapidly dissolving olanzapine pill represent further medication delivery strategies for patients in whom normal oral medication is problematic. Rapidly dissolving olanzapine may also be administered in a non-carbonated liquid.

Conclusions

Atypicals are recommended as first line agents in early psychosis since, compared to typicals, they have:

- The least adverse side effect profile
- Equal or better efficacy against symptoms
- Better effects on cognition.

There is also evidence that some atypicals may be associated with less hospitalization time, both during the index episode and during the subsequent follow-up.[210] Extra effort must be made to attend to the risks posed by atypicals regarding weight gain and neuroendocrine dysfunction. To date, the only controlled trials on early episode psychosis treated with atypicals used olanzapine and risperidone.[72,149,211] Recent research has demonstrated that doses effective for early episode psychosis tend to be smaller than the doses recommended when a new atypical comes onto the market.[13,56]

Neuroleptic-naïve patients are especially sensitive to both therapeutic and unwanted effects from antipsychotics. Doses should start low and proceed upwards slowly. Simultaneous use of two antipsychotics is discouraged. Clozapine should be reserved for treatment of refractory cases. Minimal doses are recommended for maintenance. Prescribers should become familiar with intermittent targeting procedures as an alternative for a proportion of patients. The lack of research for the majority of atypicals means there is little empirically based guidance on optimal dosing for these antipsychotics. It is hoped that studies will soon be forthcoming that demonstrate efficacy and provide better guidance regarding the use of these medications in early psychosis.

Although atypicals are effective and recommended in the acute stages of mania, their use as maintenance monotherapy cannot yet be recommended (except possibly olanzapine). The use of atypicals appears effectively to complement lithium and valproate and should be considered as viable in this context. Lithium and valproate remain the prime choices for long-term treatment of bipolar disorder. The atypicals are also recommended in cases of major depression with psychosis along with an antidepressant. The status of antidepressants both in schizophrenia and bipolar disorder after resolution of the psychosis remains unclear. It appears that depression is not effectively treated by antidepressants in most persons with these disorders. Research is certainly needed in this area. Prescribers are encouraged to facilitate psychosocial interventions for their patients when considering these limitations.

References

1. Arana GW. An overview of side effects caused by typical antipsychotics. J Clin Psychiatry 2000; **61**(Suppl 8):5–11; discussion 12–13.
2. Rosebush PI, Mazurek MF. Neurologic side effects in neuroleptic-naive patients treated with haloperidol or risperidone [see comments]. Neurology 1999; **52**(4):782–5.
3. Owens D. A guide to the extrapyramidal side effects of antipsychotic drugs. Cambridge University Press; 2000.
4. Dixon LB, Lehman AF, Levine J. Conventional

antipsychotic medications for schizophrenia. Schizophr Bull 1995; **21**(4):567–77.

5. Kapur S, Zipursky R, Jones C, et al. Relationship between dopamine D(2) occupancy, clinical response, and side effects: a double-blind PET study of first-episode schizophrenia. Am J Psychiatry 2000; **157**(4):514–20.

6. Kapur S, Seeman P. Does fast dissociation from the dopamine d(2) receptor explain the action of atypical antipsychotics?: A new hypothesis. Am J Psychiatry 2001; **158**(3):360–9.

7. de Haan L, van Bruggen M, Lavalaye J, et al. Subjective experience and D2 receptor occupancy in patients with recent-onset schizophrenia treated with low-dose olanzapine or haloperidol: a randomized, double-blind study. Am J Psychiatry 2003; **160**(2):303–9.

8. Carlson CD, Cavazzoni PA, Berg PH, et al. An integrated analysis of acute treatment-emergent extrapyramidal syndrome in patients with schizophrenia during olanzapine clinical trials: comparisons with placebo, haloperidol, risperidone, or clozapine. J Clin Psychiatry 2003; **64**(8): 898–906.

9. Ho BC, Miller D, Nopoulos P, Andreasen NC. A comparative effectiveness study of risperidone and olanzapine in the treatment of schizophrenia. J Clin Psychiatry 1999; **60**(10):658–63.

10. Leucht S, Pitschel-Walz G, Abraham D, Kissling W. Efficacy and extrapyramidal side-effects of the new antipsychotics olanzapine, quetiapine, risperidone, and sertindole compared to conventional antipsychotics and placebo. A meta-analysis of randomized controlled trials. Schizophr Res 1999; **35**(1):51–68.

11. Fenton M, Morris S, De-Silva P, et al. Zotepine for schizophrenia. Cochrane Database Syst Rev 2000; **2**:CD001948.

12. Leucht S, Pitschel-Walz G, Engel RR, Kissling W. Amisulpride, an unusual 'atypical' antipsychotic: a meta-analysis of randomized controlled trials. Am J Psychiatry 2002; **159**(2):180–90.

13. Potkin SG, Saha AR, Kujawa MJ, et al. Aripiprazole, an antipsychotic with a novel mechanism of action, and risperidone vs placebo in patients with schizophrenia and schizoaffective disorder. Arch Gen Psychiatry 2003; **60**(7):681–90.

14. Bagnall A, Lewis RA, Leitner ML, Kleijnen J. Ziprasidone for schizophrenia and severe mental illness. Cochrane Database Syst Rev 2000; **2**: CD001945.

15. Geddes J, Freemantle N, Harrison P, Bebbington P. Atypical antipsychotics in the treatment of schizophrenia: systematic overview and meta-regression analysis. BMJ 2000; **321**(7273):1371–6.

16. Carriere P, Bonhomme D, Lemperiere T. Amisulpride has a superior benefit/risk profile to haloperidol in schizophrenia: results of a multicentre, double-blind study (the Amisulpride Study Group). Eur Psychiatry 2000; **15**(5):321–9.

17. Davis JM, Chen N, Glick ID. A meta-analysis of the efficacy of second-generation antipsychotics. Arch Gen Psychiatry 2003; **60**(6):553–64.

18. Hwang TJ, Lee SM, Sun HJ, et al. Amisulpride versus risperidone in the treatment of schizophrenic patients: a double-blind pilot study in Taiwan. J Formos Med Assoc 2003; **102**(1): 30–6.

19. Martin S, Ljo H, Peuskens J, et al. A double-blind, randomised comparative trial of amisulpride versus olanzapine in the treatment of schizophrenia: short-term results at two months. Curr Med Res Opin 2002; **18**(6):355–62.

20. Van Bruggen J, Tijssen J, Dingemans P, et al. Symptom response and side-effects of olanzapine and risperidone in young adults with recent onset schizophrenia. Int Clin Psychopharmacol 2003; **18**(6):341–6.

21. Gureje O, Miles W, Keks N, et al. Olanzapine vs risperidone in the management of schizophrenia: a randomized double-blind trial in Australia and New Zealand. Schizophr Res 2003; **61**(2–3):303–14.

22. Emsley RA. Risperidone in the treatment of first-episode psychotic patients: a double-blind multi-center study. Risperidone Working Group. Schizophr Bull 1999; **25**(4):721–9.

23. Duggan L, Fenton M, Dardennes RM, et al. Olanzapine for schizophrenia. Cochrane Database Syst Rev 2003; **1**:CD001359.

24. Hunter RH, Joy CB, Kennedy E, et al. Risperidone versus typical antipsychotic medication for schizophrenia. Cochrane Database Syst Rev 2003; **2**:CD000440.

25. Mota NE, Lima MS, Soares BG. Amisulpride for schizophrenia. Cochrane Database Syst Rev 2002; **2**:CD001357.

26. Gutierrez-Esteinou R, Grebb JA. Risperidone: an analysis of the first three years in general use. Int Clin Psychopharmacol 1997; **12**(Suppl 4):S3–S10.

27. Aitchison K, Meehan K, Murray R. *First Episode Psychosis*. London: Martin Dunitz; 1999.

28. Rosenzweig P, Canal M, Patat A, et al. A review of the pharmacokinetics, tolerability and pharmaco-dynamics of amisulpride in healthy volunteers. Hum Psychopharmacol 2002; **17**(1):1–13.

29. Seeman P, Tallerico T. Antipsychotic drugs which elicit little or no parkinsonism bind more loosely than dopamine to brain D2 receptors, yet occupy high levels of these receptors. Mol Psychiatry 1998; **3**(2):123–34.

30. Seeman P, Tallerico T. Rapid release of antipsychotic drugs from dopamine D2 receptors: an explanation for low receptor occupancy and early clinical relapse upon withdrawal of clozapine or quetiapine. Am J Psychiatry 1999; **156**(6):876–84.

31. Robinson DG, Woerner MG, Alvir JM, et al. Predictors of treatment response from a first episode of schizophrenia or schizoaffective disorder [see comments]. Am J Psychiatry 1999; **156**(4): 544–9.

32. Szymanski SR, Cannon TD, Gallacher F, et al. Course of treatment response in first-episode and chronic schizophrenia. Am J Psychiatry 1996; **153**(4):519–25.

33. Kopala LC, Fredrikson D, Good KP, Honer WG. Symptoms in neuroleptic-naive, first-episode schizophrenia: response to risperidone. Biol Psychiatry 1996; **39**(4):296–8.

34. Sanger TM, Lieberman JA, Tohen M, et al. Olanzapine versus haloperidol treatment in first-episode psychosis. Am J Psychiatry 1999; **156**(1):79–87.

35. The Scottish First Episode Schizophrenia Study. II. Treatment: pimozide versus flupenthixol. The Scottish Schizophrenia Research Group. Br J Psychiatry 1987; **150**:334–8.

36. Lieberman JA, Tollefson G, Tohen M, et al. Comparative efficacy and safety of atypical and conventional antipsychotic drugs in first-episode psychosis: a randomized, double-blind trial of olanzapine versus haloperidol. Am J Psychiatry 2003;160(8):1396–404.

37. Merlo MC, Hofer H, Gekle W, et al. Risperidone, 2 mg/day vs. 4 mg/day, in first-episode, acutely psychotic patients: treatment efficacy and effects on fine motor functioning. J Clin Psychiatry 2002; **63**(10):885–91.

38. Green MF, Nuechterlein KH. Should schizophrenia be treated as a neurocognitive disorder? Schizophr Bull 1999; **25**(2):309–19.

39. Szymanski S, Masiar S, Mayerhoff D, et al. Clozapine response in treatment-refractory first-episode schizophrenia. Biol Psychiatry 1994; **35**(4): 278–80.

40. Lieberman JA, Phillips M, Gu H, et al. Atypical and conventional antipsychotic drugs in treatment-naive first-episode schizophrenia: a 52-week randomized trial of clozapine vs chlorpromazine. Neuropsychopharmacology 2003; **28**(5):995–1003.

41. Hofer A, Hummer M, Kemmler G, et al. The safety of clozapine in the treatment of first- and multiple-episode patients with treatment-resistant schizophrenia. Int J Neuropsychopharmacol 2003; **6**(3):201–6.

42. Shaw JA, Lewis JE, Pascal S. An open trial of quetiapine in adolescent patients with psychosis. In: *International Congress on Schizophrenia Research*, Whistler, Canada; 2001.

43. Tauscher-Wisniewski S, Kapur S, Tauscher J, et al. Quetiapine: an effective antipsychotic in first-episode schizophrenia despite only transiently high dopamine-2 receptor blockade. J Clin Psychiatry 2002; **63**(11):992–7.

44. Wieselgren IM, Lindstrom LH. A prospective 1–5 year outcome study in first-admitted and readmitted schizophrenic patients; relationship to heredity, premorbid adjustment, duration of disease and education level at index admission and neuroleptic treatment. Acta Psychiatr Scand 1996; **93**(1):9–19.

45. Alvir JM, Woerner MG, Gunduz H, et al. Obstetric complications predict treatment response in first-episode schizophrenia. Psychol Med 1999; **29**(3):621–7.

46. Meltzer HY, Rabinowitz J, Lee MA, et al. Age at onset and gender of schizophrenic patients in relation to neuroleptic resistance. Am J Psychiatry 1997; **154**(4):475–82.

47. Dernovsek MZ, Tavcar R. Age at onset of schizophrenia and neuroleptic dosage. Soc Psychiatry Psychiatr Epidemiol 1999; **34**(12):622–6.

48. Amminger GP, Resch F, Mutschlechner R, et al.

Premorbid adjustment and remission of positive symptoms in first-episode psychosis. Eur Child Adolesc Psychiatry 1997; **6**(4):212–18.

49. Bailer J, Brauer W, Rey ER. Premorbid adjustment as predictor of outcome in schizophrenia: results of a prospective study. Acta Psychiatr Scand 1996; **93**(5):368–77.

50. Chakos MH, Mayerhoff DI, Loebel AD, et al. Incidence and correlates of acute extrapyramidal symptoms in first episode of schizophrenia. Psychopharmacol Bull 1992; **28**(1):81–6.

51. Aguilar EJ, Keshavan MS, Martinez-Quiles MD, et al. Predictors of acute dystonia in first-episode psychotic patients. Am J Psychiatry 1994; **151**(12): 1819–21.

52. Kopala LC, Good KP, Honer WG. Extrapyramidal signs and clinical symptoms in first-episode schizophrenia: response to low-dose risperidone. J Clin Psychopharmacol 1997; **17**(4):308–13.

53. Nasrallah HA, Churchill CM, Hamdan-Allan GA. Higher frequency of neuroleptic-induced dystonia in mania than in schizophrenia. Am J Psychiatry 1988; **145**(11):1455–6.

54. Practice guidelines for the treatment of patients with schizophrenia. American Psychiatric Association [see comments]. Am J Psychiatry 1997: **154**(4 Suppl):1–63.

55. Chakos MH, Alvir JM, Woerner MG, et al. Incidence and correlates of tardive dyskinesia in first episode of schizophrenia. Arch Gen Psychiatry 1996; **53**(4):313–19.

56. Oosthuizen PP, Emsley RA, Maritz JS, et al. Incidence of tardive dyskinesia in first-episode psychosis patients treated with low-dose haloperidol. J Clin Psychiatry 2003; **64**(9):1075–80.

57. Beasley CM, Dellva MA, Tamura RN, et al. Randomised double-blind comparison of the incidence of tardive dyskinesia in patients with schizophrenia during long-term treatment with olanzapine or haloperidol [see comments]. Br J Psychiatry 1999; **174**:23–30.

58. Ghadirian AM, Chouinard G, Annable L. Sexual dysfunction and plasma prolactin levels in neuroleptic-treated schizophrenic outpatients. J Nerv Ment Dis 1982; **170**(8):463–7.

59. Lavalaye J, Linszen DH, Booij J, et al. Dopamine D2 receptor occupancy by olanzapine or risperidone in young patients with schizophrenia. Psychiatry Res 1999; **92**(1):33–44.

60. Dickson RA, Glazer WM. Neuroleptic-induced hyperprolactinemia. Schizophr Res 1999; **35**(Suppl):S75–S86.

61. Dickson RA, Seeman MV, Corenblum B. Hormonal side effects in women: typical versus atypical antipsychotic treatment. J Clin Psychiatry 2000; **61**(Suppl 3):10–5.

62. Buckman MT, Peake GT. Estrogen potentiation of phenothiazine-induced prolactin secretion in man. J Clin Endocrinol Metab 1973; **37**(6): 977–80.

63. Petty RG. Prolactin and antipsychotic medications: mechanism of action. Schizophr Res 1999; **35**(Suppl):S67–S73.

64. Bobes J, Garc APMP, Rejas J, et al. Frequency of sexual dysfunction and other reproductive side-effects in patients with schizophrenia treated with risperidone, olanzapine, quetiapine, or haloperidol: the results of the EIRE study. J Sex Marital Ther 2003; **29**(2):125–47.

65. Ghadirian AM, Annable L, Belanger MC. Lithium, benzodiazepines, and sexual function in bipolar patients. Am J Psychiatry 1992; **149**(6):801–5.

66. Correa N, Opler LA, Kay SR, Birmaher B. Amantadine in the treatment of neuroendocrine side effects of neuroleptics. J Clin Psychopharmacol 1987; **7**(2):91–5.

67. Smith S. Neuroleptic-associated hyperprolactinemia. Can it be treated with bromocriptine? J Reprod Med 1992; **37**(8):737–40.

68. Addington J, Mansley C, Addington D. Weight gain in first-episode psychosis. Can J Psychiatry 2003; **48**(4):272–6.

69. Taylor DM, McAskill R. Atypical antipsychotics and weight gain—a systematic review. Acta Psychiatr Scand 2000; **101**(6):416–32.

70. Conley RR, Meltzer HY. Adverse events related to olanzapine. J Clin Psychiatry 2000; **61**(Suppl 8): 26–9; discussion 30.

71. Zarate CA, Jr. Antipsychotic drug side effect issues in bipolar manic patients. J Clin Psychiatry 2000; **61**(Suppl 8):52–61; discussion 62–3.

72. Canadian clinical practice guidelines for the treatment of schizophrenia. The Canadian Psychiatric Association [see comments]. Can J Psychiatry 1998; **43**(Suppl 2):25S-40S.

73. Wirshing DA, Spellberg BJ, Erhart SM, et al. Novel antipsychotics and new onset diabetes. Biol Psychiatry 1998; **44**(8):778–83.

74. Werneke U, Taylor D, Sanders TA. Options for pharmacological management of obesity in patients treated with atypical antipsychotics. Int Clin Psychopharmacol 2002; **17**(4):145–60.

75. Malhi GS, Mitchell PB. Pharmacotherapy to limit weight gain caused by antipsychotic use. Expert Opin Pharmacother 2003; **4**(10):1679–86.

76. Conley RR. Risperidone side effects. J Clin Psychiatry 2000; **61**(Suppl 8):20–3; discussion 24–5.

77. Alvir JM, Lieberman JA, Safferman AZ, et al. Clozapine-induced agranulocytosis. Incidence and risk factors in the United States. N Engl J Med 1993; **329**(3):162–7.

78. Pelonero AL, Levenson JL, Pandurangi AK. Neuroleptic malignant syndrome: a review. Psychiatr Serv 1998; **49**(9):1163–72.

79. Hasan S, Buckley P. Novel antipsychotics and the neuroleptic malignant syndrome: a review and critique. Am J Psychiatry 1998; **155**(8):1113–16.

80. Gerlach J, Larsen EB. Subjective experience and mental side-effects of antipsychotic treatment. Acta Psychiatr Scand Suppl 1999; **395**:113–17.

81. Richelson E. Preclinical pharmacology of neuroleptics: focus on new generation compounds. J Clin Psychiatry 1996; **57**(Suppl 11):4–11.

82. Bollini P, Pampallona S, Orza MJ, et al. Antipsychotic drugs: is more worse? A meta-analysis of the published randomized control trials. Psychol Med 1994; **24**(2):307–16.

83. Poolsup N, Li Wan Po A, Knight TL. Pharmacogenetics and psychopharmacotherapy. J Clin Pharm Ther 2000; **25**(3):197–220.

84. Tanaka E, Hisawa S. Clinically significant pharmacokinetic drug interactions with psychoactive drugs: antidepressants and antipsychotics and the cytochrome P450 system. J Clin Pharm Ther 1999; **24**(1):7–16.

85. Sharif Z. Pharmacokinetics, metabolism and drug interactions of atypical antipsychotics in special populations. J Clin Psychiatry 2003; **5**(Suppl 6):22–25.

86. Buck M. Using atypical antipsychotics agents in children and adolescents. Pediatric Pharmacotherapy 2001; **7**(8):708–11.

87. Lyon ER. A review of the effects of nicotine on schizophrenia and antipsychotic medications. Psychiatr Serv 1999; **50**(10):1346–50.

88. Green MF. What are the functional consequences of neurocognitive deficits in schizophrenia? [see comments]. Am J Psychiatry 1996; **153**(3):321–30.

89. Harvey PD, Green MF, McGurk SR, Meltzer HY. Changes in cognitive functioning with risperidone and olanzapine treatment: a large-scale, double-blind, randomized study. Psychopharmacology (Berl) 2003; **169**(3–4):404–11.

90. Meltzer HY, McGurk SR. The effects of clozapine, risperidone, and olanzapine on cognitive function in schizophrenia. Schizophr Bull 1999; **25**(2):233–55.

91. Purdon SE, Jones BD, Stip E, et al. Neuropsychological change in early phase schizophrenia during 12 months of treatment with olanzapine, risperidone, or haloperidol. The Canadian Collaborative Group for research in schizophrenia. Arch Gen Psychiatry 2000; **57**(3):249–58.

92. Purdon SE, Malla A, Labelle A, Lit W. Neuropsychological change in patients with schizophrenia after treatment with quetiapine or haloperidol. J Psychiatry Neurosci 2001; **26**(2):137–49.

93. Spohn HE, Strauss ME. Relation of neuroleptic and anticholinergic medication to cognitive functions in schizophrenia. J Abnorm Psychol 1989; **98**(4):367–80.

94. Palmer DD, Henter ID, Wyatt RJ. Do antipsychotic medications decrease the risk of suicide in patients with schizophrenia? J Clin Psychiatry 1999; **60**(Suppl 2):100–3; discussion 111–16.

95. Reid WH, Mason M, Hogan T. Suicide prevention effects associated with clozapine therapy in schizophrenia and schizoaffective disorder. Psychiatr Serv 1998; **49**(8):1029–33.

96. Meltzer HY, Alphs L, Green AI, et al. Clozapine treatment for suicidality in schizophrenia: International Suicide Prevention Trial (InterSePT). Arch Gen Psychiatry 2003; **60**(1):82–91.

97. Coppen A. Lithium in unipolar depression and the prevention of suicide. J Clin Psychiatry 2000; **61**(Suppl 9):52–6.

98. Muller-Siecheneder F, Muller MJ, Hillert A, et al. Risperidone versus haloperidol and amitriptyline in the treatment of patients with a combined psychotic and depressive syndrome. J Clin Psychopharmacol 1998; **18**(2):111–20.

99. Tollefson GD, Sanger TM, Lu Y, Thieme ME. Depressive signs and symptoms in schizophrenia: a prospective blinded trial of olanzapine and haloperidol. Arch Gen Psychiatry 1998; **55**(3): 250–8.

100. Tollefson GD, Sanger TM, Beasley CM, Tran PV. A double-blind, controlled comparison of the novel antipsychotic olanzapine versus haloperidol or placebo on anxious and depressive symptoms accompanying schizophrenia. Biol Psychiatry 1998; **43**(11):803–10.

101. Keck PE, Strakowski SM, McElroy SL. The efficacy of atypical antipsychotics in the treatment of depressive symptoms, hostility, and suicidality in patients with schizophrenia. J Clin Psychiatry 2000; **61**(Suppl 3):4–9.

102. Peuskens J, Moller HJ, Puech A. Amisulpride improves depressive symptoms in acute exacerbations of schizophrenia: comparison with haloperidol and risperidone. Eur Neuropsychopharmacol 2002; **12**(4):305–10.

103. Cassano GB, Jori MC. Efficacy and safety of amisulpride 50 mg versus paroxetine 20 mg in major depression: a randomized, double-blind, parallel group study. Int Clin Psychopharmacol 2002; **17**(1):27–32.

104. Bowers MB, Jr., Mazure CM, Nelson JC, Jatlow PI. Psychotogenic drug use and neuroleptic response. Schizophr Bull 1990; **16**(1):81–5.

105. D'Mello DA, Boltz MK, Msibi B. Relationship between concurrent substance abuse in psychiatric patients and neuroleptic dosage. Am J Drug Alcohol Abuse 1995; **21**(2):257–65.

106. Sikich L, Hamer RM, Bashford RA, et al. A pilot study of risperidone, olanzapine, and haloperidol in psychotic youth: a double-blind, randomized, 8-week trial. Neuropsychopharmacology 2004; **29**:1133–45.

107. Voruganti LN, Heslegrave RJ, Awad AG. Neuroleptic dysphoria may be the missing link between schizophrenia and substance abuse. J Nerv Ment Dis 1997; **185**(7):463–5.

108. Buckley P, Thompson PA, Way L, Meltzer HY. Substance abuse and clozapine treatment. J Clin Psychiatry 1994; **55**(Suppl B):114–6.

109. McEvoy J, Freudenreich O, McGee M, et al. Clozapine decreases smoking in patients with chronic schizophrenia. Biol Psychiatry 1995; **37**(8):550–2.

110. Drake RE, Xie H, McHugo GJ, Green AI. The effects of clozapine on alcohol and drug use disorders among patients with schizophrenia. Schizophr Bull 2000; **26**(2):441–9.

111. Zimmet SV, Strous RD, Burgess ES, et al. Effects of clozapine on substance use in patients with schizophrenia and schizoaffective disorder: a retrospective survey. J Clin Psychopharmacol 2000; **20**(1):94–8.

112. Green AI, Salomon MS, Brenner MJ, Rawlins K. Treatment of schizophrenia and comorbid substance use disorder. Curr Drug Target CNS Neurol Disord 2002; **1**(2):129–39.

113. Smelson DA, Losonczy MF, Davis CW, et al. Risperidone decreases craving and relapses in individuals with schizophrenia and cocaine dependence. Can J Psychiatry 2002; **47**(7):671–5.

114. Albanese MJ. Safety and efficacy of risperidone in substance abusers with psychosis. Am J Addict 2001; **10**(2):190–1.

115. Littrell KH, Petty RG, Hilligoss NM, et al. Olanzapine treatment for patients with schizophrenia and substance abuse. J Subst Abuse Treat 2001; **21**(4):217–21.

116. Green AI, Burgess ES, Dawson R, et al. Alcohol and cannabis use in schizophrenia: effects of clozapine vs. risperidone. Schizophr Res 2003; **60**(1):81–5.

117. Ritsner M, Ponizovsky A, Endicott J, et al. The impact of side-effects of antipsychotic agents on life satisfaction of schizophrenia patients: a naturalistic study. Eur Neuropsychopharmacol 2002; **12**(1):31–8.

118. Rummel C, Hamann J, Kissling W, Leucht S. New generation antipsychotics for first episode schizophrenia. Cochrane Database Syst Rev 2003; **4**:CD004410.

119. Karow A, Naber D. Subjective well-being and quality of life under atypical antipsychotic treatment. Psychopharmacology (Berl) 2002; **162**(1):3–10.

120. Liddle P, Carpenter WT, Crow T. Syndromes of schizophrenia. Classic literature. Br J Psychiatry 1994; **165**(6):721–7.

121. Lehman AF, Steinwachs DM. Translating research into practice: the Schizophrenia Patient Outcomes Research Team (PORT) treatment recommendations. Schizophr Bull 1998; **24**(1):1–10.

122. Johnstone EC, Owens DG, Crow TJ, Davis JM. Does a four-week delay in the introduction of medication alter the course of functional psychosis? J Psychopharmacol 1999; **13**(3):238–44.

123. Remington G, Kapur S, Zipursky RB. Pharmacotherapy of first-episode schizophrenia. Br J Psychiatry Suppl 1998; **172**(33):66–70.

124. Zhang-Wong J, Zipursky RB, Beiser M, Bean G. Optimal haloperidol dosage in first-episode psychosis. Can J Psychiatry 1999; **44**(2):164–7.

125. Kontaxakis VP, Havaki-Kontaxaki BJ, Stamouli SS, Christodoulou GN. Optimal risperidone dose in drug-naive, first-episode schizophrenia [letter; comments]. Am J Psychiatry 2000; **157**(7): 1178–9.

126. McGorry PD. Recommended haloperidol and risperidone doses in first-episode psychosis [letter; comments]. J Clin Psychiatry 1999; **60**(11):794–5.

127. McEvoy JP, Hogarty GE, Steingard S. Optimal dose of neuroleptic in acute schizophrenia. A controlled study of the neuroleptic threshold and higher haloperidol dose. Arch Gen Psychiatry 1991; **48**(8):739–45.

128. Lambert M, Conus P, Lambert T, McGorry PD. Pharmacotherapy of first-episode psychosis. Expert Opin Pharmacother 2003; **4**(5):717–50.

129. Fabrazzo M, La Pia S, Monteleone P, et al. Is the time course of clozapine response correlated to the time course of clozapine plasma levels? A one-year prospective study in drug-resistant patients with schizophrenia. Neuropsychopharmacology 2002; **27**(6):1050–5.

130. Kronig MH, Munne RA, Szymanski S, et al. Plasma clozapine levels and clinical response for treatment-refractory schizophrenic patients. Am J Psychiatry 1995; **152**(2):179–82.

131. Practice guideline for the treatment of patients with bipolar disorder. American Psychiatric Association. Am J Psychiatry 1994; **151**(12 Suppl):1–36.

132. Wahlbeck K, Cheine MV, Gilbody S, Ahonen J. Efficacy of beta-blocker supplementation for schizophrenia: a systematic review of randomized trials. Schizophr Res 2000; **41**(2):341–7.

133. Muller-Oerlinghausen B, Berghofer A, Bauer M. Bipolar disorder. Lancet 2002; **359**(9302):241–7.

134. Bauer MS, Callahan AM, Jampala C, et al. Clinical practice guidelines for bipolar disorder from the Department of Veterans Affairs [see comments] [published erratum appears in J Clin Psychiatry 1999; **60**(5):341]. J Clin Psychiatry 1999; **60**(1):9–21.

135. Sachs GS, Printz DJ, Kahn DA, et al. The Expert Consensus Guideline Series: Medication Treatment of Bipolar Disorder 2000. Postgrad Med 2000 (Spec No):1–104.

136. Leff J, Tress K, Edwards B. The clinical course of depressive symptoms in schizophrenia. Schizophr Res 1988; **1**(1):25–30.

137. Harrow M, Yonan CA, Sands JR, Marengo J. Depression in schizophrenia: are neuroleptics, akinesia, or anhedonia involved? Schizophr Bull 1994; **20**(2):327–38.

138. Yatham LN, Kusumakar V, Parikh SV, et al. Bipolar depression: treatment options. Can J Psychiatry 1997; **42**(Suppl 2):87S–91S.

139. Kramer MS, Vogel WH, DiJohnson C, et al. Antidepressants in 'depressed' schizophrenic inpatients. A controlled trial [see comments]. Arch Gen Psychiatry 1989; **46**(10):922–8.

140. Becker RE. Depression in schizophrenia. Hosp Community Psychiatry 1988; **39**(12):1269–75.

141. Whitehead C, Moss S, Cardno A, Lewis G. Antidepressants for the treatment of depression in people with schizophrenia: a systematic review. Psychol Med 2003; **33**(4):589–99.

142. Harrison G, Hopper K, Craig T, et al. Recovery from psychotic illness: a 15- and 25-year international follow-up study. Br J Psychiatry 2001; **178**:506–17.

143. Viguera AC, Baldessarini RJ, Hegarty JD, et al. Clinical risk following abrupt and gradual withdrawal of maintenance neuroleptic treatment. Arch Gen Psychiatry 1997; **54**(1):49–55.

144. Kinon BJ, Basson BR, Gilmore JA, et al. Strategies for switching from conventional antipsychotic drugs or risperidone to olanzapine. J Clin Psychiatry 2000; **61**(11):833–40.

145. Conley RR, Tamminga CA, Kelly DL, Richardson CM. Treatment-resistant schizophrenic patients respond to clozapine after olanzapine nonresponse. Biol Psychiatry 1999; **46**(1):73–7.

146. Kane JM. Management strategies for the treatment of schizophrenia. J Clin Psychiatry 1999; **60**(Suppl 12):13–17.

147. Treatment of schizophrenia. The Expert Consensus Panel for Schizophrenia. J Clin Psychiatry 1996; **57**(Suppl 12B):3–58.

148. Miller AL, Chiles JA, Chiles JK, et al. The Texas Medication Algorithm Project (TMAP) schizophrenia algorithms. J Clin Psychiatry 1999; **60**(10):649–57.

149. *Australian Clinical Guidelines for Early Psychosis.* Melbourne: National early psychosis project, University of Melbourne; 1998.

150. AACAP official action. Summary of the practice parameters for the assessment and treatment of children and adolescents with schizophrenia. American Academy of Child and Adolescent Psychiatry. J Am Acad Child Adolesc Psychiatry 2000; **39**(12):1580–2.

151. Robinson D, Woerner MG, Alvir JM, et al. Predictors of relapse following response from a first episode of schizophrenia or schizoaffective disorder. Arch Gen Psychiatry 1999; **56**(3):241–7.

152. Schooler NR. Reducing dosage in maintenance treatment of schizophrenia. Review and prognosis [see comments]. Br J Psychiatry Suppl 1993; **22**:58–65.

153. Gaebel W. Is intermittent, early intervention medication an alternative for neuroleptic maintenance treatment? Int Clin Psychopharmacol 1995; **9**(Suppl 5):11–16.

154. Gaebel W, Janner M, Frommann N, et al. First vs multiple episode schizophrenia: two-year outcome of intermittent and maintenance medication strategies. Schizophr Res 2002; **53**(1–2):145–59.

155. Gitlin M, Nuechterlein K, Subotnik KL, et al. Clinical outcome following neuroleptic discontinuation in patients with remitted recent-onset schizophrenia. Am J Psychiatry 2001;**158**(11):1835–42.

156. Carpenter WR, Buchanan RW, Kirkpatrick B, Breier AF. Diazepam treatment of early signs of exacerbation in schizophrenia. Am J Psychiatry 1999; **156**(2):299–303.

157. Crow TJ, MacMillan JF, Johnson AL, Johnstone EC. A randomised controlled trial of prophylactic neuroleptic treatment. Br J Psychiatry 1986; **148**:120–7.

158. McClellan J, Werry J. Practice parameters for the assessment and treatment of children and adolescents with schizophrenia. American Academy of Child and Adolescent Psychiatry. J Am Acad Child Adolesc Psychiatry 1997; **36**(10 Suppl):177S–193S.

159. Kane JM. Treatment programme and long-term outcome in chronic schizophrenia. Acta Psychiatr Scand Suppl 1990; **358**:151–7.

160. Zarate CA, Jr., Tohen M. Antipsychotic drug treatment in first-episode mania: a 6–month longitudinal study. J Clin Psychiatry 2000; **61**(1):33–8.

161. Goodwin GM. Evidence-based guidelines for treating bipolar disorder: recommendations from the British Association for Psychopharmacology. J Psychopharmacol 2003; **17**(2):149–73; discussion 147.

162. American Psychiatric Association Working Group. *Practice Guidelines for the Treatment of Patients with Bipolar Disorder* (revised). Arlington: American Psychiatric Association; 2002.

163. Bowden CL, Brugger AM, Swann AC, et al. Efficacy of divalproex vs lithium and placebo in the treatment of mania. The Depakote Mania Study Group. JAMA 1994; **271**(12):918–24.

164. Kafantaris V, Coletti DJ, Dicker R, et al. Lithium treatment of acute mania in adolescents: a large open trial. J Am Acad Child Adolesc Psychiatry 2003; **42**(9):1038–45.

165. Keck PE, McElroy SL, Strakowski SM, Soutullo CA. Antipsychotics in the treatment of mood disorders and risk of tardive dyskinesia. J Clin Psychiatry 2000; **61**(Suppl 4):33–8.

166. McElroy SL, Keck PE, Jr. Pharmacologic agents for the treatment of acute bipolar mania. Biol Psychiatry 2000; **48**(6):539–57.

167. Tohen M, Jacobs TG, Grundy SL, et al. Efficacy of olanzapine in acute bipolar mania: a double-blind, placebo-controlled study. The Olanzipine HGGW Study Group. Arch Gen Psychiatry 2000; **57**(9):841–9.

168. McElroy SL, Frye M, Denicoff K, et al. Olanzapine in treatment-resistant bipolar disorder. J Affect Disord 1998; **49**(2):119–22.

169. Tohen M, Zarate CA, Jr., Centorrino F, et al. Risperidone in the treatment of mania. J Clin Psychiatry 1996; **57**(6):249–53.

170. Segal J, Berk M, Brook S. Risperidone compared with both lithium and haloperidol in mania: a double-blind randomized controlled trial. Clin Neuropharmacol 1998; **21**(3):176–80.

171. Rendell JM, Gijsman HJ, Keck P, et al. Olanzapine alone or in combination for acute mania. Cochrane Database Syst Rev 2003; **3**:CD004040.

172. Tohen M, Ketter TA, Zarate CA, et al. Olanzapine versus divalproex sodium for the treatment of acute mania and maintenance of remission: a 47–week study. Am J Psychiatry 2003; **160**(7):1263–71.

173. Baker RW, Milton DR, Stauffer VL, et al. Placebo-controlled trials do not find association of olanzapine with exacerbation of bipolar mania. J Affect Disord 2003; **73**(1–2):147–53.

174. Sachs GS, Grossman F, Ghaemi SN, et al. Combination of a mood stabilizer with risperidone or haloperidol for treatment of acute mania: a double-blind, placebo-controlled comparison of efficacy and safety. Am J Psychiatry 2002; **159**(7): 1146–54.

175. Vieta E, Reinares M, Corbella B, et al. Olanzapine as long-term adjunctive therapy in treatment-resistant bipolar disorder. J Clin Psychopharmacol 2001; **21**(5):469–73.

176. Vieta E, Goikolea JM, Corbella B, et al. Risperidone safety and efficacy in the treatment of bipolar and schizoaffective disorders: results from a 6–month, multicenter, open study. J Clin Psychiatry 2001; **62**(10):818–25.

177. Delbello MP, Schwiers ML, Rosenberg HL, Strakowski SM. A double-blind, randomized, placebo-controlled study of quetiapine as adjunctive treatment for adolescent mania. J Am Acad Child Adolesc Psychiatry 2002; **41**(10): 1216–23.

178. Soutullo CA, DelBello MP, Ochsner JE, et al. Severity of bipolarity in hospitalized manic adolescents with history of stimulant or antidepressant treatment. J Affect Disord 2002; **70**(3): 323–7.

179. DelBello MP, Carlson GA, Tohen M, et al. Rates and predictors of developing a manic or hypomanic episode 1 to 2 years following a first hospitalization for major depression with psychotic features. J Child Adolesc Psychopharmacol 2003; **13**(2):173–85.

180. Kafantaris V, Coletti DJ, Dicker R, et al. Adjunctive antipsychotic treatment of adolescents with bipolar psychosis. J Am Acad Child Adolesc Psychiatry 2001; **40**(12):1448–56.

181. Rothschild AJ, Duval SE. How long should patients with psychotic depression stay on the antipsychotic medication? J Clin Psychiatry 2003; **64**(4):390–6.

182. Goodwin GM, Jamison KR. *Manic Depressive Illness.* Oxford University Press; 1990.

183. Bowden CL, Calabrese JR, McElroy SL, et al. A randomized, placebo-controlled 12–month trial of divalproex and lithium in treatment of outpatients with bipolar I disorder. Divalproex Maintenance Study Group. Arch Gen Psychiatry 2000; **57**(5):481–9.

184. Calabrese JR, Bowden CL, Sachs G, et al. A placebo-controlled 18–month trial of lamotrigine and lithium maintenance treatment in recently depressed patients with bipolar I disorder. J Clin Psychiatry 2003; **64**(9):1013–24.

185. Faedda GL, Tondo L, Baldessarini RJ, et al. Outcome after rapid vs gradual discontinuation of lithium treatment in bipolar disorders. Arch Gen Psychiatry 1993; **50**(6):448–55.

186. Baethge C, Smolka MN, Gruschka P, et al. Does prophylaxis-delay in bipolar disorder influence outcome? Results from a long-term study of 147 patients. Acta Psychiatr Scand 2003; **107**(4): 260–7.

187. Strakowski SM, Del Bello MP, Adler CM, Keck PE, Jr. Atypical antipsychotics in the treatment of bipolar disorder. Expert Opin Pharmacother 2003; **4**(5):751–60.

188. Tohen M, Marneros A, Bowden C, et al. Olanzapine versus lithium in relapse prevention in bipolar disorder. In: *American Psychiatric Association 56th Annual Meeting*; San Francisco; 17–20 May 2003.

189. Burgess S, Geddes J, Hawton K, et al. Lithium for maintenance treatment of mood disorders. Cochrane Database Syst Rev 2001; **3**:CD003013.

190. Keck PE, Jr., McElroy SL. Carbamazepine and valproate in the maintenance treatment of bipolar disorder. J Clin Psychiatry 2002; **63**(Suppl 10):13–17.

191. Bowden CL, Calabrese JR, Sachs G, et al. A placebo-controlled 18–month trial of lamotrigine and lithium maintenance treatment in recently manic or hypomanic patients with bipolar I disorder. Arch Gen Psychiatry 2003; **60**(4):392–400.

192. Gyulai L, Bowden CL, McElroy SL, et al. Maintenance efficacy of divalproex in the prevention of bipolar depression. Neuropsychopharmacology 2003; **28**(7):1374–82.

193. Post RM, Leverich GS, Nolen WA, et al. A re-evaluation of the role of antidepressants in the treatment of bipolar depression: data from the Stanley Foundation Bipolar Network. Bipolar Disord 2003; **5**(6):396–406.

194. Altshuler L, Suppes T, Black D, et al. Impact of antidepressant discontinuation after acute

bipolar depression remission on rates of depressive relapse at 1–year follow-up. Am J Psychiatry 2003; **160**(7):1252–62.

195. Tohen M, Vieta E, Calabrese J, et al. Efficacy of olanzapine and olanzapine-fluoxetine combination in the treatment of bipolar I depression. Arch Gen Psychiatry 2003; **60**(11):1079–88.

196. Biederman J, Mick E, Spencer TJ, et al. Therapeutic dilemmas in the pharmacotherapy of bipolar depression in the young. J Child Adolesc Psychopharmacol 2000; **10**(3):185–92.

197. Lewis R. Typical and atypical antipsychotics in adolescent schizophrenia: efficacy, tolerability, and differential sensitivity to extrapyramidal symptoms. Can J Psychiatry 1998; **43**(6):596–604.

198. Kumra S, Herion D, Jacobsen LK, et al. Case study: risperidone-induced hepatotoxicity in pediatric patients. J Am Acad Child Adolesc Psychiatry 1997; **36**(5):701–5.

199. Kelly DL, Conley RR, Love RC, et al. Weight gain in adolescents treated with risperidone and conventional antipsychotics over six months. J Child Adolesc Psychopharmacol 1998; **8**(3):151–9.

200. Grothe DR, Calis KA, Jacobsen L, et al. Olanzapine pharmacokinetics in pediatric and adolescent inpatients with childhood-onset schizophrenia. J Clin Psychopharmacol 2000; **20**(2):220–5.

201. Toren P, Laor N, Weizman A. Use of atypical neuroleptics in child and adolescent psychiatry. J Clin Psychiatry 1998; **59**(12):644–56.

202. McConville BJ, Arvanitis LA, Thyrum PT, et al. Pharmacokinetics, tolerability, and clinical effectiveness of quetiapine fumarate: an open-label trial in adolescents with psychotic disorders. J Clin Psychiatry 2000; **61**(4):252–60.

203. Findling RL, McNamara NK, Youngstrom EA, et al. A prospective, open-label trial of olanzapine in adolescents with schizophrenia. J Am Acad Child Adolesc Psychiatry 2003; **42**(2):170–5.

204. Gothelf D, Apter A, Reidman J, et al. Olanzapine, risperidone and haloperidol in the treatment of adolescent patients with schizophrenia. J Neural Transm 2003; **110**(5):545–60.

205. Findling RL, McNamara NK, Gracious BL, et al. Combination lithium and divalproex sodium in pediatric bipolarity. J Am Acad Child Adolesc Psychiatry 2003; **42**(8): 895–901.

206. Allen MH, Currier GW, Hughes DH, et al. The Expert Consensus Guideline Series. Treatment of behavioral emergencies. Postgrad Med 2001(Spec No):1–88; quiz 89–90.

207. Fitzgerald P. Long-acting antipsychotic medication, restraint and treatment in the management of acute psychosis. Aust N Z J Psychiatry 1999; **33**(5):660–6.

208. Daniel DG, Potkin SG, Reeves KR, et al. Intramuscular (IM) ziprasidone 20 mg is effective in reducing acute agitation associated with psychosis: a double-blind, randomized trial. Psychopharmacology (Berl) 2001; **155**(2):128–34.

209. Tohen M, King K, Chengappa K. IM olanzapine efficacy in acute agitation. In: *12th World Congress of Psychiatry*; Yokohama; 2002.

210. Malla AK, Norman RM, Scholten DJ, et al. A comparison of long-term outcome in first-episode schizophrenia following treatment with risperidone or a typical antipsychotic. J Clin Psychiatry 2001; **62**(3):179–84.

211. Treatment of special populations with the atypical antipsychotics. Collaborative Working Group on Clinical Trial Evaluations. J Clin Psychiatry 1998; **59**(Suppl 12):46–52.

212. Oosthuizen P, Emsley RA, Turner J, Keyter N. Determining the optimal dose of haloperidol in first-episode psychosis. *J Psychopharmacol* 2001; **15**: 251–5.

7

Social and Psychological Interventions

Tom Ehmann and Laura Hanson

Psychoeducation

Psychoeducation should be provided to all persons with early psychosis and their families. The benefits are greatest when psychoeducation is ongoing and intensive. The content of psychoeducation needs to be specific to early psychosis, and should aim to promote recovery, self-management of illness, and coping abilities. Psychoeducation should be individually provided to both family and patient. Psychoeducation should be offered to all persons with a psychotic disorder, family members, spouses and partners, and other potentially supportive individuals. Group psychoeducation may be a useful adjunct to individual psychoeducation.

Goals of psychoeducation

Psychoeducation fosters the knowledge, attitudes, skills, and abilities necessary for a person to manage his or her own illness. Psychoeducation also deals with the emotional aspects of the illness experience.[1–3] Treatment adherence and relapse prevention are often considered to be the main aims of psychoeducation. However, these are embedded in the overall goal of promoting the self-management capacity needed to achieve or recover valued life goals and overall quality of life.[4] Similarly, family education is better concep-

tualized as fostering well-being of the family rather than simply preventing relapse in the patient.

Three key goals for psychoeducation in early psychosis articulated by McGorry are to help the patient:[4]

1. Negotiate 'meaning' through a constructive assimilation of the illness experience into his or her world-view.
2. Develop 'mastery' by acquiring or enhancing the subjective and objective skills needed to exert control over the disorder and its effects.
3. Protect 'self-esteem' threatened by assaults on self-identity, social roles, relationships, and future plans.

Benefits of psychoeducation

While numerous sources outline psychoeducational approaches in early psychosis,[4,5] the vast majority of research outlining the benefits of psychoeducation comes from the general literature on schizophrenia. For schizophrenia, psychoeducation has been demonstrated to lead to improved knowledge, decreased negative symptoms, improved interpersonal skills, decreased relapse rates, and shorter hospital stays.[6–9] In general, more intensive interventions and involving families in psychoeducation results in significantly better outcomes for both patient and family.[10–15] Provision of psychoeducation to both patient and family should be intensive and ongoing. Multiple studies in which psychoeducation was provided on a short-term basis (no more than 10 sessions over less than six months) failed to show convincing and long-lasting results for patient outcome,[10] although they may have some positive effects on family sense of support.[16,17] Engaging in psychoeducation over longer periods of time may lead to better outcomes by providing more opportunity to apply knowledge and skills. The risk of relapse is minimized when psychoeducation lasts at least nine months.[18] More frequent and longer involvement (e.g. closer to one year), with sessions including both patient and family, is associated with better outcomes.[10,18] For bipolar disorder, family-focused treatment consisting of psychoeducation, communications training, and problem-solving skills training has been shown to improve medication adherence and decrease relapses over a two year period.[19,20]

Research on psychoeducation in early psychosis has suggested that education may only decrease rehospitalization rates in patients who had a moderate duration of illness (4–7 years).[21] It was concluded that individuals with this duration of illness may have accepted their illness but not yet have adopted a fatalistic view of their illness. These findings may be consistent with the fact that first episode patients are less aware of having a mental illness than multiple episode patients.[22] The concept of recovery style may also have implications for psychoeducation in early psychosis. Patients appear to utilize one of two main recovery styles: (1) integration (incorporating the experience of psychosis into one's life), and (2) sealing over (isolating the experience of psychosis from the rest of one's life). In early psychosis patients, an integrative recovery style appears to be associated with better outcome,[23] while sealing over is associated with low service engagement.[24] Additionally, it appears that recov-

ery style changes over time—with a tendency to go from an early integrative style to a sealing over style within the first three months.[24] It is possible that providing psychoeducation very early in the course of the disorder may ensure that an individual maintains an integrative style. Individuals who have already adopted a sealing over recovery style may benefit from strategic psychoeducation aimed to change recovery style to one that is more integrative. A better understanding of the variables that impact psychoeducation in early psychosis is needed to allow for a more targeted approach to patient education.

Research on family psychoeducation specific to early psychosis is promising.[25] Multiple family groups may be an effective means of providing education while facilitating support across families,[30] and preliminary data demonstrate improvements in families' perceptions, knowledge and understanding of mental illness and treatments.[31]

Involving families

When psychosis develops in a close relative, the family may experience reactions ranging from fear to denial. Frequently, the family will attribute the psychotic behavior to substance abuse, adolescence, family conflicts, or other 'explanations'. These reactions suggest that the family should actively be sought out and engaged as early as possible. After the patient has made contact with mental health services, family members should be allowed time to express their feelings and relate their personal experiences. Misconceptions about psychosis and its treatments should sensitively be corrected (this part of the process can be delayed if it might threaten engagement).

Many families with a relative experiencing early psychosis will feel high levels of distress and difficulties regardless of whether their relative lives with them or not.[32] The distress experienced by family members often leads to significant social disruption and the development of psychological problems.[33,34] Psychoeducation can provide family members with the knowledge and skills necessary to help them care for their relative and increase their ability to cope. Psychoeducation that focuses on changing the family's appraisal of the impacts of psychosis may prove particularly useful as these appraisals appear to be closely linked to the level of distress experienced.[32]

If the patient seeks to limit family involvement, the basis for this request should be explored, and the importance of involving the family should be clearly explained to the patient. Clearly addressing issues of confidentiality may help alleviate some concerns about family involvement. Adequate psychoeducation for the family should always be provided, even if it must be offered in a venue apart from the patient and by other service providers. This can be accomplished even if the patient does not wish the family to be involved with, or aware of, the details of his or her care.

Psychoeducation process

Psychoeducation should occur during all phases of the illness. It may begin at the help-seeking phase when distress and dysfunction are reframed as 'illness-related', and as a reason for receiving outside help.[1] Both individuals and families benefit from an explanation of the treatment and from attempts to humanize and normalize the service. Individuals who are opposed to participating in treatment may feel that treatment is not necessary or may have concerns about stigma.[35] Explaining potential benefits of treatment and discussion of confidentiality may help to alleviate some of these concerns.

Once the patient enters into mental health services, psychoeducation can facilitate the negotiation of an initial 'rationale for treatment' with the patient and family.[4] This dialogue should be sensitive to a patient's idiosyncratic explanation regarding the disorder. Caution should be exercised about proposing other explanations before the person is ready to consider them.[36] It may be necessary to begin by framing the intervention as a response to a specific problem that has been identified as distressing by the individual.

During the early assessment phase, clinicians should convey their familiarity with the condition, the need for prompt intervention, and the message that their symptoms should respond well to treatment.[37] People will also require clear explanations about the roles of the involved professionals, treatment options, legal rights, and available supports appropriate to that phase of illness.

More formal psychoeducation should commence once the person's mental state begins to respond to medication—usually within a few weeks.[4] Psychoeducation should be paced and suitable when cognitive abilities are compromised. The ability to process information may be impaired by psychotic symptoms, cognitive deficits associated with the illness, medication side effects, or emotional reactions to the illness experience.[3,38] Furthermore, some individuals may avoid discussion as they attempt to 'seal over' their experiences. Psychoeducation may need to be delayed or tailored to accommodate the patient's inability or unpreparedness to deal with emotionally provocative issues.

Initially an individualized approach to psychoeducation is best, because people differ in their explanatory models, emotional needs, and capacities to participate.[4,37,39] Involving the family simultaneously in psychoeducation provides more opportunity for the family and patient to learn about the illness together, appreciate each other's perspective, and work out family issues.[40]

Group approaches are frequently employed, since they make efficient use of therapist time, allow members to share experiences and foster social supports. Psychoeducation to groups of early psychosis patients and families should be considered as an adjunct to individual approaches.

Peer education and learning about others who have recovered—through personal contact or media, such as stories or videotapes—can be a powerful source of hope and motivation for both patient and family members.[41]

Some studies have found that psychoeducation is more effective when performed in the home while others have found no difference in effectiveness between home and outpatient set-tings.[10,18] It may be more beneficial to hold psy-choeducation in the home, as this can be more comfortable and because learning occurs best in the context where the knowledge is to be applied. When deciding where meetings occur, consider patient and family preference. Some people are initially hesitant to attend a mental health clinic for fear of stigma and of the unknown. Other people may be reluctant to allow a mental health professional into their home due to feelings of invasion of privacy.

Content of psychoeducation

Table 7.1 shows the content areas most often covered in psychoeducation provided to patient and family. More detailed information can be found in the psychoeducational manuals for early psychosis that are listed in Chapter 10 on addi-tional early psychosis resources. It is essential to use materials that are tailored specifically to early psychosis,[4,42] because much of the self-help and patient-based literature designed for people with established chronic illnesses is inappropriate.

An important first step in providing psycho-education is to listen to the explanatory model of the patient and family. Education will be better received by the patients if the information is integrated into their own experiences.[5]

The usual framework for presenting informa-tion is the stress-vulnerability model (see Figure 7.1).

The stress-vulnerability (or diathesis-stress) model involves explaining psychosis as an under-lying vulnerability (e.g. genetic predisposition) in combination with exposure to stressors that may predispose, trigger, or serve to maintain symp-toms.[4,37] Within this context, one can present both biological strategies and psychosocial strat-egies to reduce the risk of psychosis and prevent relapse. Strategies include:[43]

- Complying with medications
- Avoiding substance use
- Managing interpersonal conflict

- Making use of peer support
- Identifying and managing environmental stressors
- Learning the 'early warning signs' of onset and relapse
- Developing and planning proactive coping and help-seeking strategies.

Analogies to the management of other ongoing health issues that fit this framework, such as dia-betes or asthma, can be drawn on as a way of nor-malizing the experience of mental illness, and as a way of promoting a sense of control.

The process of recovery (i.e. diminution of symptoms, resumption of role functioning, and improvement in quality of life) is also an import-ant organizing framework that can be utilized within both professionally based or peer-driven approaches.[44,45] By presenting recovery from a first episode as a process that is probable and occurs in recognizable stages, the individual and family are helped to normalize their experiences and to realize that they are actively participating in the steps necessary to promote recovery.

Diagnostic uncertainty in early psychosis and the potentially stigmatizing connotations associ-ated with diagnostic labels dictate that psycho-education should be 'problem-focused' rather than diagnostically focused in the early phases. The early psychosis period, with its attendant ambiguity, can be presented as an opportunity for the individual and family to take steps to mini-mize vulnerability to future episodes and maxi-mize the chances for a full recovery.

Although most psychoeducational programs initially focus on providing information about the illness and move towards enhancing coping skills, there is no predetermined series of stages through which psychoeducation has to proceed. Clinicians must remain flexible and adjust the psychoeducational process and content according to individual patient and family needs.

In a survey of first episode families, respon-dents indicated low satisfaction with the care pro-vided concerning: advice on how to handle

Table 7.1 Topics to be covered in psychoeducation

Psychosis	• Allow the patient and family time to relate their explanatory model of the psychosis and their emotional and behavioral responses. • Discuss the symptoms and associated features of psychosis. • Present the etiology of psychosis using a stress-vulnerability framework. • Communicate the expectation of recovery. • Explain why there is diagnostic ambiguity in the early phases of a psychotic illness.
Treatments	• Provide information on medications and psychosocial treatments (including possible side effects of treatment). • Help the person come to an acceptable ongoing rationale for treatment.
Recovery	• Provide information on the factors that enhance and impede recovery. • Discuss topics such as lifestyle, physical health, socialization, and drug use within this context. • For persons who have experienced a manic episode, emphasize that maintenance of circadian rhythms may help improve outcome and decrease risk of relapse.[48]
Stress management (see the section on stress management)	• Increase coping and control over symptoms and key affected areas of the person's life by teaching stress management strategies. • Foster use of social supports and services. • Explore ways of coping with persistent psychotic symptoms. • Provide practical suggestions for families coping with the behavioral and emotional changes in their family member.
Relapse prevention (see the section on relapse prevention)	• Discuss the possibility of relapse. • Provide information on early warning signs. • Develop a plan of action for dealing with impending relapse. • Help the person make lifestyle changes to reduce the likelihood of relapse.
Skills building (see the section on skills development)	• Teach skills such as structured problem solving, goal setting, and social skills (helps individuals assimilate and apply information by actively rehearsing the knowledge, skills, or strategies in question).
Normalizing the experience and addressing stigma	• Throughout psychoeducation, issues of stigma and demoralization should be addressed. • The experience of psychosis should be normalized, and the expectation of full recovery should be communicated. • Self-management of illness and social reintegration should be encouraged.
General health information	• This group is vulnerable to numerous health problems associated with lack of information, high risk behaviors, homelessness, and malnutrition. • Educational topics may include contraception, sexually transmitted diseases,[49] drugs and alcohol, hygiene, dentition, exercise, nutrition, and herbal remedies. • It is important to monitor for signs of health problems that are unreported by an individual, arrange for treatment, and provide needed education.

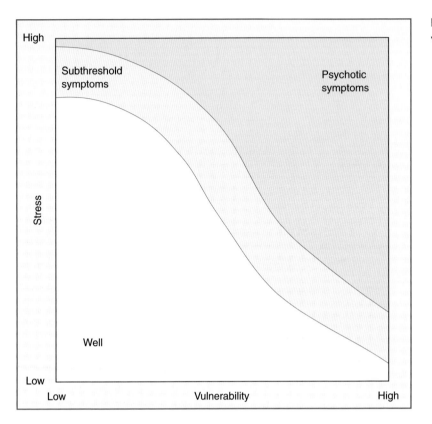

Figure 7.1 The stress-vulnerability model

specific problems—especially how to handle psychotic experiences; help with preserving or regaining social functioning; help with regaining structure and routine; information and prompt assistance preferably in the patient's own environment.[46]

Stress management

Stress and psychosis

The course of psychosis is affected by stress—higher levels of stressful life events have been associated with more severe symptoms in both schizophrenia and bipolar disorder.[47,50] In addition to external stressors, such as negative life events, internal stressors are also present and include cognitive confusion, altered perceptions, attention deficits, and impaired identity or sense of self.[51] These cognitive deficits along with high arousal levels can make adaptation to challenging situations extremely difficult.[52]

General stress management

Stress and its management may be conceptualized as consisting of four components (see Figure 7.2). Other factors, such as social support, personal resources, and general stress tolerance, will affect how a person perceives and copes with stress.

Stress management involves first ensuring that an individual is able to recognize the events and situations that are currently (or are likely to be) stressful as well as the signs and symptoms that indicate the experience of stress.

Stress management techniques can then target changing:

1. Stressors
   The reduction of responsibilities (such as work, school, etc.) can be a useful strategy when the number or degree of stressors exceeds the individual's ability to cope. This reduction of responsibilities should be done with forethought to avoid increasing stress

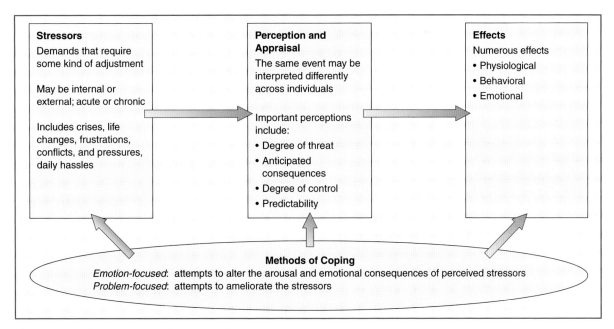

Figure 7.2 Components of stress and stress management

(e.g. losing job, or failing grades in courses). Clinicians should take steps to ensure that these negative consequences will not occur (by informing others, providing a letter, etc.). It is also important to address the individual's appraisal of this reduction of responsibilities—if the individual views this as evidence of 'failure', then taking this action will likely not have the desired beneficial effects.

Reducing daily hassles can help to reduce general stress levels. By learning time management, organizational skills, and memory aids, individuals are less likely to experience stress from more minor annoyances. Daily stressors should be assessed for and the clinician should work with the patient and family to find ways of reducing or eliminating these.

Problem solving (see the section on skills development).

2. Perception and appraisal
Appraisals are often done automatically, without taking some time to think rationally about the situation. Quite often, the appraisal of the stressor will be magnified or even irrational. Encouraging and teaching individuals to identify and challenge negative thinking patterns is an important part of stress management. Cognitive therapy provides a systematic way of evaluating and challenging these negative thoughts.

Appraisal by the person of the resources available for coping may also be distorted.

3. The subsequent physiological and behavioral responses
Teaching awareness of the early warning signs of stress is an essential part of stress management. Once the individual recognizes that stress is occurring then coping strategies can be employed.

Reduction of physiological arousal is a fundamental approach and includes relaxation, distraction, recreation, massage, hot baths, exercise, etc. Medications may also reduce physiological arousal. Additional techniques include regular sleep and a healthy diet.

Behavioral responses to stress include avoidance as well as maladaptive actions. Individuals may need coaching and instruction to rectify these tendencies. For example, frustration leading to abusive behavior could be countered by teaching more adaptive responses to the frustration.

4. Methods of coping

Multiple strategies for coping include those that are emotion-focused (e.g. relaxation, exercise, breathing techniques and/or simple distraction) and problem-focused (e.g. examining and rectifying situations in daily life, learning how to appraise internal states, and accessing available resources).

The teaching of these coping skills will entail formal instruction on both relaxation as well as problem-solving skills.

Clinicians are advised to assess patients' current and past coping styles. No single coping strategy is always effective for all individuals, problems, or situations. Discussions with the patient about the successes and limitations of their coping efforts in particular situations can prompt the initiation of a variety of strategies. Planning for the use of specific strategies in well-defined situations should be coupled with evaluation of their success. Early psychosis patients who relied more on problem-focused versus emotion-focused coping strategies reported they felt able to deal with their stressors. In turn, the use of these strategies was associated with fewer symptoms and increases in self-efficacy and perceived social support.[53,54] Despite the effectiveness of problem-focused coping, people with schizophrenia tend to use emotion-focused coping.[53] This may be related to the cognitive impairments associated with psychosis—persons with cognitive impairment may rely on emotion-focused coping even when the stressor is changeable.[52]

Teaching problem-solving skills provides individuals with a broader range of coping strategies. Targeting emotion-related information processing may also be effective and has been associated with fewer relapses and enhanced social integration.[55]

Stress management should be provided to both the patient and family and tailored to suit each individual. Families will benefit from having an explanation of the stressors they are likely to encounter when caring for their family member with psychosis, normalizing their emotional reactions, and having healthy ways of coping. Knowing that respite care is available if needed can offer significant relief for some families.

Psychosis-specific coping

A variety of coping strategies for persistent psychotic symptoms has been suggested but long-term efficacy and generalizability of these strategies have yet to be demonstrated. Techniques to reduce persistent auditory hallucinations include holding the mouth wide open,[56] quietly humming a single note,[57] wearing an ear-plug in the dominant ear,[58] and using cognitive strategies.[59] Better adaptation to the presence of psychotic symptoms has been associated with the use of strategies that are simultaneously engaging and relaxing.[60]

Clinicians are advised to explore these possible coping methods on an individualized basis.

Relapse prevention

The majority of individuals who recover from a first episode of schizophrenia or schizoaffective disorder will experience a relapse within five years.[61] Similarly, about 73% of bipolar patients maintained on lithium relapse within five years.[62] Patients experiencing a first relapse have high rates of second and third relapses. Subsequent relapses are associated with more social impairment, higher levels of secondary morbidity (e.g. depression, anxiety, substance abuse), and more residual symptomatology.[63,64]

Maintenance medication, case management, psychoeducation, and family involvement are all associated with lower relapse rates. However, even when the full range of treatments is provided, relapse still remains a real possibility. Therefore, additional efforts are necessary in order to predict and thwart an impending relapse.

Predicting relapse

The chances of a relapse after recovery from a first episode are increased if the person is not taking antipsychotic medications and if he or she had poor premorbid adjustment.[61] Stressful life events appear to increase the risk of relapse in the early phases of illness, but are less strongly associated with relapse after multiple episodes.[65]

Both retrospective,[66,67] and prospective,[68,69] studies have demonstrated the occurrence of subtle psychological changes prior to a psychotic relapse. The most common changes include both nonspecific symptoms (e.g. change in sleep pattern, anxiety, difficulties concentrating, depression) and attenuated psychotic symptoms (e.g. brief or poorly formed hallucinations, unstable ideas of reference, suspiciousness, mental confusion).[70,71] When the person is off medication, sleep disturbance may be more prominent. Also, the most robust early symptom of mania inpatients with bipolar disorder is sleep disturbance.[72] The progression from these early warning signs to the onset of psychotic relapse is fairly rapid, most often occurring over a period of less than a month.[66,69] However, the individual may be aware of these changes earlier as the interval between the onset of self-experienced vulnerability and relapse has a median duration of nine weeks.[71] In both schizophrenia and affective disorders, the family and patient are usually aware of these early changes.[67,71,73]

These changes seen prior to the re-emergence of psychosis have been referred to as both the 'relapse prodrome',[74] and 'early warning signs'.[75] Although the combination of non-specific and psychotic-like symptoms predicts relapse better than vague symptoms alone, neither approach is particularly accurate.[74,75]

The concept of a 'relapse signature' posits that individuals have their own unique profile of signs and symptoms prior to relapse. This concept of uniqueness has been questioned, since it has been demonstrated that the symptoms shown prior to relapse often change for a given individual for each relapse.[74]

Relapse prevention plans

Regardless of whether the warning signs are variable or form a consistent pattern, a relapse prevention plan for the patient and family should be developed for use when they believe a relapse may be starting. This relapse prevention plan should outline common early warning signs as well as the individualized warning signs experienced before initial onset. Working with the patient and family, the clinician should outline the steps to be taken if these early warning signs are detected. These steps might include contacting appropriate service providers, initiating stress management techniques, and/or utilizing pre-arranged medication strategies. A hard copy of this relapse prevention plan should be provided to both the individual and their family and it should include contact information for the key service providers as well as emergency services.

In bipolar patients, a program that taught recognition of early symptoms of relapse and immediate treatment seeking was associated with a significant increase in time to first manic relapse and better social and employment outcomes.[76] A manualized form of cognitive therapy for relapse prevention in bipolar disorder has also been shown to reduce the number of relapses over a one year period.[77] Disruptions in social rhythm may be related to relapses in bipolar disorder,[78] and attempts to regularize daily routines and sleep-wake cycles through social rhythm therapy may lead to lower relapse rates.[79,80] For schizophrenia, approximately half of all relapses can be predicted through the detection of early warning signs.[81] Relapse prevention involving monitoring for early warning signs, and when detected using supportive problem-solving and increasing antipsychotic medication doses, has been found successfully to reduce rates of relapse and rehospitalization for individuals with schizophrenia.[82]

If relapse does occur, this should be seen as a significant educational opportunity, both for the person and the family. A relapse should prompt re-evaluation of the person's knowledge of the illness and refinement of preventive strategies (stress management, help-seeking strategies, medication adherence, etc.).

Treatment adherence

Relapse prevention should include maintenance medication, case management, ongoing psychoeducation and family involvement, and frequent monitoring for early warning signs of relapse. In particular, maintenance medication is associated with significantly lowered relapse rates.

Non-adherence to oral medication regimes in individuals with schizophrenia has been reported to be between 39% and 60%.[83,84] Similar numbers have been reported in euthymic bipolar patients.[85] Within nine months of onset of a first episode of mania only 30% of patients were found to be consistently taking their medication.[86] One-year outcomes for non-adherence in first episode schizophrenia spectrum patients included increased rates of positive symptoms, relapse, substance use, and poorer quality of life.[87] Lack of insight, negative beliefs about the effects of medications, stigma, and side effects are major contributors to non-adherence. Studies specific to first episode patients found that non-adherence was associated with impaired executive functioning, the emergence of parkinsonian side effects, poorer premorbid functioning,[88] lower occupational status, alcohol abuse, and delusional intensity at baseline.[84] Predictors of non-adherence in the acute phase included younger age, male sex, side effects, and higher severity of non-psychotic symptoms.[89] Use of the lowest possible dose of medication improves adherence by minimizing side effects (Table 7.2).

Psychoeducation should present a rationale for treatment during the early weeks and months. Later, the benefits and drawbacks of adherence need to be explored with the patient. This discussion should be grounded in a thorough understanding of the person's attitudes towards treatment, as these will affect adherence. This exploration can take place in an unstructured or structured way, using active listening, and/or using the techniques of motivational interviewing.

Strategies that are most likely to produce improvements in treatment adherence should include both information and behavioral elements. That is, interventions need to feature aspects such as helping the person schedule medication-taking at regular, predictable times that are interwoven within the individual's daily routine, building in reminders (such as calendars or alarms), and enlisting the support of others.

Compliance therapy is an additional strategy that has been shown to enhance treatment adherence, improve insight, and decrease the risk of rehospitalization.[90] Efficacy in early psychosis still needs to be tested. This therapy is based on the strategies used in motivational interviewing and cognitive behavioral therapies. It is a brief therapy (four to six sessions) designed for acutely psychotic inpatients and consists of three phases. Phase 1 involves exploring the patient conceptualization of the psychosis; Phase 2 involves exploring ambivalence about treatment; and Phase 3 reframes treatment as a freely chosen strategy for enhancing quality of life.

Cognitive therapy

Focus of cognitive therapy

Cognitive therapy involves altering dysfunctional patterns of thinking that are linked to pathological feelings and behaviour. Cognitive therapy is not to be confused with cognitive remediation, which aims to improve specific cognitive deficits (e.g. memory and attention impairments) through cognitive retraining. Multiple forms of cognitive therapy for psychosis differ somewhat in focus and technique.[95]

Table 7.2 Treatment adherence issues[91-94]	
Common issues	**Strategies for addressing them**
Does not believe that he or she has a psychiatric disorder	• Explore the patient's conceptualization of what they experienced. • Have the individual discuss the negative impacts and social consequences that resulted from this experience. • Reframe these negative consequence as the need for continuing with treatment.
Fears about lifelong illness	• Inspire hope for recovery (e.g. by connecting the person with recovered role models). • Avoid premature 'sentencing' of person to lifelong treatment and discuss possible plans and timeframe for eventual cessation.
Stigma about taking medication	• Address stigma and misconceptions about the illness and treatment.
Medication side effects or fears about side effects	• Give information needed to recognize side effects. • Use the lowest effective dose. • Be open to negotiating treatment that minimizes side effects.
Perception that the medication does not work	• Help the person see the relationship between improvements and medication. • Monitor whether medication does in fact work. • Address the possibility of relapse and the importance of avoiding relapse or minimizing its duration.
'Feeling better'	• Help the person anticipate this feeling and see the need to maintain treatment. • Consider patient suitability for intermittent targeted approach to medication.
Complexity of treatment-taking	• Minimize polypharmacy. • Use behavioral strategies, reminders, and environmental cues (e.g. keeping medication next to the bed, using weekly pill boxes) to help the individual remember to take the medication.
Missing the euphoric mood	• Remind the person of the deleterious consequences of the behaviors that accompany the elated mood. • Explore safer activities that promote mood elevation.

The process of cognitive therapy consists of:

• Developing a collaborative working relationship between therapist and patient
• Challenging distressing thinking patterns and beliefs
• Empirically testing beliefs and developing more adaptive and rational ways of thinking.

For individuals with psychotic disorders, cognitive therapy can be used for both:

• Increasing control over and coping with psychotic symptoms (hallucination, delusions, negative symptoms)
• Treating secondary morbidity (depression, anxiety, adjustment issues, etc.).

Cognitive therapy for psychosis recognizes that biological factors have a central role in etiology but that psychological factors contribute to the expression and the experience of the psychosis. Throughout therapy, the continuum of psychotic symptoms with normal experience is emphasized.[95]

Cognitive therapy for psychosis

All studies to date have looked at the effects of cognitive therapy in medicated patients. Cognitive therapy is considered an adjunct to anti-psychotic medication, not a substitute. It has been used with patients having both early[96,97] and long-standing psychoses.[98,99] Cognitive therapy has been effectively utilized during the acute phases to improve engagement with services and promote early adjustment.[100,101] Studies that included a large proportion of early psychosis patients have reported effects similar to those seen with chronic patients.[96,97,101,102]

Some improvements associated with cognitive therapy are substantial. Four controlled trials produced an average reduction in relapse of over 50%.[103] Over and above the changes due to standard care and/or supportive counselling, cognitive therapy can result in significant reductions in the frequency of positive psychotic symptoms and improvements in general psychiatric functioning.[95,103] Additional benefits may include decreases in preoccupation and distress due to delusions,[95,101] abbreviated length of hospital stay,[104] increased insight,[101] better control over the illness,[96] and improved mood.[101]

In the literature, cognitive therapy has demonstrated limitations. A recent large-scale randomized controlled trial of cognitive therapy designed to test effectiveness in accelerating remission from acute psychosis in early schizophrenia failed to find consistent advantages over routine care or supportive counselling.[105] Additionally, another randomized controlled trial of cognitive therapy for acutely suicidal patients with early psychosis failed to demonstrate any statistically significant improvement in suicidal ideation.[106]

The use of cognitive therapy in persons with bipolar disorder is being developed.[107] As in other studies of cognitive therapy in psychosis, significant reductions in symptoms and relapse rates have been reported.[107] A particularly relevant dimension of therapy in bipolar disorder is the close attention paid to maintenance of routines and circadian rhythms.[48,108]

Cognitive therapy dropout rates are similar to those for standard care.[102] High rates of patient satisfaction with both individual and group approaches have been reported.[109,110] Generally, at follow-up periods of one year or less, most improvements with cognitive therapy continue to be superior to those seen with routine care, although the superiority of cognitive therapy over non-specific supportive therapy at follow-up is not as clear.[99,111–113] Longer-term effects and the impact of 'booster sessions' need further study.[98,100]

A more recent research application of cognitive therapy is for individuals who are deemed to be at high risk for transition to psychosis.[114,115] Only preliminary data are available at this time and further research is needed before this application can be recommended for clinical practice.

Obstacles to obtaining cognitive therapy

Cognitive therapy is a highly specialized form of therapy that is practiced by a relatively small number of practitioners. Even fewer practitioners trained in cognitive therapy are experienced with its application to psychotic disorders. It is not known how effective cognitive therapy would be when practiced by clinicians with less training or experience than therapists used in research studies.

Predictors of success

Many studies have excluded patients from trials of cognitive therapy due to intellectual deficits, severe cognitive deficits, drug or alcohol abuse, or difficulties in communicating. Therefore, the generalizability of research findings is limited. There is evidence to suggest that a patient's ability to consider hypothetical alternative explanations for delusional beliefs and paranoia, and more illness insight may predict better outcomes.[111,112] A certain degree of symptom awareness and a willingness to disclose symptoms are necessary prerequisites.

A number of controlled trials have shown that cognitive therapy benefits patients with medication-resistant symptoms, who have at least some insight into the source of their symptoms. Cognitive therapy should be offered by clinicians with demonstrated competence and should be considered a useful adjunct to traditional treatment. However, further research is needed to determine what improvements the treatment should target and the patient populations most likely to benefit from this form of treatment.

Skills development

Problem-solving skills

Deficits in problem solving are common in early psychosis.[116–118] For schizophrenia, training in structured problem solving has been associated with improvements in functioning, especially when provided to both patient and family.[14] It has also been suggested that problem-solving training may modify the course of psychotic illness,[119] although research data is not yet available to support this suggestion.

Structured problem solving involves six steps:[120]

1. Identify the problem clearly (and break it down into smaller components if necessary).
2. Brainstorm (list all possible solutions).
3. Evaluate possible solutions (list advantages and disadvantages of each).
4. Select one solution (the one that is more favorable when advantages and disadvantages were compared, and the one that the individual has the resources to carry out—e.g. time, money, skills, etc.).
5. Develop a plan to carry out the solution (break the plan into small concrete steps, set timelines for completion of steps, think ahead about likely difficulties and how they can be dealt with).
6. Carry out the plan and review progress (evaluate the progress at each step, revise the plan as necessary, continue until the problem is solved).

Problem solving is a technique that is used in conjunction with a number of different interventions, including stress management, relapse prevention, cognitive therapy, and social skills training.

Social skills

Individuals with early psychosis generally have small social networks and relatively few friends[121]—a fact that may be related to deficits in social skills.[122] Deficits in social functioning and interpersonal problem-solving skills are present early in the course of psychosis.[116] Given that non-familial social support is associated with more positive outcomes in first episode schizophrenia,[123] efforts to improve social skills and functioning early in the course of psychosis are justified.

Social skills training attempts to develop (or retrain) interpersonal skills and competencies. Interventions are based on learning theory principles, with the goal being to improve social functioning in a variety of areas (work/school, relationships, daily living). The targeted behaviors may be relatively simple motor responses (e.g. eye contact) or more complex behaviors (e.g. assertiveness, communication, social perception).

Most of the research on social skills training has been with patients who have longstanding psychotic illnesses and significant social skills deficits. The applicability of these techniques to individuals with early psychosis and/or patients with higher levels of social functioning remains to be tested. Nevertheless, problems with social skills are frequently present around the onset of psychosis, and treatment is appropriate.[116] Specific interventions have been well described in the literature,[124] and include education, modeling, role-play or behavioral rehearsal, coaching, feedback, and positive reinforcement.

Basic skills model

The basic skills training model involves the training of specific social behaviors. More complex behaviors are broken down into discrete behavioral components, making them more amenable for training. Through a combination of modeling and role-playing, the patient learns the individual components and then combines them in the appropriate sequence. The behaviors are then practiced in the patient's natural environment.

Skills training does result in acquiring the targeted social skills, as demonstrated through role-playing and naturalistic observation.[125] Additionally, these skills are generally maintained over a period of months to one year,[126,127] but appear to deteriorate over longer periods of time.[63]

Simpler types of skills (e.g. motor performance skills, such as eye contact) may generalize across situations more readily than more complex behaviors.[128] The evidence for generalizability of more complex behaviors in naturalistic settings without prompts is generally poor,[129] and tends not to lead to improvements in social adjustment.[127] This has led to the suggestion that incorporation of problem-solving techniques in social skills training is necessary.

Social problem-solving skills model

The social problem-solving skills model involves training patients to correct problems in the manner in which they receive, process, and convey information in social situations. Patients are taught to generalize these skills to apply to novel problems they might encounter. The social problem-solving model tends to target deficits within specific domains (e.g. conversation, self-care, recreation). Protocols for skills training across a number of domains have been developed.[130]

The social problem-solving model reliably enhances skills.[131,132] Additionally, there is evidence to support generalization of skills. This model has been associated with improvements in overall social adjustment,[133] independent living skills,[134] and illness self-management.[131]

> Skills training should incorporate problem solving since it appears to produce greater benefits and wider generalizability.

Cognitive skills

Cognitive functioning is frequently impaired in psychotic disorders and may precede the development of positive symptoms. Specifically, a large, generalized deficit is often present along with more specific impairment in executive function, memory, and attention.[117,118,135] These cognitive deficits appear to be related to interpersonal problem solving and social functioning,[136,137] activities of daily living, and vocational functioning.[138,139]

Cognitive rehabilitation aims to help patients function better either by directly remediating cognitive deficits or by providing strategies to help compensate for compromised cognitive abilities.

1. Remediation attempts to improve cognitive functioning by strengthening existing functions and substituting new skills for lost functions. Interventions include verbalizing and/or modifying task instructions, use of positive reinforcement, and repeated practice. The patient engages in cognitive exercises, including computer-assisted strategies, in an attempt to improve specific aspects of cognition, such as attention, memory, and executive skills.

2. Adaptation attempts to compensate for the cognitive deficit using environmental aids and other strategies. Interventions include the use of visual prompts or memory aids, printed schedules, and memory books. These strategies do not attempt to rectify cognitive deficits but to alter the environment and utilize cognitive strengths in ways that make the consequences of the cognitive deficits easier to manage.

Neuropsychological assessment guides the efforts at rehabilitation by identifying cognitive strengths and weaknesses.

Cognitive remediation in schizophrenia has been associated with enhanced performance on neuropsychological tests in a number of studies.[140–142] However, a recent review located only three randomized controlled studies and concluded that there was no evidence of improved cognitive functioning.[143] Additionally, there is little evidence that cognitive remediation can lead to improvements in social functioning. When cognitive remediation was provided prior to social skills training there were fewer benefits than when the training was provided in the opposite order (social skills training and then cognitive remediation).[144] A randomized controlled trial of daily one hour sessions of cognitive remediation of executive functioning deficits (i.e. cognitive flexibility, working memory, and planning) resulted in improvements in cognitive ability and self-esteem, but did not result in any direct improvements in social functioning.[141]

It has been argued that until there is more evidence supporting the efficacy of cognitive remediation, adaptive or compensatory strategies should be used as the primary rehabilitation strategy for people with serious mental illness.[145,146] The use of adaptive strategies has been found to improve global functioning as well as reduce symptomatology and relapse rates in schizophrenia.[138,147] Nevertheless, a number of groups are, quite rightly, pursuing cognitive remediation techniques in the context of training in activities such as social perception and interpersonal behavior.[148]

Family communication training

Deficits in communication skills (e.g. difficulties facilitating interactions, tendency to acquiesce) are amenable to social skills training (see the previous section on social skills). This section discusses the use of communication retraining designed to decrease expressed emotion between family members and patient. 'Expressed emotion'

is a term used to describe a pattern of communication that involves hostility, emotional over-involvement, and critical comments.[149] More recently, the concept of covert criticism has been suggested as an important component of expressed emotion.[150]

It has been consistently demonstrated that patients with chronic schizophrenia and major depression, living with families rated high in expressed emotion, are more likely to experience relapse.[151,152] Family work that reduces expressed emotion (such as communications retraining) reduces relapse rates.[153]

There is, however, less evidence to suggest that expressed emotion is predictive of relapse in patients with early psychosis,[154–158] or that family work designed to decrease expressed emotion is effective at reducing relapse in that group.[159,160] A transactional model has been proposed in which expressed emotion develops over time in families that have difficulties adjusting to the psychotic illness.[161] However, there are data inconsistent with this proposed model. One study comparing first episode to chronic schizophrenia found that expressed emotion status of families was independent of chronicity of psychosis[162]—and this was true regardless of whether covert criticism was included as a criterion of expressed emotion.

The majority of evidence to date suggests that key interventions during the early phases of the psychotic illness would be constructive problem solving, development of better coping mechanisms, and increasing social networks, as opposed to strategies specific to lowering expressed emotion.[2]

Promoting community functioning

Community reintegration

Symptomatic recovery in first episode psychosis appears to be greater than functional recovery,[163,164] and this finding remains true even within early psychosis services.[165] Approximately 40–60% of individuals with early psychosis are unemployed after one year.[163,165] Additional efforts and resources may be required in order to improve functional outcome for these patients.

Reintegration readiness

'Reintegration readiness' refers to a stage that comes after basic needs (e.g. stabilization, housing, income) have been taken care of and psychosocial strengths begin to rebuild (self-esteem, ability to relate socially, etc.). The length of time until readiness will depend upon the speed of recovery, the duration of untreated psychosis, the extent that community roles have been disrupted, and on psychological factors such as the individual's confidence. Poor premorbid function, negative symptoms, and cognitive dysfunction are significantly associated with unemployment in schizophrenia.[139]

Readiness for reintegration depends upon whether the recovery process is relatively quick or prolonged. Despite the laudable goals of quick reintegration, interviews with patients suggest that many people try to resume normal community activities too quickly.[41] In retrospect, patients reported that a period of convalescence of several months would have been more appropriate.

The person's interests, strengths, and values in relation to work and school should be explored before setting social and vocational goals. After discussion with the patient and family, the clinician may make contact with guidance counselors, human resource personnel, teachers, or employers. The clinician can help the patient disclose the nature of the disability, negotiate accommodations and support within the setting (e.g. modifications to the curricula, study aids, time accommodations), and monitor his or her ability to manage the stresses of the situation. The ultimate goal is to help the individual negotiate his or her support needs on an independent basis.

Cognitive functioning is a better predictor of success in rehabilitation programs and community functioning than psychiatric symptoms.[166] Cognitive assessment can provide important information on a patient's profile of strengths and weaknesses. The ability to determine a person's learning potential through neuropsychological testing is an exciting area that has implications both for placing persons in suitable programs and for customizing learning and performance situations. Occupational therapy is very useful in evaluating functional abilities, undertaking analyses of the requisite skills needed to perform a task, and then assisting a person to perform the task—either through direct training or modification of the task to suit the person's abilities.

Job retraining or alternative schooling

Individualized training plans and/or alternative schooling should be considered if necessary. Unfortunately, schooling methodology appropriate for students experiencing early psychosis is in its infancy. When broaching the topic of job retraining, care must be taken not to communicate the message that the clinician is giving up on the person's previous goals, or that the clinician holds low expectations of the person. Lowering expectations must be communicated as something that will enable the individual to achieve success and to explore personal interests.

Role of peer support in reintegration

Peer-based education and support groups provide an opportunity for people to practice social skills and achieve a sense of belonging and social support.[7] In general, when people in early psychosis meet or learn about people who have 'been where they've been, and gotten to where they want to be', this offers a powerful source of inspiration, as well as a rich source of knowledge about how to achieve their own goals.[41]

Housing and finances

All patients should be asked about their current living arrangements, finances, and housing. Although most early psychosis patients live with their parents, many do not or will cease to do so. It is essential that safe and affordable housing be available to patients whose current living environment is detrimental to their mental or physical well-being. If the individual's housing situation is poor or unsafe, his or her mental state might improve upon placement in a safe, clean, and calm environment. If a person needs housing, the type of placement should be determined after an assessment of:

- The individual's level of functioning (e.g. ability to perform activities of daily living, routine, independence, social interactions)
- Risk behavior (e.g. medication adherence, suicide risk, drug/alcohol use, self-organization)
- Family needs and concerns (e.g. care-giving, safety concerns, functioning, availability)
- Goals of the patient (e.g. promotion of independence, learning of life skills, socialization)
- Financial resources.

The use of small therapeutic houses populated with people of about the same age and at the same stage of recovery appears promising.[167] These settings might help to reduce length of hospitalization (especially when housing is an issue) and facilitate group recovery and reintegration. When shared accommodations are considered, efforts should be made to place the patient with others who are of approximately the same age and level of functioning. For individuals who are not able to return to work, application for disability benefits may be considered. The positive and negative aspects of receiving disability benefits should be discussed with the patient prior to making the decision to apply. This includes explaining the application and cancellation process, monies provided versus financial need, coverage of other expenses if any, other income sources allowed, as well as a discussion of patient concerns, such as possible fears of stigma and dependency.

Summary of social and psychological interventions

All patients and their families should be provided with comprehensive and prolonged individualized psychoeducation, including relapse prevention because these interventions are associated with greater improvements in clinical outcome and quality of life. In order to enhance the effectiveness of these interventions clinicians should: (1) actively engage the client and family throughout the process; (2) thoroughly assess for client and family strengths and weaknesses and methods of coping; and (3) provide education that is age- and stage-appropriate. A relapse prevention plan should be developed for patients and families at the beginning of treatment. This plan should be evaluated regularly throughout the course of care and modified as needed. Positive and negative aspects of treatment adherence should be discussed in a collaborative and non-judgmental manner. Strategies employing both information and behavioral elements may help ensure better treatment adherence. Clinicians should regularly assess for medication side effects as these may contribute greatly to medication non-adherence. For patients who are unwilling to continue with medication, close monitoring along with the use of intermittent targeted medication approaches may be most appropriate.

Other social and psychological interventions, such as group education, cognitive therapy, skills training, peer support, and appropriate housing, appear to be associated with improved outcomes. However, the availability of these types of interventions may be limited due to lack of resources and/or expertise. Where these interventions are available, they should be undertaken only after an assessment of readiness and suitability. Where these interventions are unavailable, clinicians should endeavor to develop the competence they require and/or advocate for these types of resources in their community.

References

1. Gleeson J. Family intervention in early psychosis. In: McGorry PD, Jackson HJ (eds). *The Recognition and Managment of Early Psychosis.* Cambridge University Press; 1999.

2. Birchwood M. The critical period for early intervention. In: Birchwood M, Jackson C (eds). *Early Intervention in Psychosis: A Guide to Concepts, Evidence and Interventions.* Chichester: Wiley; 2000.

3. Jackson CIZ. Psychological adjustment to early psychosis. In: Birchwood M, Jackson C (eds). *Early Intervention in Psychosis: A Guide to Concepts, Evidence and Interventions.* Chichester: Wiley; 2000.

4. McGorry PD. Psychoeducation in first-episode psychosis: a therapeutic process. Psychiatry 1995; **58**(4):313–28.

5. Kilkku N, Munnukka T, Lehtinen K. From information to knowledge: the meaning of information-giving to patients who had experienced first-episode psychosis. J Psychiatr Ment Health Nurs 2003; **10**(1):57–64.

6. Goldman CR, Quinn FL. Effects of a patient education program in the treatment of schizophrenia. Hosp Community Psychiatry 1988; **39**(3): 282–6.

7. Atkinson JM, Coia DA, Gilmour WH, Harper JP. The impact of education groups for people with schizophrenia on social functioning and quality of life. Br J Psychiatry 1996; **168**(2):199–204.

8. Merinder LB. Patient education in schizophrenia: a review. Acta Psychiatr Scand 2000; **102**(2): 98–106.

9. Pekkala E, Merinder L. Psychoeducation for schizophrenia (Cochrane Review). Cochrane Database Syst Rev 2000;4.

10. Barbato A, D'Avanzo B. Family interventions in schizophrenia and related disorders: a critical review of clinical trials. Acta Psychiatr Scand 2000; **102**(2):81–97.

11. Pharoah FM, Mari JJ, Streiner D. Family intervention for schizophrenia. Cochrane Database Syst Rev 2000;2.

12. Dyck DG, Short RA, Hendryx MS, et al. Management of negative symptoms among patients with schizophrenia attending multiple-family groups. Psychiatr Serv 2000; **51**(4):513–19.

13. Falloon IR, Boyd JL, McGill CW, et al. Family management in the prevention of morbidity of schizophrenia. Clinical outcome of a two-year longitudinal study. Arch Gen Psychiatry 1985; **42**(9):887–96.

14. Falloon IR, Pederson J. Family management in the prevention of morbidity of schizophrenia: the adjustment of the family unit. Br J Psychiatry 1985; **147**:156–63.

15. Falloon IR, McGill CW, Boyd JL, Pederson J. Family management in the prevention of morbidity of schizophrenia: social outcome of a two-year longitudinal study. Psychol Med 1987; **17**(1): 59–66.

16. Cozolino LJ, Goldstein MJ, Nuechterlein KH, et al. The impact of education about schizophrenia on relatives varying in expressed emotion. Schizophr Bull 1988; **14**(4):675–87.

17. Tarrier N, Barrowclough C, Vaughn C, et al. The community management of schizophrenia. A controlled trial of a behavioural intervention with families to reduce relapse. Br J Psychiatry 1988; **153**:532–42.

18. Dixon L, Adams C, Lucksted A. Update on family psychoeducation for schizophrenia [see comments]. Schizophr Bull 2000; **26**(1):5–20.

19. Miklowitz DJ, George EL, Richards JA, et al. A randomized study of family-focused psychoeducation and pharmacotherapy in the outpatient management of bipolar disorder. Arch Gen Psychiatry 2003; **60**(9):904–12.

20. Rea MM, Tompson MC, Miklowitz DJ, et al. Family-focused treatment versus individual treatment for bipolar disorder: results of a randomized clinical trial. J Consult Clin Psychol 2003; **71**(3):482–92.

21. Feldmann R, Hornung WP, Prein B, et al. Timing of psychoeducational psychotherapeutic interventions in schizophrenic patients. Eur Arch Psychiatry Clin Neurosci 2002; **252**(3):115–19.

22. Thompson KN, McGorry PD, Harrigan SM. Reduced awareness of illness in first-episode psychosis. Compr Psychiatry 2001; **42**(6):498–503.

23. Thompson KN, McGorry PD, Harrigan SM. Recovery style and outcome in first-episode psychosis. Schizophr Res 2003; **62**(1–2):31–6.

24. Tait L, Birchwood M, Trower P. Predicting engagement with services for psychosis: insight, symptoms and recovery style. Br J Psychiatry 2003; **182**:123–8.

25. Gleeson J, McGorry PD (eds). *Psychological Interventions in Early Psychosis: A Practical Treatment Handbook*. Chichester: Wiley; 2004.

30. McFarlane WR, Lukens E, Link B, et al. Multiple-family groups and psychoeducation in the treatment of schizophrenia. Arch Gen Psychiatry 1995; **52**(8):679–87.

31. Mullen A, Murray L, Happell B. Multiple family group interventions in first episode psychosis: Enhancing knowledge and understanding. Int J Ment Health Nurs 2002; **11**(4):225–32.

32. Addington J, Coldham EL, Jones B, et al. The first episode of psychosis: the experience of relatives. Acta Psychiatr Scand 2003; **108**(4):285-9.

33. Fadden G, Bebbington P, Kuipers L. The burden of care: the impact of functional psychiatric illness on the patient's family. Br J Psychiatry 1987; **150**:285–92.

34. Anderson CM, Hogarty G, Bayer T, Needleman R. Expressed emotion and social networks of parents of schizophrenic patients. Br J Psychiatry 1984; **144**:247–55.

35. de Haan L, Peters B, Dingemans P, et al. Attitudes of patients toward the first psychotic episode and the start of treatment. Schizophr Bull 2002; **28**(3):431–42.

36. Garety PA, Fowler D, Kuipers E. Cognitive-behavioral therapy for medication-resistant symptoms. Schizophr Bull 2000; **26**(1):73–86.

37. Williams CA. Patient education for people with schizophrenia. Perspect Psychiatr Care 1989; **25**(2):14–21.

38. Macpherson R, Jerrom B, Hughes A. A controlled study of education about drug treatment in schizophrenia. Br J Psychiatry 1996; **168**(6):709–17.

39. Wilson JH, Hobbs H. The family educator: a professional resource for families. J Psychosoc Nurs Ment Health Serv 1999; **37**(6):22–7.

40. Goldstein MJ. Psycho-education and family treatment related to the phase of a psychotic disorder. Int Clin Psychopharmacol 1996; **11**(Suppl 2):77–83.

41. Macnaughton E. *The BC Early Intervention Study: Report of findings*. Vancouver: Canadian Mental Health Association, BC Division; 1999.

42. Edwards J, Cocks J, Bott J. Preventive case management in first-episode psychosis. In: McGorry PD, Jackson, HJ (eds). *The Recognition and Management of Early Psychosis*. Cambridge University Press; 1999.

43. Falloon IR, Held T, Roncone R, et al. Optimal treatment strategies to enhance recovery from schizophrenia [see comments]. Aust N Z J Psychiatry 1998; **32**(1):43–9.

44. Hobbs H, Wilson JH, Archie S. The Alumni program: redefining continuity of care in psychiatry. J Psychosoc Nurs Ment Health Serv 1999; **37**(1):23–9.

45. McGorry P. Psychotherapy and recovery in early psychosis: A core clinical and research challenge. In: Martindale AB, Crowe M, Margison F (eds). *Psychosis: Psychological Approaches and their Effectiveness*. London: Gaskell; 2000:266–92.

46. de Haan L, Kramer L, van Raay B, et al. Priorities and satisfaction on the help needed and provided in a first episode of psychosis. A survey in five European Family Associations. Eur Psychiatry 2002; **17**(8):425–33.

47. Norman RM, Malla AK. Stressful life events and schizophrenia: I. A review of the research. Br J Psychiatry 1993; **162**:161–6.

48. Miklowitz DJ, Simoneau TL, George EL, et al. Family-focused treatment of bipolar disorder: 1-year effects of a psychoeducational program in conjunction with pharmacotherapy. Biol Psychiatry 2000; **48**(6):582–92.

49. Mason SE, Miller R. Safe sex and first-episode schizophrenia. Bull Menninger Clin 2001; **65**(12):179–93.

50. Swendsen J, Hammen C, Heller T, Gitlin M. Correlates of stress reactivity in patients with bipolar disorder. Am J Psychiatry 1995; **152**(5):795–7.

51. Hatfield AB. Patients' accounts of stress and coping in schizophrenia [see comments]. Hosp Community Psychiatry 1989; **40**(11):1141–5.

52. Gispen-de Wied CC. Stress in schizophrenia: an integrative view. Eur J Pharmacol 2000; **405**(1–3):375–84.

53. Macdonald EM, Pica S, McDonald S, et al. Stress and coping in early psychosis. Role of symptoms, self-efficacy, and social support in coping with stress. Br J Psychiatry Suppl 1998; **172**(33):122–7.

54. Leclerc C, Lesage AD, Ricard N, et al. Assessment of a new rehabilitative coping skills module for persons with schizophrenia. Am J Orthopsychiatry 2000; **70**(3):380–8.

55. Hodel B, Brenner HD, Merlo MC, Teuber JF. Emotional management therapy in early

psychosis. Br J Psychiatry Suppl 1998; **172**(33):128–33.

56. Bick PA, Kinsbourne M. Auditory hallucinations and subvocal speech in schizophrenic patients. Am J Psychiatry 1987; **144**(2):222–5.

57. Green MF, Kinsbourne M. Subvocal activity and auditory hallucinations: clues for behavioral treatments? Schizophr Bull 1990; **16**(4):617–25.

58. Done DJ, Frith CD, Owens DC. Reducing persistent auditory hallucinations by wearing an ear-plug. Br J Clin Psychology 1986; **25**:151–2.

59. Jenner JA, van de Willige G, Wiersma D. Effectiveness of cognitive therapy with coping training for persistent auditory hallucinations: a retrospective study of attenders of a psychiatric outpatient department. Acta Psychiatr Scand 1998; **98**(5):384–9.

60. Falloon IR, Talbot RE. Persistent auditory hallucinations: coping mechanisms and implications for management. Psychol Med 1981; **11**(2):329–39.

61. Robinson D, Woerner MG, Alvir JM, et al. Predictors of relapse following response from a first episode of schizophrenia or schizoaffective disorder. Arch Gen Psychiatry 1999; **56**(3):241–7.

62. Gitlin MJ, Swendsen J, Heller TL, Hammen C. Relapse and impairment in bipolar disorder. Am J Psychiatry 1995; **152**(11):1635–40.

63. Hogarty GE, Anderson CM, Reiss DJ, et al. Family psychoeducation, social skills training, and maintenance chemotherapy in the aftercare treatment of schizophrenia: II. Two-year effects of a controlled study on relapse and adjustment. Environmental–Personal Indicators in the Course of Schizophrenia (EPICS) Research Group [see comments]. Arch Gen Psychiatry 1991; **48**(4):340–7.

64. Wiersma D, Nienhuis FJ, Slooff CJ, Giel R. Natural course of schizophrenic disorders: a 15-year follow-up of a Dutch incidence cohort. Schizophr Bull 1998; **24**(1):75–85.

65. Castine MR, Meador-Woodruff JH, Dalack GW. The role of life events in onset and recurrent episodes of schizophrenia and schizoaffective disorder. J Psychiatr Res 1998; **32**(5):283–8.

66. Birchwood M, Smith J, Macmillan F, et al. Predicting relapse in schizophrenia: the development and implementation of an early signs monitoring system using patients and families as observers, a preliminary investigation. Psychol Med 1989; **19**(3):649–56.

67. Keitner GI, Solomon DA, Ryan CE, et al. Prodromal and residual symptoms in bipolar I disorder. Compr Psychiatry 1996; **37**(5):362–7.

68. Tarrier N, Barrowclough C, Bamrah JS. Prodromal signs of relapse in schizophrenia. Soc Psychiatry Psychiatr Epidemiol 1991; **26**(4):157–61.

69. Jorgensen P. Early signs of psychotic relapse in schizophrenia. Br J Psychiatry 1998; **172**:327–30.

70. Heinrichs DW, Carpenter WT, Jr. Prospective study of prodromal symptoms in schizophrenic relapse. Am J Psychiatry 1985; **142**(3):371–3.

71. Bechdolf A, Schultze-Lutter F, Klosterkötter J. Self-experienced vulnerability, prodromal symptoms and coping strategies preceding schizophrenic and depressive relapses. Eur Psychiatry 2002; **17**(7):384–93.

72. Jackson A, Cavanagh J, Scott J. A systematic review of manic and depressive prodromes. J Affect Disord 2003; **74**(3):209–17.

73. Herz MI, Glazer W, Mirza M, et al. Treating prodromal episodes to prevent relapse in schizophrenia. Br J Psychiatry Suppl 1989(5):123–7.

74. Norman RM, Malla AK. Prodromal symptoms of relapse in schizophrenia: a review. Schizophr Bull 1995; **21**(4):527–39.

75. Bustillo J, Buchanan RW, Carpenter WT, Jr. Prodromal symptoms vs. early warning signs and clinical action in schizophrenia. Schizophr Bull 1995; **21**(4):553–9.

76. Perry A, Tarrier N, Morriss R, et al. Randomised controlled trial of efficacy of teaching patients with bipolar disorder to identify early symptoms of relapse and obtain treatment [see comments]. BMJ 1999; **318**(7177):149–53.

77. Lam DH, Watkins ER, Hayward P, et al. A randomized controlled study of cognitive therapy for relapse prevention for bipolar affective disorder: outcome of the first year. Arch Gen Psychiatry 2003; **60**(2):145–52.

78. Kadri N, Mouchtaq N, Hakkou F, Moussaoui D. Relapses in bipolar patients: changes in social rhythm? Int J Neuropsychopharmacol 2000; **3**(1):45–49.

79. Frank E, Swartz HA, Kupfer DJ. Interpersonal and social rhythm therapy: managing the chaos of bipolar disorder. Biol Psychiatry 2000; **48**(6):593–604.

80. Miklowitz DJ, Richards JA, George EL, et al. Integrated family and individual therapy

for bipolar disorder: results of a treatment development study. J Clin Psychiatry 2003; **64**(2): 182–91.

81. Marder SR, Meibach RC. Risperidone in the treatment of schizophrenia [see comments]. Am J Psychiatry 1994; **151**(6):825–35.

82. Herz MI, Lamberti JS, Mintz J, et al. A program for relapse prevention in schizophrenia: a controlled study. Arch Gen Psychiatry 2000; **57**(3):277–83.

83. Kissling W. Compliance, quality assurance and standards for relapse prevention in schizophrenia. Acta Psychiatr Scand Suppl 1994; **382**:16–24.

84. Verdoux H, Lengronne J, Liraud F, et al. Medication adherence in psychosis: predictors and impact on outcome. A 2–year follow-up of first-admitted subjects. Acta Psychiatr Scand 2000; **102**(3):203–10.

85. Colom F, Vieta E, Martinez-Aran A, et al. Clinical factors associated with treatment noncompliance in euthymic bipolar patients. J Clin Psychiatry 2000; **61**(8):549–55.

86. Miklowitz DJ, Goldstein MJ, Nuechterlein KH, et al. Family factors and the course of bipolar affective disorder. Arch Gen Psychiatry 1988; **45**(3):225–31.

87. Coldham EL, Addington J, Addington D. Medication adherence of individuals with a first episode of psychosis. Acta Psychiatr Scand 2002; **106**(4): 286–90.

88. Robinson DG, Woerner MG, Alvir JM, et al. Predictors of medication discontinuation by patients with first-episode schizophrenia and schizoaffective disorder. Schizophr Res 2002; **57**(2–3): 209–19.

89. Kampman O, Laippala P, Vaananen J, et al. Indicators of medication compliance in first-episode psychosis. Psychiatry Res 2002; **110**(1): 39–48.

90. Kemp R, Kirov G, Everitt B, et al. Randomised controlled trial of compliance therapy. 18-month follow-up [see comments]. Br J Psychiatry 1998; **172**:413–19.

91. Kulkarni J, Power P. Initial treatment of first episode psychosis. In: McGorry P, Jackson H, Perris C (eds). *Recognition and Management of Early Psychosis*. Cambridge: Cambridge University Press; 1999.

92. Spencer E, Murray E, Plaistow J. Relapse prevention in early psychosis. In: Birchwood M, Fowler D, Jackson C (eds). *Early Intervention in Psychosis: A Guide to Concepts, Evidence and Interventions.* Chichester: Wiley; 2000.

93. Hayward P, Kemp R, David A. Compliance therapy: a collaborative approach to medication. In: Martinedale B, Bateman A, Crowe M, Margison F (eds). *Psychosis: Psychological Approaches and their Effectiveness.* London: Gaskell; 2000.

94. de Haan L, van Der Gaag M, Wolthaus J. Duration of untreated psychosis and the long-term course of schizophrenia. Eur Psychiatry 2000; **15**(4):264–7.

95. Dickerson FB. Cognitive behavioral psychotherapy for schizophrenia: a review of recent empirical studies. Schizophr Res 2000; **43**(2–3): 71–90.

96. Jackson H, McGorry P, Edwards J, et al. Cognitively-oriented psychotherapy for early psychosis (COPE). Preliminary results. Br J Psychiatry Suppl 1998; **172**(33):93–100.

97. Haddock G, Morrison AP, Hopkins R, et al. Individual cognitive-behavioural interventions in early psychosis. Br J Psychiatry Suppl 1998; **172**(33):101–6.

98. Tarrier N, Kinney C, McCarthy E, et al. Two-year follow-up of cognitive-behavioral therapy and supportive counseling in the treatment of persistent symptoms in chronic schizophrenia. J Consult Clin Psychol 2000; **68**(5):917–22.

99. Sensky T, Turkington D, Kingdon D, et al. A randomized controlled trial of cognitive-behavioral therapy for persistent symptoms in schizophrenia resistant to medication. Arch Gen Psychiatry 2000; **57**(2):165–72.

100. Drury V, Birchwood M, Cochrane R. Cognitive therapy and recovery from acute psychosis: a controlled trial: 3. Five-year follow-up. Br J Psychiatry 2000; **177**:8–14.

101. Drury V, Birchwood M, Cochrane R, Macmillan F. Cognitive therapy and recovery from acute psychosis: a controlled trial. I. Impact on psychotic symptoms [see comments]. Br J Psychiatry 1996; **169**(5):593–601.

102. Haddock G, Tarrier N, Morrison AP, et al. A pilot study evaluating the effectiveness of individual inpatient cognitive-behavioural therapy in early psychosis. Soc Psychiatry Psychiatr Epidemiol 1999; **34**(5):254–8.

103. Jones C, Cormac I, Mota J, Campbell C. Cognitive behaviour therapy for schizophrenia. Cochrane Database Syst Rev 2000;2.

104. Drury V, Birchwood M, Cochrane R, Macmillan F. Cognitive therapy and recovery from acute psychosis: a controlled trial. II. Impact on recovery time [see comments]. Br J Psychiatry 1996; **169**(5):602–7.

105. Lewis S, Tarrier N, Haddock G, et al. Randomised controlled trial of cognitive-behavioural therapy in early schizophrenia: acute-phase outcomes. Br J Psychiatry Suppl 2002; **43**:S91–S97.

106. Power PJ, Bell RJ, Mills R, et al. Suicide prevention in first episode psychosis: the development of a randomised controlled trial of cognitive therapy for acutely suicidal patients with early psychosis. Aust N Z J Psychiatry 2003; **37**(4): 414–20.

107. Scott J, Garland A, Moorhead S. A pilot study of cognitive therapy in bipolar disorders. Psychol Med 2001; **31**(3):459–67.

108. Scott J. Cognitive therapy as an adjunct to medication in bipolar disorder. Br J Psychiatry 2001; **178**(Suppl 41):S164–8.

109. Kuipers E, Garety P, Fowler D, et al. London-East Anglia randomised controlled trial of cognitive-behavioural therapy for psychosis: I. Effects of the treatment phase. Br J Psychiatry 1997; **171**:319–27.

110. Chadwick P, Sambrooke S, Rasch S, Davies E. Challenging the omnipotence of voices: group cognitive behavior therapy for voices. Behav Res Ther 2000; **38**(10):993–1003.

111. Tarrier N, Wittkowski A, Kinney C, et al. Durability of the effects of cognitive-behavioural therapy in the treatment of chronic schizophrenia: 12–month follow-up. Br J Psychiatry 1999; **174**:500–4.

112. Garety P, Fowler D, Kuipers E, et al. London-East Anglia randomised controlled trial of cognitive-behavioural therapy for psychosis: II. Predictors of outcome. Br J Psychiatry 1997; **171**:420–6.

113. Kuipers E, Fowler D, Garety P, et al. London-east Anglia randomised controlled trial of cognitive-behavioural therapy for psychosis: III. Follow-up and economic evaluation at 18 months. Br J Psychiatry 1998; **173**:61–8.

114. Morrison AP, Bentall RP, French P, et al. Randomised controlled trial of early detection and cognitive therapy for preventing transition to psychosis in high-risk individuals. Study design and interim analysis of transition rate and psychological risk factors. Br J Psychiatry Suppl 2002; **43**:S78–S84.

115. McGorry PD, Yung AR, Phillips LJ, et al. Randomized controlled trial of interventions designed to reduce the risk of progression to first-episode psychosis in a clinical sample with subthreshold symptoms. Arch Gen Psychiatry 2002; **59**(10):921–8.

116. Grant C, Addington J, Addington D, Konnert C. Social functioning in first- and multiepisode schizophrenia. Can J Psychiatry 2001; **46**(8): 746–9.

117. Hutton SB, Puri BK, Duncan LJ, et al. Executive function in first-episode schizophrenia. Psychol Med 1998; **28**(2): 463–73.

118. Riley EM, McGovern D, Mockler D, et al. Neuropsychological functioning in first-episode psychosis—evidence of specific deficits. Schizophr Res 2000; **43**(1):47–55.

119. Falloon IR. Problem solving as a core strategy in the prevention of schizophrenia and other mental disorders. Aust N Z J Psychiatry 2000; **34**(Suppl):S185–S90.

120. D'Zurilla T. *Problem Solving Therapy*. New York: Springer; 1986.

121. Macdonald EM, Hayes RL, Baglioni AJ, Jr. The quantity and quality of the social networks of young people with early psychosis compared with closely matched controls. Schizophr Res 2000; **46**(1):25–30.

122. Macdonald EM, Jackson HJ, Hayes RL, et al. Social skill as determinant of social networks and perceived social support in schizophrenia. Schizophr Res 1998; **29**(3):275–86.

123. Erickson DH, Beiser M, Iacono WG. Social support predicts 5–year outcome in first-episode schizophrenia. J Abnorm Psychol 1998; **107**(4):681–5.

124. Bellack A, Meuser K, Gingerich S, Agresta J. *Social Skills Training for Schizophrenia: A Step by Step Guide*. Guilford. New York Press; 1997.

125. Scott JE, Dixon LB. Psychological interventions for schizophrenia. Schizophr Bull 1995; **21**(4): 621–30.

126. Donahue C, Driesanga S. A review of social skills training with chronic mental patients. In: Eisler

R, Miller P (eds). *Progress in Behavior Modification.* Newbury Park: Sage; 1988.

127. Bellack AS, Mueser KT. Psychosocial treatment for schizophrenia. Schizophr Bull 1993; **19**(2): 317–36.

128. Wallace CJ, Nelson CJ, Liberman RP, et al. A review and critique of social skills training with schizophrenic patients. Schizophr Bull 1980; **6**(1):42–63.

129. Lauriello J, Bustillo J, Keith SJ. A critical review of research on psychosocial treatment of schizophrenia. Biol Psychiatry 1999; **46**(10):1409–17.

130. Wallace CJ, Liberman RP, MacKain SJ, et al. Effectiveness and replicability of modules for teaching social and instrumental skills to the severely mentally ill. Am J Psychiatry 1992; **149**(5):654–8.

131. Eckman TA, Wirshing WC, Marder SR, et al. Technique for training schizophrenic patients in illness self-management: a controlled trial. Am J Psychiatry 1992; **149**(11):1549–55.

132. Wallace CJ, Liberman RP. Social skills training for patients with schizophrenia: a controlled clinical trial. Psychiatry Res 1985; **15**(3):239–47.

133. Marder SR, Wirshing WC, Mintz J, et al. Two-year outcome of social skills training and group psychotherapy for outpatients with schizophrenia. Am J Psychiatry 1996; **153**(12):1585–92.

134. Liberman RP, Wallace CJ, Blackwell G, et al. Skills training versus psychosocial occupational therapy for persons with persistent schizophrenia. Am J Psychiatry 1998; **155**(8):1087–91.

135. Bilder RM, Goldman RS, Robinson D, et al. Neuropsychology of first-episode schizophrenia: initial characterization and clinical correlates. Am J Psychiatry 2000; **157**(4):549–59.

136. Addington J, Addington D. Neurocognitive and social functioning in schizophrenia. Schizophr Bull 1999; **25**(1):173–82.

137. Addington J, Addington D. Neurocognitive and social functioning in schizophrenia: a 2.5 year follow-up study. Schizophr Res 2000; **44**(1):47–56.

138. Velligan DI, Bow-Thomas CC, Huntzinger C, et al. Randomized controlled trial of the use of compensatory strategies to enhance adaptive functioning in outpatients with schizophrenia. Am J Psychiatry 2000; **157**(8):1317–23.

139. McGurk SR, Meltzer HY. The role of cognition in vocational functioning in schizophrenia. Schizophr Res 2000; **45**(3):175–84.

140. Bell M, Bryson G, Greig T, et al. Neurocognitive enhancement therapy with work therapy: effects on neuropsychological test performance. Arch Gen Psychiatry 2001; **58**(8):763–8.

141. Wykes T, Reeder C, Corner J, et al. The effects of neurocognitive remediation on executive processing in patients with schizophrenia. Schizophr Bull 1999; **25**(2):291–307.

142. Stratta P, Mancini F, Mattei P, et al. Remediation of Wisconsin Card Sorting Test performance in schizophrenia. A controlled study. Psychopathology 1997; **30**(2):59–66.

143. Hayes RL, McGrath JJ. Cognitive rehabilitation for people with schizophrenia and related conditions. Cochrane Database Syst Rev 2000; **3**:CD000968.

144. Hodel B, Brenner HD. Cognitive therapy with schizophrenic patients: conceptual basis, present state, future directions. Acta Psychiatr Scand Suppl 1994; **384**:108–15.

145. Bellack AS. Cognitive rehabilitation for schizophrenia: is it possible? Is it necessary? Schizophr Bull 1992; **18**(1):43–50.

146. Bellack AS, Gold JM, Buchanan RW. Cognitive rehabilitation for schizophrenia: problems, prospects, and strategies. Schizophr Bull 1999; **25**(2):257–74.

147. Velligan DI, Mahurin RK, True JE, et al. Preliminary evaluation of cognitive adaptation training to compensate for cognitive deficits in schizophrenia. Psychiatr Serv 1996; **47**(4):415–17.

148. Hogarty GE, Flesher S. Practice principles of cognitive enhancement therapy for schizophrenia. Schizophr Bull 1999; **25**(4):693–708.

149. Brown GW, Birley JL, Wing JK. Influence of family life on the course of schizophrenic disorders: a replication. Br J Psychiatry 1972; **121**(562):241–58.

150. Leeb B, Mundt C, Fiedler P, et al. ['Covert criticism'—a new criterion for determining the expressed emotion index in a five-minute speech sample of partners of depressed patients]. Nervenarzt 1993; **64**(11):727–9.

151. Kavanagh DJ. Recent developments in expressed emotion and schizophrenia. Br J Psychiatry 1992; **160**:601–20.

152. Kuipers L. The measurement of expressed emotion: Its influence on research and clinical practice. Int Rev Psychiatry 1994; **6**:187–99.

153. Leff J, Kuipers L, Berkowitz R, et al. A controlled trial of social intervention in the families of schizophrenic patients. Br J Psychiatry 1982; **141**:121–34.

154. Macmillan JF, Crow TJ, Johnson AL, Johnstone EC. Expressed emotion and relapse in first episodes of schizophrenia. Br J Psychiatry 1987; **151**:320–3.

155. Stirling J, Tantam D, Thomas P, et al. Expressed emotion and schizophrenia: the ontogeny of EE during an 18–month follow-up. Psychol Med 1993; **23**(3):771–8.

156. Barrelet L, Ferrero F, Szigethy L, et al. Expressed emotion and first-admission schizophrenia. Nine-month follow-up in a French cultural environment. Br J Psychiatry 1990; **156**:357–62.

157. Rund BR, Oie M, Borchgrevink TS, Fjell A. Expressed emotion, communication deviance and schizophrenia. An exploratory study of the relationship between two family variables and the course and outcome of a psychoeducational treatment programme. Psychopathology 1995; **28**(4):220–8.

158. Huguelet P, Favre S, Binyet S, et al. The use of the Expressed Emotion Index as a predictor of outcome in first admitted schizophrenic patients in a French speaking area of Switzerland. Acta Psychiatr Scand 1995; **92**(6):447–52.

159. Zastowny TR, Lehman AF, Cole RE, Kane C. Family management of schizophrenia: a comparison of behavioral and supportive family treatment. Psychiatr Q 1992; **63**(2):159–86.

160. Linszen D, Dingemans P, Van der Does JW, et al. Treatment, expressed emotion and relapse in recent onset schizophrenic disorders. Psychol Med 1996; **26**(2):333–42.

161. Birchwood M, Smith J. Expressed emotions and first episodes of schizophrenia. Br J Psychiatry 1987; **151**:859–60.

162. Bachmann S, Bottmer C, Jacob S, et al. Expressed emotion in relatives of first-episode and chronic patients with schizophrenia and major depressive disorder—a comparison. Psychiatry Res 2002; **112**(3):239–50.

163. Gupta S, Andreasen NC, Arndt S, et al. The Iowa Longitudinal Study of Recent Onset Psychosis: one-year follow-up of first episode patients. Schizophr Res 1997; **23**(1):1–13.

164. Tohen M, Strakowski SM, Zarate C, Jr, et al. The McLean-Harvard first-episode project: 6-month symptomatic and functional outcome in affective and nonaffective psychosis. Biol Psychiatry 2000; **48**(6):467–76.

165. Addington J, Young J, Addington D. Social outcome in early psychosis. Psychol Med 2003; **33**(6):1119–24.

166. Green MF. What are the functional consequences of neurocognitive deficits in schizophrenia? [see comments]. Am J Psychiatry 1996; **153**(3):321–30.

167. Newman SJ. Housing attributes and serious mental illness: implications for research and practice. Psychiatr Serv 2001; **52**(10):1309–17.

8

Special Populations

Tom Ehmann, Laura Hanson and Robin Friedlander

'At risk' prodromal states

The prodrome is a period of disturbance that represents a deviation from a person's previous experience and behavior prior to the development of florid features of psychosis.[1,2] The term 'prodrome' has been used to describe both the period prior to the first episode of psychosis (initial prodrome) and the period prior to relapse of psychosis (relapse prodrome).

Here, the term 'prodrome' is used to describe the period of non-specific symptoms and disruption before the individual became psychotic for the first time. The prodrome is diagnosed retrospectively (i.e. is identified only after the development of florid features of psychosis). Retrospective assessment for the presence of a prodrome carries implications for diagnosis and treatment.

Other terms that have been used to describe the disturbances that may precede onset include 'at-risk mental state',[3] and 'precursor syndrome'.[4] When an individual has experienced a decline but is not yet psychotic, it is preferable to describe this as an 'at-risk mental state' rather than a prodrome. The pre-relapse period is better referred to as 'early warning signs of relapse' or 'signs and symptoms of impending relapse'.[5]

Features of the prodrome

Prodromes occur prior to the development of numerous psychotic disorders including schizophrenia and bipolar disorder. The average prodrome lasts 12 to 24 months.[6] However, it may range in length from days to decades, with a median of about one year for schizophrenia.[1,2,7]

DSM-III-R described the schizophrenia prodrome with nine features that encompassed behavioral, affective, perceptual, thinking, and deficit features. However, raters failed to agree consistently on the presence of specific symptoms and their stability over time, and the symptoms did not reliably precede the onset of schizophrenia.[8–11] DSM-IV now simply refers to the prodrome as consisting of negative symptoms and/or attenuated psychotic symptoms.[12]

The most frequent prominent prodromal symptoms include:[2,13]

- Social isolation or withdrawal
- Marked impairment in role functioning
- Odd or bizarre ideation
- Decreased drive and energy
- Blunting of affect.

Other frequent symptoms are:

- School difficulties
- Somatic complaints

- Perceptual abnormalities
- Changes in sense of the self, others, or the world
- Fatigue
- Sleep disturbance
- Suspiciousness
- Anxiety
- Irritability
- Depression
- Aggression
- Speech abnormalities
- Concentration and memory problems.

Symptoms associated with the prodrome are common to other mental disorders and are frequently seen as part of normal developmental phases, responses to stress, and interpersonal problems.

Diagnostic implications of assessing for a prodrome

It is important to establish whether a prodrome was present before onset of psychosis, since diagnostic clarity may depend upon its presence. For example, differentiation of schizophrenia from schizophreniform or other psychoses depends upon a longitudinal assessment of changes in the patient. The presence of a prodrome may also help clarify the role of substance abuse in the etiology of the psychosis. Sometimes, an error is made by attributing the psychosis to recent substance use, thus ignoring or failing to elicit a history of years of prodromal symptoms and functional impairment.

Predictive validity of prodromal-like symptoms

The non-specific changes associated with the prodrome may be thought of as a precursor or risk factor. Individuals exhibiting changes suggestive of a prodrome may be considered at risk for developing psychosis. The long established search for risk factors in schizophrenia has revealed numerous associations with genetic, environmental, and developmental variables. However,

each of these variables carries limited predictive value. For example, persons at fairly high genetic risk may have less than a 20% chance of developing psychosis. Therefore, strategies have been developed to better predict the likelihood a person will become psychotic in the near future. These strategies generally combine prodromal symptoms with other risk factors, such as a family history of psychosis, transient psychotic symptoms, 'basic symptoms' or schizotypal personality traits.[14–18] However, a substantial risk of falsely predicting psychosis still occurs when utilizing these strategies. Even using this more sophisticated approach to identifying individuals in an ultra at-risk state, about 41% actually made the transition to psychosis within one year.[19]

Appropriate interventions

It has been reported that it may be possible to prevent or reduce the severity of psychosis by intervening in the at-risk mental state.[20] Research projects currently underway should help determine whether interventions during an at-risk state may be beneficial in preventing onset or otherwise modifying the course of the psychotic disorder if it develops. Some research groups focus more on low dose atypical antipsychotic medications,[21] while others also examine psychological treatments.[22] Yet others are adopting a more naturalistic approach to gathering intervention data.[23]

Despite these research efforts, several effects must be considered before embracing medication as an intervention in persons identified as at risk. First, the proportion of false positives is high, with many individuals falsely identified as being in the prodrome. These falsely identified individuals are then placed at risk for unnecessary treatment, stress, turmoil, labeling, and stigma. Furthermore, the type(s) of effective treatment to be given along with their timing, intensity, and duration all remain unknown. These ethical and scientific concerns have prompted a lively debate in the literature.[24,25] The level of technical and clinical expertise currently required to pursue at-risk intervention is beyond that found in most treatment settings.

Such concerns have led some to recommend prudently that interventions for those in possible prodromal states be symptomatic and problem-focused.[26] The inability to predict accurately transition to psychosis together with a lack of knowledge about the ability of interventions to prevent onset of psychosis or provide other benefits suggests precluding the use of psychosis-specific treatments until psychosis is definitely present. In general clinical practice, the prediction of psychosis or initiation of treatment for psychosis should not be made either on the basis of symptoms interpreted as prodromal or on the basis that risk factors for psychosis are present. Individuals who appear to be at very high risk for psychosis (possible prodromal) should be thoroughly assessed, engaged, treated for presenting complaints (i.e. depression, anxiety, insomnia), and closely monitored. Stressors that could exacerbate the condition should be ameliorated. Standard approaches include modification or avoidance of stressors, shifting perception of the stressor to render it less threatening, and decreasing attendant physiological arousal. Treatment specific for psychosis (e.g. provision of antipsychotic medications, education about psychosis) should be initiated only upon emergence of florid psychosis.

Substance abuse

Extent and consequences of substance abuse in psychosis

One year and point-prevalence estimates of comorbid substance abuse in early psychosis range from approximately 20% to 30%.[27,28] The rates of comorbidity in first episode affective versus nonaffective psychosis appear to be similar.[29] In early psychosis, cannabis and alcohol appear to be the two most frequently abused substances.[27,28] The prevalence of stimulant (amphetamines and cocaine) and hallucinogen abuse is also relatively high, while sedative and opiate use

is less common.[28,30] Risk factors for the development of comorbidity include male gender,[27,28] and antisocial behavior.[27] Substance abuse has been associated with an earlier age of onset of psychosis.[27,28,31]

Although substance abuse does not appear to be related to the severity of psychopathology in the early phases of psychosis,[27,32] there is evidence that substance abuse in early psychosis is associated with impairments in functioning, lower quality of life, and increased risk of hospital readmission.[31] Longstanding psychotic illness coupled with comorbid substance abuse is associated with higher rates of negative outcomes (e.g. poor money management, homelessness, medication non-adherence, relapse and rehospitalization, violence, legal problems and incarceration, depression and suicide, as well as sexually transmitted disease).[33]

Explanations of comorbidity

The high prevalence of substance abuse in individuals with psychosis raises questions about the relationship between psychosis and substance use. Three causal relationships might explain comorbidity:

1. Substance abuse causes psychosis.
2. Psychopathology and distress cause the substance abuse ('self-medication').
3. A third variable accounts for the development of both (e.g. personality, environment, genetics).

There does not appear to be a single pattern to the emergence of substance abuse in relation to the onset of psychosis. For first episode schizophrenia, three temporal patterns were seen with approximately equal frequency—substance abuse pre-dated the onset of psychosis, emerged at the same time as the psychosis, or developed after psychosis.[30] Literature reviews on the question of etiology have generally concluded that there is no solid evidence that clearly demonstrates the nature of the relationship between substance abuse and psychosis.[34,35] The relationship between substance abuse and psychosis is probably multi-dimensional and dependent upon numerous mitigating factors.

Integrated treatment

Integrated programs provide treatment for both substance abuse and mental illness by the same clinician or team of clinicians. This helps to ensure consistency of information and coherence of treatment framework. Integrated programs differ to some degree in the specific treatment components they offer. However, there are many common elements across approaches including comprehensive assessment, group and individual counseling, education, mediation management, stress management, and relapse prevention.[36,37]

The emphasis of integrated treatment tends to be on:[36,37]

Long-term treatment vs short-term fixes

- Time is allowed to foster engagement before active treatment.
- Motivating patients to alter current substance use is considered crucial and often constitutes a considerable portion of treatment.
- A gradual reduction of substance use is sought to allow for the setting of small goals and to foster self-efficacy.
- Time is needed for the patient to learn how the psychosis and substance abuse interact.
- Ongoing strategies need to be provided to enhance recovery from both psychosis and substance abuse (e.g. enhancing coping skills or social skills).

Harm reduction vs abstinence

- Abstinence is unimaginable to many patients, and it is often exceptionally difficult motivating them towards this goal.
- The main goal is to reduce harm due to substance use.
- Changing consumption patterns is portrayed as a means to a different goal that is desirable to the patient (e.g. 'reducing your use will help you stay out of hospital, improve your relationship with your girlfriend, help with your financial problems, and allow you to rent a nicer apartment').
- Because of their emphasis on abstinence, attendance at groups, such as Alcoholics Anonymous or Narcotics Anonymous, is usually not recommended (unless desired by the patient).

Motivational interventions vs confrontational counseling

- Motivating patients to reduce current substance use is of primary importance.
- Confrontation is counter to the goals of engaging and motivating patients.
- Confrontational interactions may even exacerbate stress and psychotic symptoms.

Effectiveness of treatments
Early psychosis

Although a number of early psychosis programs have integrated substance abuse treatments, data documenting their effectiveness remain limited.[38] Given the paucity of treatment outcome data specific to early psychosis, most conclusions must be based on research for comorbidity present in those with more longstanding psychotic disorders.

Outpatient integrated treatment

Several reviews concluded that integrated treatment confers superior benefits compared to other treatment models.[36,39] Studies comparing differing models of integrated treatment generally found that the addition of motivational and behavioral interventions could lead to better outcomes.[40,41] However, a review of six randomized controlled outpatient treatment approaches concluded that there is no convincing evidence that integrating substance misuse programs within psychiatric care produced better outcomes than standard psychiatric care and there is insufficient evidence to conclude that any single approach to integrated treatment is superior.[42]

The paucity of well controlled effectiveness research is surprising, given the number of treatment programs that have developed in recent years. Fortunately, the publication of the review described above[42] appears to have acted as a catalyst, stimulating better controlled research in this area. Some of this more recent evidence has demonstrated that integrated treatment programs have lower attrition rates (50% lower than standard programs), decrease abuse severity, and decrease psychiatric symptoms.[43,44]

'Dual-diagnosis'* groups

To address the need to provide treatment for patients with comorbid psychosis and substance abuse, many mental health systems have incorporated 'dual-diagnosis' groups into existing mental health services. Professionals who are not part of the patient's clinical team usually lead these groups. Groups vary in structure and content covered but tend to address substance abuse through a combination of education, skills training, and support.

Adding a dual-diagnosis' group onto existing outpatient mental health services may be effective if patients attend regularly. However, the dropout rate appears to be high, even when patients are motivated to reduce their substance use.[45] Given the very high attrition rate, dual diagnosis group interventions appear to be insufficient for the majority of patients and may better be regarded as adjunctive.[46]

Intensive integrated treatment

Intensive integrated treatment is usually provided on an inpatient basis or within residential programs. It consists of daily treatment for several hours per day for weeks or months. Interventions usually consist of education, skills building, individual and group counseling, and medication

*The term 'dual-diagnosis' has multiple meanings including the following: (1) Axis I diagnosis plus mental retardation. (2) Axis I diagnosis plus personality disorder. (3) Axis I diagnosis plus substance abuse or dependence. In this context, it is used to refer to an Axis I diagnosis of severe mental illness and substance abuse or dependence.

management.[36] Studies that have investigated the efficacy of intensive treatment of this nature often report high dropout rates.[47,48] Those patients who do not drop out appear to have either little change in overall substance use or a high rate of return to their prior level of substance abuse.[47,49]

The poor outcomes associated with intensive integrated treatment may result from:

- Patients' inability to tolerate such intensive interventions
- The fact that the patients' access to substances is only limited while they are in active treatment
- The artificial environment patients are in during active treatment—return to their normal environment exposes them to social pressures and environmental cues that trigger use and hence relapse.

Given the relative lack of effectiveness and the expense associated with intensive treatment programs, hospitalization and residential programs are probably best reserved for withdrawal and detoxification.

Motivational interventions

One of the core features of integrated treatment programs is the focus on motivational interventions. Lack of motivation for reducing substance abuse appears to be a significant obstacle to successful treatment. Based on motivational interviewing techniques,[50] motivational interventions for substance abuse treatment for psychiatric patients have been developed.[51,52] Matching motivational interventions to stage of recovery is viewed as crucial to outcome.[36,53,54]

Core principles of motivational interviewing include:[50]

- Expressing empathy and avoiding confrontation to foster engagement
- Supporting self-efficacy by focusing on successes
- Developing a sense of the discrepancy between current and more attractive behaviors.

The motivational model consists of discrete stages of recovery that correspond well to the stages of treatment for psychosis. In integrated treatment, the substance abuse and psychosis interventions are usually blended together according to the stage of treatment. Evidence is accumulating that the incorporation of motivational techniques produces better outcomes.[44,55]

Assessment

Clinicians often do not adequately assess current substance use, consequences of use, and development of the problem.[56] Essential elements of the assessment of both current and past use include:

- Drugs used
- Frequency and duration of use
- Dose and method of administration
- Availability, assurance of quality, and financial cost
- Positive and negative effects as triggers and consequences
- Effect of use on psychiatric symptoms
- Preferred times, situations, and other prompts for use
- Attempts to quit (successful and unsuccessful)
- Motivations for reducing and continuing use
- Impact on functioning
- Dangerous behavior.

Behavioral analysis (assessing antecedents, substance use behavior, and consequences) may uncover variables that prompt drug use and that could then be modified or avoided. Stimulus control, skills training—especially drug refusal skills, adaptive behavioral alternatives, and motivational interventions—may all be guided by the assessment.

Reassessment at regular intervals helps evaluate treatment progress. Outcome measures often used include frequency, quantity, high risk use, and cravings. Relatively few instruments or rating scales have been validated for patients with comorbidity.[57]

Substance-induced psychosis

Although there is no consensus on whether substance use can cause a longstanding psychotic illness (such as schizophrenia),[35] certain substances (e.g. amphetamines) certainly can induce a brief acute episode of psychosis.[58]

Biochemical methods of detecting substances in the blood, breath, or urine may be most useful upon hospital admission to help determine whether psychotic symptoms might be substance-induced. Self-report regarding substance abuse tends to be less valid for inpatients than for outpatients and biochemical screens may identify substance use that otherwise would have gone undetected.[59] Emergency treatment should involve detoxification, supportive measures, and brief use of benzodiazepines if indicated.[58] An antipsychotic-free period during this time may help to clarify diagnosis.

In outpatient settings, the clinician may best be able to make a differential diagnosis by:[57,58]

- Determining the temporal relationship between substance use and onset of psychosis
- Noting if the symptoms are characteristic of substance intoxication/withdrawal (e.g. tactile hallucinations are characteristic of amphetamine intoxication; visual distortions are characteristic of LSD intoxication)
- Observing for the persistence or remission of psychotic symptoms during periods of abstinence.

Developmental disabilities

Developmental disability and early psychosis

Developmental disability loosely refers to individuals with neurodevelopmental disorders, such as mental retardation, autism, and cerebral palsy. In this section, the term 'developmental disability' refers to individuals with mental retardation (intellectual disability), defined as an IQ of less than 70 along with deficits in adaptive functioning and onset before age 18.

Low average intellectual functioning is a consistent finding in schizophrenia research with 10–20% of those with early onset schizophrenia having an IQ of less than 80.[60] In some patients with first episode psychosis, the second diagnosis of developmental disability may not be recognized. It may also be difficult to know what role schizophrenia has played in cognitive deterioration since many individuals experience a drop in IQ of about one standard deviation after onset. This decline has also been reported in those with mild developmental disability at the onset of schizophrenia.[61]

The prevalence of developmental disability is about 3% although the number of those receiving appropriate services is considerably lower.[62] The rate of schizophrenia appears elevated in those with developmental disability.[63] In adults with mild or moderate developmental disability a significantly increased rate of psychosis (5.5%), particularly schizophrenia (4.4%), has been reported.[64]

Presentation of psychosis in individuals with developmental disability

In individuals with mild developmental disability, the presentation of psychosis appears similar to that found in the general population. There is nothing unique or esoteric in the symptomatology of schizophrenia,[65] although delusions may be bland and unremarkable.[66] Hallucinations, especially auditory, appear to be the most frequently reported positive symptom in schizophrenia, followed by persecutory delusions and formal thought disorder.[63,67]

Inappropriate affect and affective blunting, although common, are non-specific symptoms in the developmental disability population.[68] Increasing severity of developmental disability brings an inability to use language and reduced accessibility to inner mental states, thereby making assessment more difficult.

Assessment

The assessment of psychosis in individuals with limited intellectual abilities requires ongoing consideration of several additional factors. The following suggestions and comments are to assist clinicians avoid some of the problems of interpretation that can easily arise.

- Look for a change in a person's baseline/premorbid functional level or behavior. Symptoms that are part of developmental disability or due to a concurrent disorder, such as autism, tend to be longstanding and stable.[61,69]
- Give weight to observable phenomena in low verbal patients, such as reports of a change in behavior that appears bizarre and is sustained in different environments. However, these observed phenomena are not necessarily reliable symptoms of psychosis. For example, the observation 'seems to be hallucinating' could be indicative of abnormal interest in peripheral stimuli or autism.
- Avoid diagnostic overshadowing that may lead to under-diagnosis of concurrent mental illness. Overshadowing refers to the assumption that observed aberrant behavior is a manifestation of developmental disability rather than a possible reflection of comorbid psychosis.[70] Conversely, because individuals may have difficulty communicating their feelings and thoughts, a clinician may misinterpret as psychopathology behaviors that are quite understandable responses to environmental or internal variables (e.g. noise or pain).
- Recognize phenomena that may be developmentally appropriate in individuals with developmental delays. Thinking out loud, talking to him/herself or having imaginary friends may be normal in adults with developmental disability.[71,72]
- Wish fulfilment and fantasy may lead to the appearance of false beliefs that are not always open to persuasion and argument. Generally, these ideas tend to be ephemeral and are not held with intensity for any length of time.[73]
- Recognize the tendency of individuals with developmental disability to acquiesce when they do not understand a question. Avoid

questions that are closed as well as questions that are too open. Multiple choice questions may be helpful (such as 'Are the voices inside your head or are they coming from outside of you?').

- When inquiring about hallucinations, ask questions in different ways on different occasions to check for consistency of the symptom.[69]
- Concentration problems may necessitate frequent reiteration of questions and breaks during the interview.
- Corroborate information from a reliable informant. Where large discrepancies exist between patient and informant reports, experience from child psychiatry suggests the following:
  - Informants are more likely to give clear accounts of worries, loss of interest, irritability, and social withdrawal.
  - Patients are more likely to report hallucinations, delusions, and autonomic symptoms.
- Sensory impairments, such as vision and hearing, are common in developmental disability and should always be assessed as they may be an aggravating factor in psychosis.[69]
- Aggression is a non-specific symptom that commonly leads to referral and may be misinterpreted as reflecting psychosis. There is no evidence to suggest that psychosis is specifically associated with aggression in developmental disability. Aggression is often due to communication problems or a provocative environment. Some people have a long history of aggression that is elicited or exacerbated by their particular personality structure but such behavior does not reflect psychosis.

Diagnostic considerations

High rates of initial misdiagnosis of psychosis in children and youth[74] may also be found in the developmental disability population across all ages.[69,75] Communication difficulties that make diagnosis difficult,[70] along with concerns regarding overuse of antipsychotic medications in developmental disability patients, have prompted

some authors to caution against over-diagnosing psychosis in those with developmental disability.[76] Some experts argue it is not possible reliably to diagnose schizophrenia in those with an IQ of less than 50.[69,75] Exceptions to this rule include catatonic posturing and responding to observable hallucinations, especially if these signs have never been seen before.[77]

Although there has been recent interest in modifying ICD-10 and DSM-IV criteria for this population, criteria changes may be more useful for mood and anxiety disorders than psychotic disorders. Psychotic disorder not otherwise specified (NOS) has been the recommended diagnosis for patients with clear psychotic symptoms and IQ<50.[75] However, studious reviews of patient files, repeated interviews, and prolonged observation often, but not always, clarify the diagnosis.[78] Using a careful extended observation approach, schizophrenia has been reliably diagnosed in patients with IQ scores of less than 50.[61] When the diagnosis remains unclear, the default diagnosis of psychosis NOS should be used.

Schizophrenia is the most frequent psychotic disorder diagnosed in individuals with developmental disability.[65,67] However, any psychotic disorder may occur.[63,66,69] In a large study of early-onset schizophrenia in children with IQ>70, approximately one third did not have schizophrenia and were found to be multidimensionally impaired with traumatic personal histories, cognitive impairment, mood lability, and subclinical or atypical psychotic symptoms.[79] Thus, it may be difficult to decide whether psychotic symptoms are part of a primary mood disorder or schizophrenia.[79] One small study found that youth with schizoaffective disorder had the most severe symptoms and the worst outcome of all psychotic disorders.[80]

Autism may present with flat or inappropriate affect, posturing, disorganized speech, alogia, and avolition. However, age of onset is much earlier than in schizophrenia. The risk of schizophrenia developing later in people with autistic disorder probably remains the same as in the general population.[81] To prevent misdiagnosis of schizophrenia in individuals with autism, DSM-IV recommends that prominent hallucinations or delusions be present for at least one month (in the presence of underlying autism), for a diagnosis of concurrent schizophrenia to be made.

High rates of epilepsy are noted in the developmental disability population.[82] Temporal lobe epilepsy increases risk of psychosis and the hallucinatory phenomena may be misidentified as psychosis.

Finally, the diagnostic formulation should consider genetic syndromes that increase the risk for developmental delays and psychoses. Investigations should rule out the following: 22q 11 deletion syndrome, Lujan-Fryns syndrome, Fragile X syndrome, Prader-Willi syndrome, Wolfram syndrome and Usher syndrome.

Treatment
Pharmacotherapy

Reviews on appropriate antipsychotic use in persons with developmental disability and psychosis have been published.[83,84] However, current clinical practice is guided by evidence from trials of those with schizophrenia and IQ>70 because of a paucity of research on antipsychotics in persons with developmental disability and psychosis.[85] For individuals with mild developmental disability, mental health team members with competence in psychotic disorders and knowledge of early intervention should be suitable clinicians. For individuals with IQ<50, consultation, if not direct treatment, with a specialized mental health team is advised.

Antipsychotic medication remains the first line treatment of psychosis. As for all patients with a psychotic disorder, a 'start low, go slow' approach is recommended.[75] The use of antipsychotics in this population is associated with greater risk of developing movement disorders (especially tardive dyskinesia and tardive akathisia) and cognitive impairment.[86–88]

Psychosocial interventions

Psychoeducation, especially for families and caregivers, is of paramount importance.

Adaptation of existing psychoeducational materials is needed and should include topics relevant to developmental disability and the consequences of this comorbidity. Although social skills training can be valuable, there are no guidelines for delivering this treatment to patients with both developmental disability and psychosis.[73]

The overall level of care needed for individuals with developmental disability and mental illness is higher than for patients with normal IQs.[89] Although the percentage of individuals with developmental disability requiring psychiatric hospitalization is similar to those with an IQ>70, their average length of stay is significantly longer.[89] More residential treatment facilities and intensive case management services are needed for this population. Provision of these specialized services should provide better supports for those in the community and prevent unnecessary hospitalization. There is a need for specialized day treatment programs because many of these individuals are not able to cope with generic day programs for psychosis offered by community mental health teams.

Summary

In summary, psychotic disorders appear to be increased threefold in persons with developmental disabilities. Assessment must be careful to avoid either over- or under-diagnosis of psychosis. Treatment follows guidelines for the general population, but with an awareness of possible increases in the required level of care and vulnerability to neuroleptic side effects. People with developmental disability and concurrent psychotic disorders are an underserved population. Skilled psychiatric care is greatly appreciated by the patients and families, which makes the clinical work particularly rewarding. The co-occurrence of developmental disability, psychosis, genetic syndromes, and perinatal brain injury also makes this field of study particularly relevant for clinicians involved in understanding psychosis.

References

1. Beiser M, Erickson D, Fleming JA, Iacono WG. Establishing the onset of psychotic illness. Am J Psychiatry 1993; **150**(9):1349–54.

2. Yung AR, McGorry PD. The initial prodrome in psychosis: descriptive and qualitative aspects. Aust N Z J Psychiatry 1996; **30**(5):587–99.

3. Yung AR, McGorry PD. The prodromal phase of first-episode psychosis: past and current conceptualizations. Schizophr Bull 1996; **22**(2): 353–70.

4. Eaton WW, Badawi M, Melton B. Prodromes and precursors: epidemiologic data for primary prevention of disorders with slow onset. Am J Psychiatry 1995; **152**(7):967–72.

5. Bustillo J, Buchanan RW, Carpenter WT, Jr. Prodromal symptoms vs. early warning signs and clinical action in schizophrenia. Schizophr Bull 1995; **21**(4):553–9.

6. Sheitman BB, Lee H, Strauss R, Lieberman JA. The evaluation and treatment of first-episode psychosis. Schizophr Bull 1997; **23**(4):653–61.

7. Moller P, Husby R. The initial prodrome in schizophrenia: searching for naturalistic core dimensions of experience and behavior. Schizophr Bull 2000; **26**(1):217–32.

8. Jackson HJ, McGorry PD, Dakis J, et al. The inter-rater and test-retest reliabilities of prodromal symptoms in first-episode psychosis. Aust N Z J Psychiatry 1996; **30**(4):498–504.

9. Jackson HJ, McGorry PD, Dudgeon P. Prodromal symptoms of schizophrenia in first-episode psychosis: prevalence and specificity [published erratum appears in Compr Psychiatry 1996; **37**(1):75]. Compr Psychiatry 1995; **36**(4):241–50.

10. Jackson HJ, McGorry PD, McKenzie D. The reliability of DSM-III prodromal symptoms in first-episode psychotic patients. Acta Psychiatr Scand 1994; **90**(5):375–8.

11. McGorry PD, McKenzie D, Jackson HJ, et al. Can we improve the diagnostic efficiency and predictive power of prodromal symptoms for schizophrenia? Schizophr Res 2000; **42**(2):91–100.

12. American Psychiatric Association (APA). *Diagnostic and Statistical Manual of Mental Disorders* (4th edn). Washington, DC: American Psychiatric Association; 1994.

13. Creel SM. Prodromal psychosocial behaviors in soldiers with schizophrenic and schizophreniform disorder. Mil Med 1988; **153**(3):146–50.

14. McGlashan TH. Early detection and intervention of schizophrenia: rationale and research. Br J Psychiatry Suppl 1998; **172**(33):3–6.

15. Yung AR, McGorry PD, McFarlane CA, et al. Monitoring and care of young people at incipient risk of psychosis. Schizophr Bull 1996; **22**(2):283–303.

16. Gross G. The onset of schizophrenia. Schizophr Res 1997; **28**(2–3):187–98.

17. Meehl PE. Schizotaxia revisited. Arch Gen Psychiatry 1989; **46**(10):935–44.

18. Miller P, Byrne M, Hodges A, et al. Schizotypal components in people at high risk of developing schizophrenia: early findings from the Edinburgh High-Risk Study. Br J Psychiatry 2002; **180**:179–84.

19. Yung AR, Phillips LJ, Yuen HP, et al. Psychosis prediction: 12-month follow up of a high-risk ('prodromal') group. Schizophr Res 2003; **60**(1):21–32.

20. Falloon IR. Early intervention for first episodes of schizophrenia: a preliminary exploration [see comments]. Psychiatry 1992; **55**(1):4–15.

21. McGlashan TH, Zipursky RB, Perkins D, et al. The PRIME North America randomized double-blind clinical trial of olanzapine versus placebo in patients at risk of being prodromally symptomatic for psychosis: I. Study rationale and design. Schizophr Res 2003; **61**(1):7–18.

22. McGorry PD, Yung AR, Phillips LJ, et al. Randomized controlled trial of interventions designed to reduce the risk of progression to first-episode psychosis in a clinical sample with subthreshold symptoms. Arch Gen Psychiatry 2002; **59**(10):921–8.

23. Cornblatt B, Lencz T, Obuchowski M. The schizophrenia prodrome: treatment and high-risk perspectives. Schizophr Res 2002; **54**(1–2):177–86.

24. Cornblatt BA, Lencz T, Kane JM. Treatment of the schizophrenia prodrome: is it presently ethical? Schizophr Res 2001; **51**(1):31–8.

25. McGlashan TH. Psychosis treatment prior to psychosis onset: ethical issues. Schizophr Res 2001; **51**(1):47–54.

26. *Australian Clinical Guidelines for Early Psychosis*. Melbourne: National early psychosis project, University of Melbourne; 1998.

27. Rabinowitz J, Bromet EJ, Lavelle J, et al. Prevalence and severity of substance use disorders and onset of psychosis in first-admission psychotic patients. Psychol Med 1998; **28**(6):1411–19.

28. Cantwell R, Brewin J, Glazebrook C, et al. Prevalence of substance misuse in first-episode psychosis. Br J Psychiatry 1999; **174**:150–3.

29. Malik N, Singh MM, Pradhan SC. Substance misuse in first-episode psychosis [letter; comment]. Br J Psychiatry 2000; **176**:195.

30. Hambrecht M, Hafner H. Substance abuse and the onset of schizophrenia. Biol Psychiatry 1996; **40**(11):1155–63.

31. Addington J, Addington D. Effect of substance misuse in early psychosis. Br J Psychiatry Suppl 1998; **172**(33):134–6.

32. Sevy S, Robinson DG, Holloway S, et al. Correlates of substance misuse in patients with first-episode schizophrenia and schizoaffective disorder. Acta Psychiatr Scand 2001; **104**(5):367–74.

33. Drake RE, Brunette MF. Complications of severe mental illness related to alcohol and drug use disorders. Recent Dev Alcohol 1998; **14**:285–99.

34. Mueser KT, Drake RE, Wallach MA. Dual diagnosis: a review of etiological theories. Addict Behav 1998; **23**(6):717–34.

35. Phillips P, Johnson S. How does drug and alcohol misuse develop among people with psychotic illness? A literature review. Soc Psychiatry Psychiatr Epidemiol 2001; **36**(6):269–76.

36. Drake RE, Mercer-McFadden C, Mueser KT, et al. Review of integrated mental health and substance abuse treatment for patients with dual disorders. Schizophr Bull 1998; **24**(4):589–608.

37. Minkoff K. Program components of a comprehensive integrated care system for seriously mentally ill patients with substance disorders. New Dir Ment Health Serv 2001; **91**:17–30.

38. Addington J, Addington D. Impact of an early psychosis program on substance use. Psychiatr Rehabil J 2001; **25**(1):60–7.

39. Drake RE, Mueser KT. Psychosocial approaches to dual diagnosis. Schizophr Bull 2000; **26**(1):105–18.

40. Jerrell JM, Ridgely MS. Comparative effectiveness of three approaches to serving people with severe mental illness and substance abuse disorders. J Nerv Ment Dis 1995; **183**(9):566–76.

41. Jerrell JM, Ridgely MS. Impact of robustness of program implementation on outcomes of clients in dual diagnosis programs. Psychiatr Serv 1999; **50**(1):109–12.

42. Ley A, Jeffery DP, McLaren S, Siegfried N. Treatment programmes for people with both severe mental illness and substance misuse. Cochrane Database Syst Rev 2000;4.

43. Hellerstein DJ, Rosenthal RN, Miner CR. Integrating services for schizophrenia and substance abuse. Psychiatr Q 2001; **72**(4):291–306.

44. Barrowclough C, Haddock G, Tarrier N, et al. Randomized controlled trial of motivational interviewing, cognitive behavior therapy, and family intervention for patients with comorbid schizophrenia and substance use disorders. Am J Psychiatry 2001; **158**(10):1706–13.

45. Hellerstein DJ, Rosenthal RN, Miner CR. A prospective study of integrated outpatient treatment for substance-abusing schizophrenic outpatients. Am J Addictions 1995; **4**:33–42.

46. Kofoed L, Kania J, Walsh T, Atkinson RM. Outpatient treatment of patients with substance abuse and coexisting psychiatric disorders. Am J Psychiatry 1986; **143**(7):867–72.

47. Bartels SJ, Drake RE. A pilot study of residential treatment for dual diagnoses. J Nerv Ment Dis 1996; **184**(6):379–81.

48. Hanson M, Kramer TH, Gross W. Outpatient treatment of adults with coexisting substance use and mental disorders. J Subst Abuse Treat 1990; **7**(2):109–16.

49. Bachmann KM, Moggi F, Hirsbrunner HP, et al. An integrated treatment program for dually diagnosed patients. Psychiatr Serv 1997; **48**(3):314–16.

50. Miller WR, Rollnick S. *Motivational interviewing: Preparing people to change addictive behavior*. New York: Guildford Press; 1991.

51. Carey KB. Substance use reduction in the context of outpatient psychiatric treatment: a collaborative, motivational, harm reduction approach. Community Ment Health J 1996; **32**(3):291–306; discussion 307–10.

52. Carey KB, Purnine DM, Maisto SA, Carey MP. Enhancing readiness-to-change substance abuse in persons with schizophrenia. A four-session motivation-based intervention. Behav Modif 2001; **25**(3):331–84.

53. Ziedonis DM, Trudeau K. Motivation to quit using substances among individuals with schizophrenia: implications for a motivation-based treatment model. Schizophr Bull 1997; **23**(2):229–38.

54. Drake RE, Essock SM, Shaner A, et al. Implementing dual diagnosis services for clients with severe mental illness. Psychiatr Serv 2001; **52**(4):469–76.

55. Lehman AF, Herron JD, Schwartz RP, Myers CP. Rehabilitation for adults with severe mental illness and substance use disorders. A clinical trial. J Nerv Ment Dis 1993; **181**(2):86–90.

56. Ananth J, Vandewater S, Kamal M, et al. Missed diagnosis of substance abuse in psychiatric patients. Hosp Community Psychiatry 1989; **40**(3): 297–9.

57. Carey KB, Correia CJ. Severe mental illness and addictions: assessment considerations. Addict Behav 1998; **23**(6):735–48.

58. Bacon A, Granholm E, Withers N. Substance-induced psychosis. Semin Clin Neuropsychiatry 1998; **3**(1):70–79.

59. Galletly CA, Field CD, Prior M. Urine drug screening of patients admitted to a state psychiatric hospital. Hosp Community Psychiatry 1993; **44**(6): 587–9.

60. McClellan J, McCurry C. Neurodevelopmental pathways in schizophrenia. Semin Clin Neuropsychiatry 1998; **3**(4):320–332.

61. Lee P, Moss S, Friedlander R, et al. Early-onset schizophrenia in children with mental retardation: diagnostic reliability and stability of clinical features. J Am Acad Child Adolesc Psychiatry 2003; **42**(2):162–9.

62. Roeleveld N, Zielhuis GA, Gabreels F. The prevalence of mental retardation: a critical review of recent literature. Dev Med Child Neurol 1997; **39**(2):125–32.

63. Clarke D. Functional psychoses in people with mental retardation. In: Bouras N (ed). *Psychiatric and Behavioural Disorders in Developmental Disabilities and Mental Retardation.* Cambridge University Press; 1999:188–99.

64. Deb S, Thomas M, Bright C. Mental disorder in adults with intellectual disorder. J Intellect Disabil Res 2001; **45**(6):495–505.

65. Reid AH. Schizophrenia in mental retardation: clinical features. Res Dev Disabil 1989; **10**:241–249.

66. Sovner R. Limiting factors in the use of DSM-III criteria with mentally ill/mentally retarded persons. Psychopharmacol Bull 1986; **22**(4): 1055–9.

67. Meadows G, Turner T, Campbell L, et al. Assessing schizophrenia in adults with mental retardation. A comparative study. Br J Psychiatry 1991; **158**:103–5.

68. Moss S, Prosser H, Goldberg D. Validity of the schizophrenia diagnosis of the psychiatric assessment schedule for adults with developmental disability (PAS-ADD). Br J Psychiatry 1996; **168**(3): 359–67.

69. Deb S, Matthews T, Holt G, Bouras N. *Practice Guidelines for the Assessment and Diagnosis of Mental Health Problems in Adults with Intellectual Disability.* London: Pavilion Press; 2001.

70. Reiss S, Szyszko J. Diagnostic overshadowing and professional experience with mentally retarded persons. Am J Mental Deficiency 1983; **87**:396–402.

71. Hurley AD. The misdiagnosis of hallucinations and delusions in persons with mental retardation: A neurodevelopmental perspective. Semin Clin Neuropsychiatry 1996; **1**(2):122–133.

72. McGuire D, et al. Life issues of adolescents and adults with Down syndrome. In: Hassold TJ, Patterson D (eds). *Down Syndrome: A Promising Life Together.* Chichester: Wiley; 1998.

73. Tyrer SP, Dunstan JA. Schizophrenia in those with learning disability. In: Read SG (ed). *Psychiatry in Learning Disability.* London: WB Saunders; 1997:185–215.

74. McClellan J, McCurry C, Snell J, DuBose A. Early-onset psychotic disorders: course and outcome over a 2–year period. J Am Acad Child Adolesc Psychiatry 1999; **38**(11):1380–8.

75. Szymanski L, King BH. Practice parameters for the assessment and treatment of children, adolescents, and adults with mental retardation and comorbid mental disorders. American Academy of Child and Adolescent Psychiatry Working Group on Quality Issues. J Am Acad Child Adolesc Psychiatry 1999; **38**(12 Suppl):5S-31S.

76. Robertson J, Emerson E, Gregory N, et al. Receipt of psychotropic medication by people with intellectual disability in residential settings. J Intellect Disabil Res 2000; **44**(Pt 6):666–76.

77. Stavrakaki C. The DSM-IV and how it applies to persons with developmental disabilities. In: Griffiths D, Stavrakaki C, Summers J (eds). *Dual Diagnosis. An Introduction to the Mental Health Needs of Persons with Developental Disabilities.* Sudbury, Ontario: Habilitative Mental Health Resource Network; 2002:115–49.

78. Cain NN, Davidson PW, Burhan AM, et al. Identifying bipolar disorders in individuals with intellectual disability. J Intellect Disabil Res 2003; **47**(Pt 1):31–8.

79. McKenna K, Gordon CT, Lenane M, et al. Looking for childhood-onset schizophrenia: the first 71

cases screened. J Am Acad Child Adolesc Psychiatry 1994; **33**(5):636–44.

80. Friedlander R, Donnelly T. Early onset psychosis in youth with intellectual disability. J Intellect Disabil Res. (in press).

81. Volkmar FR, Cohen DJ. Comorbid association of autism and schizophrenia. Am J Psychiatry 1991; **148**(12):1705–7.

82. Goulden KJ, Shinnar S, Koller H, et al. Epilepsy in children with mental retardation: a cohort study. Epilepsia 1991; **32**(5):690–7.

83. Connor D, Posever T. A brief review of atypical antipsychotics in individuals with developmental disability. Mental Health Aspects of Developmental Disabilities 1998; **1**(4):93–102.

84. Gualtieri CT. *Brain Injury and Mental Retardation: Psychopharmacology and Neuropsychiatry.* Philadelphia: Lippincott, Williams & Wilkins; 2002.

85. Duggan L, Brylewski J. Effectiveness of antipsychotic medication in people with intellectual disability and schizophrenia: a systematic review. J Intellect Disabil Res 1999; **43**(Pt 2):94–104.

86. Gualtieri CT, Schroeder SR, Hicks RE, Quade D. Tardive dyskinesia in young mentally retarded individuals. Arch Gen Psychiatry 1986; **43**(4): 335–40.

87. Gingell K, Nadarajah J. A controlled community study of movement disorder in people with learning difficulties on anti-psychotic medication. J Intellect Disabil Res 1994; **38**(Pt 1):53–9.

88. Friedlander R, Lazar S, Klancnik J. Atypical antipsychotic use in treating adolescents and young adults with developmental disabilities. Can J Psychiatry 2001; **46**(8):741–5.

89. Lunsky Y, Bradley E, Durbain J, et al. *Dual Diagnosis in Provincial Psychiatric Hospitals: A Population-based Study. Year 1 Summary Report.* Toronto: Centre for Addiction and Mental Health; 2003.

9

Measuring the Effectiveness of Care

Tom Ehmann and Laura Hanson

The following tables are a selection of instruments that may be useful for clinical, research, and administrative purposes in early psychosis.

Generic symptoms scales

Table 9.1 Scales for assessing general symptoms	
Positive and Negative Syndrome Scale (PANSS)[1,2]	A comprehensive observer rating scale that can be combined with a structured interview schedule
Brief Psychiatric Rating Scale (BPRS)[3]	A widely used observer rating scale embedded in the PANSS It has a smaller number of items than the PANSS

Specific symptoms

Table 9.2 Scales for assessing specific symptoms	
Calgary Depression Scale[4,5]	Specifically assesses depression in schizophrenia
Beck Depression Inventory (BDI)[6,7]	A popular 21 item self-report measure of depression severity
Beck Hopelessness Scale (BHS)[8]	A self-report measure to assess suicidal risk
Scale for the Assessment of Positive Symptoms (SAPS)	Observer rating of positive symptoms
Scale for the Assessment of Negative Symptoms (SANS)[9]	Observer rating of negative symptoms
Young Mania Rating Scale[10]	Widely used measure of manic symptoms
Clinician Administered Rating Scale for Mania[11]	Newer mania rating scale

Inpatient scales

Table 9.3 Inpatient scales	
Routine Assessment of Patient Progress (RAPP)[12,13]	A validated measure of symptoms and function completed by nursing staff
Nurses' Observation of Inpatient Evaluation (NOSIE)[14]	A widely used nurse rating scale

Global rating scales

Table 9.4 Global rating scales	
Global Assessment of Functioning (GAF)[15]	A quick measure that utilizes both symptoms and functioning; the GAF represents axis V of the DSM-IV multi-axial diagnostic system
Scale of Occupational and Functional Assessment (SOFAS)[15]	Derivation of the GAF that omits symptoms as a basis for the rating
Clinical Global Impression (CGI)[16]	Clinician rating of severity of illness
Clinical Global Scale of Improvement (CGI-Imp)[16]	Clinician improvement rating—users need to establish the baseline when doing repeated assessments

Quality of life and functioning scales

Table 9.5 Quality of life/functioning scales	
Quality of Life Interview[17]	A comprehensive scale specifically formulated for schizophrenia
MOS 36-item short form health survey (SF-36)[18]	A generic quality of life scale widely employed in many healthcare areas
Role Functioning Scale[19]	A simple four-item scale with specific anchor points assessing four areas of functioning
Life Functioning Questionnaire[15]	A 14-item self-report scale assessing role function over the preceding month in four domains—validated for bipolar disorder
Life Skills Profile[20,21]	A measure of function and disability focused on schizophrenia
Bay Area Functional Performance Evaluation (BaFPE)[22]	Frequently used in occupational therapy as a measure of functional status

Miscellaneous instruments

Table 9.6 Miscellaneous assessment tools	
Social Rhythm Metric[23]	Focuses on daily social rhythms—to assist planning in bipolar disorder
2-COM[24]	Self-report measure of perceived needs
Symptom Onset in Schizophrenia[25]	Retrospective assessment to date onset
Interview for the Retrospective Assessment of the Onset of Schizophrenia (IRAOS)[26]	Dates onset of the first episode of schizophrenia
Drug Attitude Inventory[27–29]	A measure of subjective response that may be useful to predict adherence to medication
Social Functioning Scale[30]	Assesses effectiveness of family interventions
Experience of Caregiving Inventory[31]	Assesses family burden

Intelligence and cognitive abilities

Intelligence testing may only be performed by psychologists. Many neuropsychological instruments are also restricted. Therefore, consultation with a qualified practitioner should be undertaken regarding these types of assessments.

References

1. Kay SR, Opler LA, Spitzer RL, et al. SCID-PANSS: two-tier diagnostic system for psychotic disorders. Compr Psychiatry 1991; **32**(4):355–61.
2. Kay SR, Opler LA, Lindenmayer JP. The Positive and Negative Syndrome Scale (PANSS): rationale and standardisation. Br J Psychiatry Suppl 1989; **7**:59–67.
3. Overall J, Gorham D. The Brief Psychiatric Rating Scale: Recent developments in ascertainment and scaling. Psychopharmacol Bull 1988; **24**:97–99.
4. Addington D, Addington J, Maticka-Tyndale E. Assessing depression in schizophrenia: the Calgary Depression Scale. Br J Psychiatry Suppl 1993; **22**:39–44.
5. Addington D, Addington J, Maticka-Tyndale E. Specificity of the Calgary Depression Scale for schizophrenics. Schizophr Res 1994; **11**(3):239–44.
6. Beck AT, Rush AJ, Shaw BF, Emery G. *Cognitive Therapy of Depression*. New York: Guilford Press; 1979.
7. Beck AT, Beamesderfer A. Assessment of depression: the depression inventory. Mod Probl Pharmacopsychiatry 1974; **7**:151–69.
8. Beck AT, Weissman A, Lester D, Trexler L. The measurement of pessimism: the hopelessness scale. J Consult Clin Psychol 1974; **42**(6):861–5.
9. Andreasen NC. Methods for assessing positive and negative symptoms. Mod Probl Pharmacopsychiatry 1990; **24**:73–88.
10. Young RC, Biggs JT, Ziegler VE, Meyer DA. A rating scale for mania: reliability, validity and sensitivity. Br J Psychiatry 1978; **133**:429–35.
11. Altman EG, Hedeker DR, Janicak PG, et al. The Clinician-Administered Rating Scale for Mania (CARS-M): development, reliability, and validity. Biol Psychiatry 1994; **36**(2):124–34.
12. Ehmann TS, Higgs E, Smith GN, et al. Routine assessment of patient progress: a multiformat, change-sensitive nurses' instrument for assessing psychotic inpatients. Compr Psychiatry 1995; **36**(4):289–95.

13. Ehmann TS, Holliday SG, MacEwan GW, Smith GN. Multidimensional assessment of psychosis: A factor-analytic validation study of the routine assessment of patient progress. Compr Psychiatry 2001; **42**(1):32–38.

14. Honigfeld G, Gillis RD, Klett CJ. NOSIE-30: a treatment-sensitive ward behavior scale. Psychol Rep 1966; **19**(1):180–2.

15. American Psychiatric Association (APA). *Diagnostic and Statistical Manual of Mental Disorders* (4th edn). Washington, DC: American Psychiatric Association; 1994.

16. Guy W. ECDEU Assessment manual for psychopharmacology, revised. In: *U.S Department of Health, Education and Welfare publication 76–338.* Rockville, MD: National Institute of Mental Health; 1976.

17. Lehman AF. Measures of quality of life among persons with severe and persistent mental disorders. Soc Psychiatry Psychiatr Epidemiol 1996; **31**(2):78–88.

18. Ware J. The MOS 36-item short form health survey (SF-36). In: Sederer L, Dickey B (eds). *Outcomes Assessment in Clinical Practice.* Baltimore: Williams & Wilkins; 1996.

19. Goodman SH, Sewell DR, Cooley EL, Leavitt N. Assessing levels of adaptive functioning: the Role Functioning Scale. Community Ment Health J 1993; **29**:119–131.

20. Parker G, Rosen A, Emdur N, Hadzi-Pavlov D. The Life Skills Profile: psychometric properties of a measure assessing function and disability in schizophrenia. Acta Psychiatr Scand 1991; **83**(2):145–52.

21. Rosen A, Hadzi-Pavlovic D, Parker G. The life skills profile: a measure assessing function and disability in schizophrenia. Schizophr Bull 1989; **15**(2):325–37.

22. Houston D, Williams SL, Bloomer J, Mann WC. The Bay Area Functional Performance Evaluation: development and standardization. Am J Occup Ther 1989; **43**(3):170–83.

23. Monk TH, Flaherty JF, Frank E, et al. The Social Rhythm Metric. An instrument to quantify the daily rhythms of life. J Nerv Ment Dis 1990; **178**(2):120–6.

24. van Os J, Altamura AC, Bobes J, et al. 2–COM: an instrument to facilitate patient-professional communication in routine clinical practice. Acta Psychiatr Scand 2002; **106**(6):446–52.

25. Perkins DO, Leserman J, Jarskog LF, et al. Characterizing and dating the onset of symptoms in psychotic illness: the Symptom Onset in Schizophrenia (SOS) inventory. Schizophr Res 2000; **44**(1):1–10.

26. Hafner H, Riecher-Rossler A, Hambrecht M, et al. IRAOS: an instrument for the assessment of onset and early course of schizophrenia. Schizophr Res 1992; **6**(3):209–23.

27. Awad AG, Voruganti LN, Heslegrave RJ, Hogan TP. Assessment of the patient's subjective experience in acute neuroleptic treatment: implications for compliance and outcome. Int Clin Psychopharmacol 1996; **11**(Suppl 2):55–9.

28. Awad AG, Hogan TP, Voruganti LN, Heslegrave RJ. Patients' subjective experiences on antipsychotic medications: implications for outcome and quality of life. Int Clin Psychopharmacol 1995; **10**(Suppl 3):123–32.

29. Hogan TP, Awad AG. Subjective response to neuroleptics and outcome in schizophrenia: a re-examination comparing two measures. Psychol Med 1992; **22**(2):347–52.

30. Birchwood M, Smith J, Cochrane R, et al. The Social Functioning Scale. The development and validation of a new scale of social adjustment for use in family intervention programmes with schizophrenic patients. Br J Psychiatry 1990; **157**:853–9.

31. Szmukler GI, Burgess P, Herrman H, et al. Caring for relatives with serious mental illness: the development of the Experience of Caregiving Inventory. Soc Psychiatry Psychiatr Epidemiol 1996; **31**(3–4):137–48.

10

A Compendium of Early Psychosis Resources

Tom Ehmann and Laura Hanson

The following resources may help readers find additional information useful to developing and delivering educational and clinical services. The list is not comprehensive and resources are growing at a rapid rate. Nevertheless, this sampling provides a fairly thorough overview of the main sources available in English at this time. Many of the listed websites provide excellent lists of links to other sites concerning early psychosis.

Books

Recognition and Management of Early Psychosis: A Preventative Approach
McGorr PD, Jackson HJ, Perris C (editors)
1999, Cambridge University Press.

Early Intervention in Psychosis: A Guide to Concepts, Evidence and Interventions
Birchwood M, Fowler D, Jackson C (editors)
2000, John Wiley: Chichester, UK.

First Episode Psychosis
Aitchison KJ, Meehan K, Murray RM
1999, Martin Dunitz: London.

Implementing Early Intervention in Psychosis: A Guide to Establishing Early Psychosis Services
Edwards J, McGorry PD
2002, Martin Dunitz: London.

The Early Stages of Schizophrenia
Zipursky RB, Schulz S (editors)
2002, American Psychiatric Publishing: Washington, DC.

Systematic Treatment of Persistent Psychosis: A Psychological Approach to Facilitating Recovery in Young People with First Episode Psychosis
Herrmann-Doig T, Maude D, Edwards J
2003, Martin Dunitz: London.

Psychological Interventions in Early Psychosis: A Practical Treatment Handbook
Gleeson J, McGorry PD (editors)
2004, John Wiley: Chichester, UK.

Guidelines, manuals, and videos

Early Psychosis Prevention and Intervention Centre (EPPIC), Australia
http://www.eppic.org.au/
The Australian Clinical Guidelines for Early Psychosis (1999/2000).
Case Management in Early Psychosis: A Handbook.
Prolonged Recovery Package. *Prolonged Recovery in Early Psychosis: A Treatment Manual, and The Next Step* video (package only, not sold separately).

Cannabis and Psychosis: An Early Psychosis Treatment Manual.
Cognitively Oriented Psychotherapy for First Episode Psychosis (COPE): A Practitioner's Manual.
The Early Psychosis Training Pack (10 Modules).
Manual for Psychoeducation in Early Psychosis
Manual for Working with Families in Early Psychosis.
Community video—*A Stitch in Time: Psychosis . . . Get Help Early.*
Video for general practitioners—*A Stitch in Time: Psychosis . . . Get Help Early*
Video for mental health professionals—*Sally's Story.*
Video—*The Next Step Part of the Prolonged Recovery Package.*
Video—*Back to Reality Cannabis and Psychosis: An Early Psychosis Video.*
Video—*Getting Real.*

Canadian Schizophrenia Society

http://www.schizophrenia.ca/
High school curriculum resource: *Reaching Out: The Need For Early Treatment.*
Video for school and community health: *Reaching Out.*
Video for physicians and mental health Professionals: *Reaching Out.*

Sainsbury Centre for Mental Health, UK

http://www.scmh.org.uk/
A Window of Opportunity—A Practical Guide for Developing Early Intervention in Psychosis Services (2003).

Initiative to Reduce the Impact of Schizophrenia (IRIS), UK

http://www.iris-initiative.org.uk/guidelines.htm
Clinical guidelines and service frameworks.

Canadian Mental Health Association

http://www.cmha.ca/english/intrvent/
Early psychosis parent video—*One Day at a Time.*

Additional websites for early psychosis projects and/or educational materials

International Early Psychosis Association (IEPA) Melbourne, Australia
http://www.iepa.org.au

British Columbia Schizophrenia Society (BCSS), Canada
http://www.bcss.org

European Early Prediction of Psychosis Study
http://www.epos5.org/

The Prevention and Early Intervention Program for Psychoses (PEPP)
London Health Sciences Centre/University of Western Ontario, Ontario, Canada
http://www.pepp.ca

The Early Psychosis Initiative (EPI) Mental Health Evaluation and Community Consultation Unit, British Columbia, Canada
http://www.mheccu.ubc.ca/

Singapore Early Psychosis Program (EPIP)
http://www.epip.org.sg/

Early Psychosis Intervention (EPI) Program, Fraser South, British Columbia, Canada
http://www.psychosissucks.ca

TIPS—An Early Intervention Program for Psychosis, Norway
http://www.tips-info.com

Early Psychosis Program University of Calgary/ Foothills Hospital, Alberta, Canada
http://www.ucalgary.ca/cdss/epp

National Early Psychosis Project (NEPP), Melbourne, Australia
http://ariel.ucs.unimelb.edu.au/~nepp

Helping Overcome Psychosis Early (HOPE), Vancouver/Richmond EPI Demonstration Project, British Columbia, Canada
http://www.hope.vancouver.bc.ca

Swiss Early Psychosis Project (SWEPP), Switzerland
http://www.rehab-infoweb.net/swepp/

Rethink—National Schizophrenia Fellowship
http://www.rethink.org/

World Fellowship for Schizophrenia and Allied Disorders
http://www.world-schizophrenia.org/

SANE
http://www.sane.org.uk/

New Zealand Mental Health Commission
http://www.mhc.govt.nz/

For a list of some non-English sites, see:
http://www.debuterendepsykose.fa.dk/links.htm

Section II Systems of Care Around the World

11

Early Intervention in Psychosis in the UK: A Radical Plan for Nationwide Service Reform

Jenny Bywaters, Max Birchwood, David Shiers, Jo Smith, and Eric Davis

The case for radical service reform

The British government has recently embarked upon a radical plan for nationwide reform of its mental health services, a key feature of which is the implementation of 50 early intervention services by December 2004. The aim is that by that time, every young person with a first episode of psychosis will receive the early and intensive support they need from a specialist team, which will continue to help them through the first three years of their illness.[1] By 31 March 2004, 48 early intervention teams were in place. Beginning with the UK Northwick Park Study of First Episodes of Schizophrenia in 1986,[2] a number of studies have demonstrated the frequently long interval between onset of psychosis and treatment, averaging approximately a year.[3] This period of untreated psychosis is frequently associated with severe behavioral disturbance, sometimes including harm to self or others, and family difficulties.[2] This in itself is enough to justify a government focus on this group of young people with a major mental illness.

However, the scientific rationale for earlier intervention is overwhelming. A great deal is now known about the long-term trajectories of psychosis and their biological and psychosocial influences. Delay in first treatment is robustly linked to poor early outcome,[3] and long-term follow-up studies show clearly that the outcome at 2/3 years strongly predicts outcome 20 years later,[4] and that disability 'plateaus' by this time: the early phase is indeed a 'critical period'.[5] Not only is the potential human benefit enormous, but it has been calculated that the annual cost of schizophrenia in England is £2.6 billion,[6] so there is also a health economic case for pursuing policies which may reduce the lifetime costs of care. Perhaps the more powerful case for the UK service reform has, however, come from consumers of mental healthcare.

RETHINK (formerly known as the National Schizophrenia Fellowship, a campaigning UK mental health charity), launched their campaign 'Reaching People Early' in 2002, in order to bring to wider attention the poor state of services for the young severely mentally ill.[7] They described a catalogue of concerns. They highlight the delay of 12 months between the onset of the positive symptoms and first treatment;[3] their members described how some of this delay occurs due to problems at the interface of primary and secondary care, including the lack of an 'assertive' response when the diagnosis is first raised. Long delays increase the chance of use of the Mental Health Act (which is high at the first episode, over one half in many settings),[8] and its use breeds service disengagement and treatment reluctance. In many routine service settings over 50% are lost to services within 12 months.[9] Early use of the Mental Health Act increases the likelihood of its further use, with young black males being particularly at risk.[10] Suicide remains high and young people in the early phase are particularly at risk.[1] RETHINK point out that the incidence of schizophrenia begins to rise during the 15–18 age range and does not respect the often impermeable service boundaries between child and adolescent mental health services (CAMHS) and adult services. Young people surveyed by RETHINK found services stigmatizing, therapeutically pessimistic, and youth insensitive (access to employment and training are high on their priorities). They invite us to consider: 'Would we be happy with our children receiving care from our services? My impression is that many mental health professionals are also dissatisfied with the current quality of care but provide a caring and professional service within the constraints that service pressure and resources allow. These are reasons enough to 'rethink' our services to the young severely mentally ill. Imagine the uproar if, instead of early psychosis, these observations were made about youth cancer services!'

This combination of consumer dissatisfaction and failure to provide evidence-based care at such a critical period in the evolution of the illness has brought about the zeitgeist in the UK that paved the way for radical service reform, which we now consider.

The National Service Framework for mental health

The specific proposal for 50 early intervention services built upon earlier developments in mental health policy which had been set out in the *National Service Framework for Mental Health* (NSF), published in 1999.[11] Its intention is to set national standards based on the best available evidence, supported by new investment of resources and backed by new legislation suited to

Table 11.1 The National Service Framework (NSF) standards
1. Mental health promotion and reduction of stigma
2 and 3. Primary care and access to services
4 and 5. Effective services for people with severe mental illness
6. Caring for carers
7. Suicide prevention

modern patterns of service delivery. It describes the kind of services that will be needed to meet the standards, and sets target dates for achieving milestones on the way to meeting all the standards over a 10 year period (see Table 11.1).

All these standards are relevant to the issue of first episode psychosis. Raising awareness of mental health issues through health promotion programs and reducing the stigma surrounding mental health increases the chance of early signs of illness being recognized, and of young people and their families being willing to approach services for help. Improvements in primary care will mean that general practitioners (GPs) are more likely to refer possible cases early for expert assessment, rather than adopting a policy of 'wait and see' until the severity of symptoms makes the diagnosis unmistakable, thereby prolonging the duration of untreated psychosis. Effective services for those with severe illness are obviously vital; their families or other carers need support, and these young people are a vulnerable group for suicide, which may be prevented by appropriate early intervention with intensive and sustained support. In general terms, the practice of early intervention fits well with these seven national standards.

Awareness of this evidence and the poor state of services for the young severely mentally ill was first promoted in England by the efforts of the Initiative to Reduce the Impact of Schizophrenia (IRIS) group formed in the West Midlands, UK in

1994.[12] Members of the IRIS group included Professor Max Birchwood, who developed the UK's first early intervention service in Birmingham in 1989,[13] Dr Fiona MacMillan, one of the researchers involved in the Northwick Park study, Dr David Shiers, a GP and carer whose daughter developed schizophrenia, the National Schizophrenia Fellowship (now called RETHINK), and other clinicians and service users, who shared a vision of how services should be improved for young people with schizophrenia. This group also included Professor Antony Sheehan, at that time the West Midlands' regional mental health head, but now Director of Care Services in the Department of Health. The IRIS group made presentations all over England, and organized two major conferences at which international experts in early psychosis presented their work. Among others, Professor Patrick McGorry described the work of the Melbourne Early Psychosis Prevention and Intervention Centre (EPPIC) service, and the impact of the international network on opinion in the UK was very significant in securing the inclusion of early psychosis services in the National Service Framework for significant investment.

Implementation of the NSF has been carried forward in a number of ways. The document itself highlighted specific services as examples of good practice from which others could learn. The government also established a 'Beacon' award program, under which good services were recognized as standards of excellence, and awarded additional funds to support teaching programs for visiting practitioners. The Early Intervention Service in Birmingham was awarded Beacon status under this scheme, and has received over 500 visitors through its 'site visit' programs, organised within the Beacon program.

The NHS Plan

The next important step forward was taken in July 2000, when the government published *The NHS Plan*, setting out its intentions for the next three years.[1] Much of the plan concerned structural and cultural changes for services as a whole, but it identified three clinical priorities: coronary heart disease, cancer, and mental health. The government announced in the plan additional annual funds of over £300 million by 2003/2004 to 'fast-forward' the National Service Framework for Mental Health. Commitments on early intervention became more specific. The plan stated:

- Fifty early intervention teams will be established over the next three years to provide treatment and active support in the community to these young people and their families.
- By 2004 all young people with a first episode of psychosis, such as schizophrenia, will receive the early and intensive support they need. This will benefit 7500 young people each year.

There are a number of models for delivering early intervention, ranging from the 'specialized services' model adopted in the NHS plan to the 'mainstream services' model in which appropriate interventions are delivered by staff entirely integrated within mainstream psychiatric services, and various alternatives in between.

The specialized team approach has a number of advantages, which are described by Initiative to Reduce the Impact of Schizophrenia (IRIS) as follows:[12]

Staff expertise and team coherence are encouraged by the consistent experience of managing similar clients and the informal supervision and sharing of ideas that occur when a team is housed on one site; the creation of a concrete 'service' allows easy identification of the service by the referrers (who might include other clients and families): it is possible to create a separate point of entry for direct referrals, thus increasing ease of referral; the existence of a concrete team with a physical location allows the creation of an actual youth-friendly space which may promote client engagement.

An additional advantage, from the government's perspective, is that the creation of separate and identifiable teams is a clear target, the delivery of which is easily monitored.

NHS mapping

When the NHS plan was published, there was no national picture of what services were available where. During the summer of 2000, a national mapping exercise was undertaken, which is now updated annually.[14] As part of this process the following definition of early intervention was issued: 'Early intervention in psychosis services provide quick diagnosis of the first onset of a psychotic disorder and appropriate treatment including intensive support in the early years. Best practice is early treatment with low dose neuroleptics in addition to cognitive behavioral therapy and psychosocial interventions including family work.'

Sixteen teams were identified as meeting basic requirements, which was felt to be very encouraging, given how recently early intervention had become official NHS policy. However, no information was collected on the numbers of staff or the number of young people covered, so it is likely that these teams fell short of full fidelity to the ideal model.

Mental Health Policy Implementation Guide

In March 2001, the Department of Health published more detailed guidance for local services, the *Mental Health Policy Implementation Guide* (MHPIG), which includes a model service specification for early intervention in psychosis.[15] This drew extensively on the advice of the IRIS group, and reflects the community assertive outreach model developed by the Birmingham Early Intervention Service. The MHPIG sets out *who* the early intervention service is for, *what* it is intended to achieve, and what it does; it outlines *management and operational procedures*; and gives refer-

ences to the evidence. The government investment in new services for early psychosis has been welcomed by consumer organizations in the UK (but not by all professionals).[16] The MHPIG is intended to address the problems raised by RETHINK; it states, for example, that a case manager is to be provided and remain with each case of actual or possible psychosis (with a staff: client ratio of 1:12). The Government has set targets for reducing duration of untreated psychosis (DUP) to a median of three months, with no one waiting more than six months, and for reducing use of the Mental Health Act by 50%. 'Social inclusion' of service users is a major priority of these new services, setting an ambitious target of achieving employment and training on a par with those of their peers in the same district. The new services will also provide an important opportunity to address key research questions and the research infrastructure provided by the UK's new National Institute for Mental Health in England (NIMHE) will provide a unique opportunity to conduct major large-scale research in this area.

In June 2002, these aspirations for the new services were crystallized and restated in the 'Newcastle Declaration'. This joint declaration by consumers, professionals, and government, sets basic standards for services, social inclusion, stigma, and illness outcome (see www.rethink.org.uk/newcastledeclaration). In September 2002, this was developed further with the International Early Psychosis Association (IEPA) and more recently with the World Health Organization (WHO). On 19 May 2004 at the NIMHE/Rethink National Early Intervention Conference in Bristol, UK, the Newcastle Early Psychosis Declaration was released as an International Consensus Statement about Early Intervention and Recovery for Young People with Early Psychosis, jointly issued by the WHO and the IEPA.

Planning locations and catchment populations

The NHS Plan target of 50 services for a population of 50 million people assumes an average catchment population for each service of 1 million. It is no coincidence that the EPPIC service in Melbourne serves a population of this size, and that the Birmingham Early Intervention Service will soon extend its coverage to include the whole city (population approx. 1.1 m.) The Nottingham Centre of the Determinants of Severe Mental Illness and Disability (DOSMD) study,[17] found 24 new cases/100 000/year of 'broad' diagnosis schizophrenia. Therefore, given that about 85% of these cases will be in the age group 14–35 years, this leads to a predicted 7500 new cases per annum in England in the target age band for the new early intervention services. Each of the teams that comprise a service will manage about 150 new cases. They will provide support for about three years, giving a total caseload of around 450 per service. However, these are only average figures. The incidence of first episode psychosis varies across the country, with higher rates in areas of social deprivation. It is important, therefore, that the planning of the new teams takes this into account. On this basis, the number of teams required in each Strategic Health Authority (SHA) has been calculated.

This information has been made available to the SHAs and their local implementation teams to facilitate planning of service development.

Service delivery: potential obstacles and solutions

Service delivery reform is a hugely challenging agenda for local services, and mental health professionals are by no means unanimous in accepting the need for it. The national strategy is to continue to actively disseminate the evidence, both scientific- and consumer-based, and to put forward the argument that, even if the long-term benefits of early intervention are controversial, there is an overwhelming case for intervening early to prevent the problems that are known to occur in the early phase of psychosis. After all, intensive mental health services for the severely mentally ill (e.g. Assertive Community Treatment (ACT), rehabilitation) kick in far too late, long after the horse has bolted: we need to ensure that our best treatments and service configurations are available early, when the long-term trajectories and disabilities develop.[17]

Through its national research and development program, the Department of Health has commissioned an independent expert review of the evidence, and agreed that the national program of early intervention should be the subject of long-term evaluation.

Some critics are concerned about the potential fragmentation of services with the development of the separate teams specified in the NHS Plan, which includes assertive outreach teams and crisis resolution/home treatment teams, as well as early intervention teams. The Department of Health is responding to this genuine concern by amplifying the *Mental Health Policy Implementation Guide* (MHPIG), making it clearer how the various types of specialist teams work together as a whole system, with community mental health teams being at its heart.

Other practitioners are concerned about how the new teams will interface with child and adolescent mental health services (CAMHS). A national working group has been established on early intervention and CAMHS threshold issues, which also includes representation from the CAMHS section of the Royal College of Psychiatrists. This group took the lead in the organization of a conference in September 2002, which brought together the key players from each of the 50 sites where early intervention services were developing, including, crucially, psychiatrists treating both adults *and* adolescents, so that these issues could be explored. One outcome of this conference was the establishment of an early intervention network which will enable sharing of good practice and mutual support in resolving areas of difficulty.

Another concern is that there may not be enough skilled staff to deliver all the new services outlined in the National Service Framework and the NHS Plan. The Department of Health has established a Mental Health Care Group Workforce Team to consider and plan for the recruitment, training, and retention of the skilled staff who will be needed. In Birmingham, the Birmingham Early Intervention Service and the mental health charity, RETHINK, have developed a joint scheme enabling the employment and training of non-professional case managers, including service users themselves, to work initially under the supervision of conventionally trained staff. A training and placement program is underway to support this and to pave the way for a large-scale program.

Finally, there remains the challenge of sustaining support for this radical reform program and, in particular, of trying to ensure that funding intended for mental health is not diverted elsewhere. In 2002/2003, the government earmarked £75 million of the NHS allocation specifically for new service developments in mental health (assertive outreach, crisis resolution, and early intervention teams). In subsequent years, funding intended for mental health has been included in general NHS allocations. The main lever is not ring-fencing of funds, but performance management of targets.

Conclusions

The national reforms of services for the young severely mentally ill are radical, create major challenges for implementation, and, when completed, will totally transform the consumer experience of services. They will set the stage for research to determine *which kind* of early intervention is appropriate for achieving the outcomes that are possible with our current and developing range of treatments.[17] It is important to emphasize that the early intervention reforms described in this chapter were not driven by the randomized controlled trial. They arose out of consumer involve-

ment in service reform and a recognition that there is a failure to engage service users in a sustained way in current service structures, at what is a critical phase in the development of the illness. Service engagement and consumer satisfaction are key outcomes of the UK service reforms in early psychosis.

References

1. Department of Health (DoH). *The NHS Plan.* London: DoH; 2000
2. Johnstone EC, Crow TJ, Johnson AL, MacMillan JF. The Northwick Park Study of First Episodes of Schizophrenia 1. Presentation of the illness and problems relating to admission. Br J Psychiatry 1986; **148:**115–20.
3. Norman RM, Malla AK. Duration of untreated psychosis: a critical examination of the concept and its importance. Psychol Med 2001; **31:**381–400.
4. Harrison G, Hopper K, Craig T, et al. Recovery from psychotic illness: a 15- and 25-year international follow-up study. Br J Psychiatry 2001; **178:** 506–17.
5. Birchwood M, McGorry P, Jackson H. Early intervention in schizophrenia. Br J Psychiatry 1997; **170:**2–5.
6. Knapp M. Costs of schizophrenia. Br J Psychiatry 1997; **171:**509–18.
7. RETHINK. Reaching people early (www.rethink.org/reachingpeopleearly) 2002.
8. Burnett R, Mallett R, Bhugra D, et al. The first contact of patients with schizophrenia with psychiatric services: social factors and pathways to care in a multi-ethnic population. Psychol Med 1999; **29:**475–83.
9. McGovern D, Hemmings P, Cope R. Long-term follow-up of young Afro-Caribbean Britons and White Britons with a 1st admission diagnosis of schizophrenia. Soc Psychiatry Psychiatr Epidemiol 1994; **29:**8–19.
10. Harrison G. Ethnic minorities and the Mental Health Act. Br J Psychiatry 2002; **180:**198–9.
11. Department of Health (DoH). *A National Service Framework for Mental Health.* London: DoH; 1999.
12. Initiative to Reduce the Impact of Schizophrenia. Early intervention in psychosis: clinical guidelines and service frameworks; 2000. Available at: www.iris-initiative.org.uk

13. Spencer E, Birchwood M, McGovern D. Management of first episode psychosis. *Advances in Psychiatric Treatment* 2001; **7:**133–40.

14. Barnes D, Dyer W, Glover G. *Mental Health Service Provision for Working Age Adults in England.* Centre for Public Mental Health, University of Durham; 2000, unpublished. Available at: www.dur.ac.uk/service.mapping

15. Department of Health (DoH). *Mental Health Policy Implementation Guide* (MHPIG). www.doh.gov.uk/mentalhealth/impementationguide.htm London: DoH; 2001.

16. Pelosi AJ, Birchwood M. Is early intervention for psychosis a waste of valuable resources? Br J Psychiatry 2003; **182:**196–8.

17. Harrison G, Croudcae T, et al. Predicting the long-term outcome of schizophrenia. Psychol Med 1996; **26:**697–705

12

Implementing Treatment for Early Psychosis: Evolution from Specialist to Generalist Services in Australia

John Gleeson, Swagata Bapat, Kerryn Pennell, Helen Krstev, Annemarie Wright, Steve Haines, and Patrick D McGorry

Introduction

This chapter outlines the development of a specialist, statewide, early psychosis consultation and training service which evolved from the clinical and research infrastructure of the Early Psychosis Prevention and Intervention Centre (EPPIC), based in Melbourne in the state of Victoria, Australia.[1] Victoria, situated on the tip of the Australian east coast, extends across 227 600 square kilometers, which is roughly the size of the British Isles, and has a total population of approximately 5 million people. According to the Australian Bureau of Statistics, 70% of Victoria's population is based in Melbourne, the state's capital.[2]

The Victoria EPPIC Statewide Services provide a case example of how the principles and practice of a specialist mental health program can be disseminated, especially in a sparsely populated country like Australia. Since its establishment in 1995, the work of EPPIC Statewide Services has progressed in its model of training and consultation. This can roughly be divided into two phases, both of which were influenced by the broader national and state policy and reform context. In addition to funding support, this progression was predicated upon the presence of a mature and evolving clinical and research infrastructure at EPPIC.[3]

EPPIC: the essential context for the statewide initiative

EPPIC commenced operation in 1992.[1] Nested within a broader youth mental health service,[4] EPPIC continues to provide a separate stream of treatment, comprising a comprehensive service for adolescents, young adults, and their families experiencing the first onset of a psychotic illness. EPPIC aims to address early detection, prevent secondary morbidity, and maintain social and occupational functioning during the early 'critical period'.[5] Its service area includes a population of approximately 850 000 people in the western area of Melbourne, an area served by two public psychiatric hospitals and five adult community mental health centres. The average number of new cases accepted into the service has been 260 with a standing caseload of approximately 340 as of June 2004.

The core components of the EPPIC program have been detailed elsewhere,[6] but, in brief, include a mobile community-based assessment and treatment team, an outpatient case-management program, a group program, a family worker, and an acute 15 bed inpatient unit. Additional specialist review and treatment options for patients at risk for treatment resistance also form a core of the service.[7] Recent initiatives also include the development of specific treatment pathways for mania,[8] and intensive relapse prevention for patients who reach remission.[9]

Other specialist activities have addressed liaison with general practitioners (GPs), comorbid substance abuse (especially cannabis abuse), vocational rehabilitation, and suicide prevention.[10] Service evaluation has been integral to the program, consistent with a philosophy of combining research and clinical practice.[11] However, most of the state of Victoria is not serviced by specialist first episode clinical programs—one solution was for EPPIC to take a lead role in providing support to the broader generalist mental health service structure. The evolution of this model needs to be understood alongside the broader national policy framework and the process of reform which was initiated in the early 1990s within Victoria.

The national policy context: the National Mental Health Strategy and early psychosis

The National Mental Health Strategy was launched in 1992 as a joint initiative of the federal, five state, and two territory governments.[12] The strategy set policy directions and priorities for mental health until mid 1998. The main thrust of the strategy included an expansion of the community-based, case-management sector of mental health services and reduced reliance on inpatient services.

Early intervention was identified as a fundamental strategy, with AU$3 million allocated for special projects in the area of early intervention in mental health. The National Early Psychosis Project, described below, was funded under this program.

The Second National Mental Health Plan (NMHP) was subsequently formulated to cover the period 1998–2003.[13] The second plan focused on promoting mental health, reducing the incidence and prevalence of mental disorders, and addressing associated disability. Priority areas for reform were mental health promotion and illness prevention, the development of partnerships in

service reform, and ensuring the quality and effectiveness of service delivery. As part of the plan, state and territory governments accepted a range of responsibilities including the organization and funding of specialized public mental health initiatives, and the support of mental health research and evaluation. A further iteration of the plan (2003–2008) was endorsed by all Australian Health Ministers in July 2003.[14] Drawing upon the evaluation of the second NMHP and broad consultations within the mental health sector and the community, the NMHP 2003–2008 defined four key themes:

1. Promoting mental health and preventing mental health problems and mental illness
2. Increasing service responsiveness
3. Strengthening quality
4. Fostering research, innovation, and sustainability.

The National Early Psychosis Project

The National Early Psychosis Project (NEPP) (1996–1998) was funded by the Commonwealth, state and territory governments,[15] and was conducted under the auspices of EPPIC Statewide Services. The project had four core areas: development and promotion of best practice; service and policy development; professional education and training; and information dissemination. In addition, the NEPP also initiated a number of national projects such as development of an early psychosis resource centre, production of a series of newsletters, and development of the *Australian Clinical Guidelines for Early Psychosis*.[16] Increased awareness of issues related to early psychosis and early intervention, and the professional training provided by the project, were seen as major achievements.[15]

Victoria's mental health services and the establishment of statewide programs

Following a landmark 1994 report, *Victoria's Mental Health Service: The Framework for Service Delivery*,[17] Victoria's government released a policy statement in 1996 that established the current structure of area mental health services in Victoria.[18] Changes flowing from the initial 1994 report led to the expansion of community-based services, and the relocation of stand-alone psychiatric hospitals into community-based services or services co-located with general hospitals. Other changes included the introduction of consistent approaches to case management across the state. A separate policy statement addressed the particular mental health needs of children and adolescents.[19]

The framework defined 22 Area Mental Health Services throughout Victoria. Each service had the elements necessary to respond to the needs of people with mental illness in their catchment area, but were supplemented by a range of statewide services dealing with specialized issues, such as forensic, transcultural, and postnatal psychiatry; the mental health needs of Aborigines and patients with HIV/AIDS or brain trauma; and neuropsychiatry.

The framework defined three specific objectives for EPPIC Statewide Service:

1. To undertake and evaluate early psychosis projects in two mental health service areas with a view to subsequent statewide implementation
2. To develop and implement a model of statewide secondary consultation to staff in area mental health services
3. To produce a range of resources to assist clinicians working with people experiencing early onset psychosis.

The development of consultation and training models

Since 1995, EPPIC Statewide Services have been funded by the Mental Health Branch (MHB) of the Victorian Department of Human Services (DHS). The first phase of the service included the development and delivery of a training program, a primary and secondary consultation service, and a number of intensive projects within defined areas of the state.

Consultation

EPPIC Statewide Services initially provided primary, secondary, and tertiary consultation on issues related to early psychosis. Secondary consultation involved the provision of clinical advice and support to clinical teams within mental health services across Victoria.[20,21] Services included second opinions on diagnosis or management (a form of primary consultation), case discussion, and clinical consultation. Secondary consultation was designed to assist mental health professionals develop skills and knowledge. This was of particular benefit to rural and remote mental health workers who had difficulty in accessing this specialized knowledge locally. Video conferencing was used frequently to improve access in rural areas.[22] Since the establishment of the service 48 secondary consultations have been provided to Victoria's mental health services, although demand has lessened with the commencement of the early intervention worker initiative, described below.

Tertiary consultation as undertaken by EPPIC Statewide Services refers to strategies provided to mental health agencies to assist them in developing appropriate and responsive services for young people with emergent psychosis.[20] Support for community mental health agencies in Victoria was facilitated by intensive work with discrete regional sectors in a model of service delivery known as 'early psychosis projects'. A total of six early psychosis projects were completed, with three urban and three rural Area Mental Health Services, with the final project completed in June 2002. EPPIC Statewide Services worked intensively with each of the six Area Mental Health Services for a minimum period of six months, in order to develop structures focused on the needs of young people with early psychosis. Follow-up was provided where possible via participation in ongoing local early psychosis reference groups. Early psychosis projects aimed to involve all components of the local clinical program, including child and adolescent mental health service, non-government organizations, family/carer groups, youth sector-specific groups, and local GPs. The specific aims of each project reflected local priorities and resources, but usually included:

- Ensuring early identification and treatment of the primary symptoms of psychotic illness by improving access to specialized services and reducing delays in initial treatment[23,24]
- Reducing secondary morbidity in the post-psychotic phase of illness[25]
- Reducing disruption in social and vocational functioning and in psychosocial development in the critical early years following onset of illness[5]
- Reducing the burden for carers and promoting well-being among family members.[26]

Steering groups were formed which included senior management from the Area Mental Health Service and EPPIC Statewide Services. A reference group consisting of interested workers was convened to address the day-to-day issues of the project and define its aims and key activities. Responsibility for activities was devolved to working parties, commonly addressing issues such as:

1. Professional education and training
2. Local clinical guidelines for early psychosis
3. Provision of specialized family services
4. Development of group-based interventions[27]
5. Development of local education campaigns to reduce delays in treatment.

Box 12.1 shows an example of an early psychosis project.

Funding was provided by the Mental Health Branch of the DHS to evaluate early psychosis projects as a model of service delivery. This involved mapping the symptomatic and functional domains, over a 15 month period, of all young people who presented with psychosis to the Northern and Central East Area Mental Health Services (in metropolitan Melbourne) in 1997, before and after the projects were implemented.[28]

Box 12.1 An early psychosis project

An urban early psychosis project was undertaken in the Northern Area Mental Health Service, involving the Child and Adolescent Mental Health Service, the North East Alliance for the Mentally Ill (a psychiatric disability service), and the Richmond Fellowship. A series of working parties was established. Some of the activities undertaken within the project included:

- A recovery phase psychoeducation group for young people with early psychosis
- Two groups for families and carers including an initial psychoeducation group and an ongoing support group
- Development of a local clinicians' guide
- A series of resource materials, including pamphlets and posters, developed to raise awareness amongst general practitioners and primary healthcare providers regarding the early warning signs of psychosis in young people
- A resources kit for carers
- A regular supervision group for case management staff focused on cognitively orientated psychotherapy for the recovery phase, facilitated by an experienced cognitive therapist from EPPIC.

Training

Since its inception, training and skill development for mental health workers in Victoria has been provided by EPPIC Statewide Services through workshops, conferences, a structured site visit service, and a graduate diploma. EPPIC Statewide Services continue to provide a yearly calendar of one day workshops at the EPPIC campus. In 2003, for example, 201 clinicians attended workshops on topics including introduction to early psychosis, acute phase assessment and treatment, recovery in early psychosis, prolonged recovery, family work, cannabis and early psychosis, and psychological interventions in early psychosis.

However, from 2002 training has increasingly been provided on-site and tailored to specific services. Figure 12.1 shows the number of clinicians from rural and metropolitan mental health services who attended these center-based workshops between 2001 and the end of 2003, and the number of clinicians from rural and metropolitan services who accessed training provided by EPPIC Statewide Services at their place of work. This highlights the increasing accessibility of training over this period, especially with respect to rural services.

Access has also been maximized by providing a distance education program. The Graduate Diploma in Mental Health Sciences (Young People's Mental Health) is a significant educational program developed and implemented by EPPIC Statewide Services. This two year postgraduate course is offered via distance education by the Department of Psychiatry at the University of Melbourne and EPPIC Statewide Services. Spanning the 'youth' developmental phase from 14 to 25 years, the course integrates a developmental perspective with an emphasis on early detection, intensive intervention, and secondary prevention across a range of serious mental illnesses including early psychosis, eating disorders, and depression. As of June 2004, 126 students had enrolled in the course since it was launched in 1998.

Resource development

EPPIC Statewide Services also developed, produced, and promoted a range of training and educational resources. They include:

- A series of four EPPIC information sheets for patients and their families
- A range of video-based educational resources for consumers and professionals[11]
- Early psychosis manuals for clinicians on topics such as family work, psychoeducation, cannabis and psychosis, and cognitively orientated psychosis
- The EPPIC website located at: http://www.eppic.org.au attracts over 500 new visitors a week and has been used to launch the early intervention message internationally
- The National Early Psychosis Resource Center's website at http://www.earlypsychosis.org.au which is a clearinghouse for new information and research on early psychosis
- *Trips and Journeys*, an anthology of first-person accounts of psychosis.[29]

Editorial support was also provided for:

- *The Recognition and Management of Early Psychosis: A Preventative Approach*, a text published by Cambridge University Press.[30] The book has become established as a reference work for clinicians.
- The *Early Psychosis Kit*. Developed with the support of Janssen Cilag, the kit consists of 10 modules providing a comprehensive introduction to clinical work in early psychosis. The kit has been endorsed by the World Psychiatric Association, and translated into Norwegian, Swedish, Dutch, French, Flemish, German, Spanish, and Portuguese.[31]

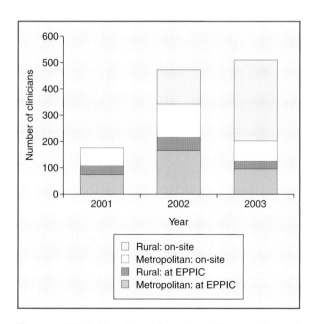

Figure 12.1 Number of metropolitan and rural clinicians attending training workshops, delivered by EPPIC Statewide Services, at EPPIC and on-site at their service during 2001–2003

The early intervention worker network

A number of limitations became apparent with the initial model of statewide service delivery.[28] Resources devoted to early psychosis were time-limited. Informal feedback indicated that Area Mental Health Services held concerns about the sustainability of project initiatives beyond the formal involvement of EPPIC Statewide Services.

Partly in response to this, a statewide early intervention strategy deploying early intervention workers was launched by Victoria's Department of Human Services in 2002 as an improved model for implementing best practice in early psychosis. Early intervention workers, linked to 18 of the Area Mental Health Services, provide limited direct care for a number of patients, in addition to training in phase-specific treatment for staff. Early intervention workers are also committed to enhancing the capacity of the primary care sector and specialist care services for early identification and assessment of mental health disorders. The overall aim is to enhance early recognition and timely and appropriate treatment.[32]

Key steps taken by EPPIC Statewide Services in supporting this initiative have included:

- Orientation and training of early intervention workers
- Formation of networks of early psychosis special interest groups
- Ensuring access for the early intervention workers to early psychosis resource materials
- Continuing consultation for the early intervention workers in planning and implementing local projects.

In 2003, four workshops were provided to early intervention workers, including a two day forum in July which showcased the work of early intervention workers across the state of Victoria. In addition, a total of 351 consultation contacts were recorded, which included one-to-one consultation meetings with the early intervention workers to assist them with the development of local strategic plans and the implementation of local initiatives.

Already a challenge to this initiative has become the difficulty of stretching these scarce additional resources across the primary health-care sector, in addition to Area Mental Health Services. Concerns have been raised that this 'capacity-building' model may produce incremental and unsustainable change when more significant structural reform is required which guarantees access for first episode patients to specialist service structures.[33]

Future directions for the service include ensuring greater input from carers and consumers in the training, and availability of introductory workshops on-line. Advanced workshops, which were piloted in 2003, will be further developed, to be followed up with supervision groups, as a means of maximizing integration of learning into clinical practice. The *New Directions for Victoria's Mental Health Services* document highlights 'extended prevention and early intervention' as one of six key directions for the next five years.[34] The Mental Health Branch has announced a special budget initiative of AU$1.8 million to expand early psychosis programs for young people in Victoria, including a commitment to replicating specialized early psychosis programs in one metropolitan and one rural area. This initiative is likely to impact significantly on the strategic directions and future service provision of EPPIC Statewide Services.

Conclusions

EPPIC Statewide Services provide one example of how skills, experience, research findings, and resources relating to the detection and treatment of early psychosis can be disseminated from a specialist unit. Consultation, professional development, and the development of resources have been the cornerstones of the services' activities. However, the question remains to be answered: are recent developments and the future directions enough to impact significantly upon the well-being of Victoria's young people and their families facing a critical point in their lives?

References

1. McGorry PD, Edwards J, Mihalopoulos C, et al. EPPIC: An evolving system of early detection and optimal management. Schizophr Bull 1996; **22**(2):305–26.

2. Australian Bureau of Statistics. *Melbourne: A Social Atlas.* Canberra: Australian Bureau of Statistics; 2001.

3. McGorry PD, Edwards J, Pennell K. Sharpening the focus: Early intervention in the real world. In: McGorry PD, Jackson HJ (eds). *The Recognition and Management of Early Psychosis: A Preventive Approach.* Cambridge University Press; 1999: 441–70.

4. McGorry P. Beyond adolescent psychiatry: The logic of a youth mental health model. *Aust N Z J Psychiatry* 1998; **32**(1):138–9.

5. Birchwood M. The critical period for early psychosis. In: Birchwood M, Fowler D (eds). *Early intervention in psychosis.* Chichester: Wiley; 2000.

6. Edwards J, Harris M, Herman A. The early psychosis prevention and intervention centre, Melbourne, Australia: An overview, November 2001. In: Ogura C (ed). *Recent Advances in Early Intervention and Prevention in Psychiatric Disorders.* Tokyo: Seiwa Shoten; 2002: 26–33.

7. Edwards J, Maude D, Herrmann-Doig T, et al. A service response to prolonged recovery in early psychosis. Psychiatr Serv 2002; **53**(9):1067–9.

8. Conus P, McGorry PD. First-episode mania: A neglected priority for early intervention. Aust N Z J Psychiatry 2002; **36**(2):158–72.

9. Gleeson JF. Early warning signs and predictors of relapse following early psychosis (PhD). Melbourne: University of Melbourne; 2001.

10. Power PJR, Bell RJ, Mills R, et al. Suicide prevention in first episode psychosis: The development of a randomised controlled trial of cognitive therapy for acutely suicidal patients with early psychosis. Aust N Z J Psychiatry 2003; **37**(4):414–20.

11. Edwards J, McGorry PD. Implementing early intervention in psychosis: A guide to establishing early psychosis services. Aust N Z J Psychiatry 2003; **37**(2):247.

12. Australian Health Ministers. *National Mental Health Plan.* Canberra: Commonwealth Department of Health and Family Services; 1993.

13. Australian Health Ministers. *Second National Mental Health Plan.* Canberra: Commonwealth Department of Health and Family Services; 1998.

14. Australian Health Ministers. *National Mental Health Plan, 2003–2008.* Canberra: Commonwealth Department of Health and Family Services; 2003.

15. Pennell K, McGorry, PD. *Australian National Early Psychosis Project: Its Activities, Outcomes and Recommendations.* Melbourne: University of Melbourne; 2001.

16. National Early Psychosis Project Clinical Guidelines Working Party. *Australian Clinical Guidelines for Early Psychosis.* Melbourne: National Early Psychosis Project, University of Melbourne; 1998.

17. Department of Health and Community Services Victoria. *Victoria's Mental Health Service: The Framework for Service Delivery.* Melbourne: Department of Health and Community Services Victoria; 1994.

18. Department of Health and Community Services Victoria. *The Framework for Service Delivery. Better Outcomes Through Area Mental Health Services.* Melbourne: Department of Health and Community Services; 1996.

19. Department of Health and Community Services Victoria. *Victoria's Mental Health Service. The Framework for Service Delivery. Child and Adolescent Services.* Melbourne: Department of Health and Community Services; 1996.

20. Luntz J. What is mental health consultation? Child Australia 1999; **24**(3):28–33.

21. Luntz J. Mental health consultation: Stages in the consultation process. Child Australia 2000; **25**(1):21–6.

22. Hilty D, Luo J, Morache C, et al. Telepsychiatry: An overview for psychiatrists. CNS Drugs 2000; **168**(8):527–48.

23. Harrigan SM, McGorry PD, Krstev H. Does treatment delay in first-episode psychosis really matter? Psychol Med 2003; **33**(1):97–110.

24. Larsen T, McGlashan T, Johannessen J, et al. Shortened duration of untreated early first episode of psychosis: Changes in patient characteristics at treatment. Am J Psychiatry 2001; **158**:1917–19.

25. Jackson H, Edwards J, Hulbert C, McGorry PD. Recovery from psychosis: Psychological interventions. In: McGorry PD, Jackson HJ (eds). *The Recognition and Management of Early Psychosis: A Preventive Approach.* Cambridge University Press; 1999: 265–307.

26. Gleeson J, Jackson H, Stavely H, Burnett P. Family intervention in early psychosis. In: McGorry PD, Jackson HJ, (eds). *The Recognition and Management of Early Psychosis: A Preventive Approach.* Cambridge University Press; 1999: 376–406.

27. Albiston D, Francey S, Harrigan S. Group programmes for recovery from early psychosis. Br J Psychiatry 1998; **172**(Suppl 33):177–21.

28. Krstev H, Gleeson J, McGorry P, et al. Evaluation of an early psychosis within an adult area mental health service. (in press).

29. Early Psychosis Prevention and Intervention Centre. *Trips and Journeys – Personal Accounts of Early Psychosis.* Melbourne: Early Psychosis Prevention and Intervention Centre; 2000.

30. McGorry PD, Jackson HJ (eds). *The Recognition and Management of Early Psychosis: A Preventive Approach.* Cambridge University Press; 1999.

31. McGorry P, Edwards J. *Early Psychosis Training Pack.* Macclesfield, UK: Gardiner-Caldwell; 1997.

32. Edwards J, McGorry PD. *Implementing Early Intervention in Psychosis.* London: Martin Dunitz; 2002.

33. McGorry PD, Yung AR. Early intervention in psychosis: An overdue reform. Aust N Z J Psychiatry 2003; **37**(4):393–8.

34. Department of Human Services Victoria. *New Directions for Victoria's Mental Health Services. The Next Five Years.* Melbourne: Department of Human Services Victoria; 2002.

13

Developing an Early Intervention Service in Hong Kong

Eric Chen

Introduction

This chapter describes the development of an early intervention program in Hong Kong, illustrating the various decision points and key issues that occurred in the process. The purpose is to use this as a case example to reflect on some general principles that might be useful in planning the development of a new service. The first section provides the background context for the development of the service. Then, some of the key processes in setting up the service are discussed. This is followed by a description of the structure and the processes in the Hong Kong program. In this review some of the important factors that shaped the service, whether planned or evolved, will be highlighted.

Background

Hong Kong is a well-defined geographic region with a population of 7.5 million. Within Hong Kong, over 95% of the population is Han Chinese and the primary language is Cantonese. The Hong Kong population has a fair degree of international exposure through education and commerce. Population density is high. Importantly, young people usually live with their parents until they start their own families.

Public healthcare delivery in Hong Kong is coordinated by the Hospital Authority. In addition, there is a substantial private sector primarily providing outpatient care. The primary care system (family medicine) is less comprehensive and is mainly consumer-driven.

Psychiatric services originally consisted of inpatient, outpatient, and community care. There were two major psychiatric hospitals each with about 1500 beds. In recent years there has been a move to develop psychiatric units in general hospitals. Rehabilitation work is often managed by nongovernmental organizations (NGOs) providing half-way houses, sheltered workshops, and day care facilities. Each NGO runs its own program. Also, community services are limited and mainly consist of monitoring visits by community psychiatric nurses (CPNs) and occasional crisis assessments. Outpatient psychiatry is characterized by a high service volume (20–30 patients per three hour session) and a lack of subspecialty clinics. Referral to psychiatry requires a prior assessment by a physician and an outpatient appointment usually has a waiting time of at least several weeks (at times months). Patients with psychosis often present in crisis situations involving risks of self-harm or violence. Such presentations often involve the accident and emergency department, and sometimes necessitate police escorts as well as compulsory admission.

There is a relatively high level of stigmatization for psychiatric disorders. This has been fueled by sensational media reporting of any incident of violence involving individuals with abnormal mental states. Plans to set up half-way houses have repeatedly evoked public protests from the affected neighborhood.

There has been no recent epidemiological survey to provide incidence figures for psychiatric disorders. Public knowledge of mental illness is also limited. A study based on case vignette assessment showed that the majority of the general public could not distinguish symptoms of stress from symptoms of a psychotic disorder.[1]

Preparation for the service

Identifying a core interest group

Initial interest in early onset psychosis originated from research work on first episode schizophrenia as well as exposure to international projects. The Hong Kong Schizophrenia Research Society is an informal organization that promotes local research. Early psychosis was identified as one of its focuses. This resulted in the formation of a core group which met to discuss the strategy for developing early intervention.

Raising local awareness

The Hong Kong Schizophrenia Research Society organized seminars and training workshops for local professionals. Other activities included publishing articles in local general medical journals and presentations at local conferences for general medical practitioners.[2] These efforts spread awareness beyond the psychiatric profession. Media coverage also raised the hazards of treatment delay at the community level.

Initial research

In Hong Kong, a comprehensive first episode psychosis study has been underway since 1998 and initial data on duration of untreated psychosis (DUP) was particularly important for planning.[3] In general, it is particularly advantageous if research addresses DUP and pathways to care, as well as the outcome of first episode psychosis. DUP and pathway to care data are very important in service planning and in strengthening a service development proposal. Availability of outcome data in a representative first episode cohort can potentially be employed as baseline data for evaluating the efficacy of the future program.

Key planning decisions

More detailed planning began with communications with administrators advising that funding support would be in the form of personnel rather than infrastructure. This constraint led us to consider a primarily outpatient-based service. Available funding provided for eight clinicians, 12 nursing staff, and one clinical psychologist. It was necessary to attempt an estimation of the workload. We resorted to international data for age-specific incidence from recent reports. Based on this calculation we realized that with our resources we could not handle all of the cases of first episode psychosis in Hong Kong. There were three options. The first was to choose a smaller region within Hong Kong for implementation. The second approach was to provide a service for a specific age range. The third option was to provide a less intensive service. We ruled out the third option as a diluted intervention defeated the purpose of early detection. The first approach was attractive as this left open the possibility of comparison between regions with and without early onset intervention services. However, in Hong Kong it was impossible to limit the media campaign to a specific region. With the population exposed to media education, not having access to services would have been hard to justify. This left us with the second option of setting an age limit to the program. We decided to focus on the younger patients as they usually have poorer outcomes[4,5] and have more developmental tasks which could be disrupted by psychosis. Setting the upper age limit at 25 years corresponds to an estimated annual incidence caseload of around 700.

This would cover around 40% of all psychosis cases.

In considering the length of the service provided after a patient entered the program, the general principle is that the patient should be managed by the same team for as long as possible. The optimal length relates to the critical period hypothesis which suggests that the first few years in the course of a psychotic illness exert a much stronger influence on long-term outcome.[6–9] We have therefore opted for the provision for intensive keyworker contact for the first two years. The third year in the program is a transitional period with decreased keyworker input while medical follow-up is maintained. This transition prepares towards the transfer to a general psychiatry service after the third year.

Services that potentially interface with the early psychosis program include child psychiatry, general psychiatry, substance abuse, learning disability, and community psychiatry. Discussion of boundary issues with representatives from the relevant specialties facilitated the definition of the primary target group of patients without severe learning disability and not having a drug-induced psychosis.

We also had to decide whether there should be one team covering the whole of Hong Kong or whether there should be several teams. With one large team, there would have been more consistency in approach and the administrative structure would be simpler. However, the contact of the team with other services and other sectors at the local level could be compromised. On the other hand, with several teams, there would be more flexibility in local adaptation. We opted for having four teams working under a central steering committee. Each team covers a geographic defined catchment area. The four intervention teams each consist of two psychiatrists and three psychiatric nurses, and each is flexible in applying its mode of operation, adapting as much as possible to the needs and practices of the local clinics, NGOs, and communities.

Key preparation processes

The steering committee

The steering committee consists of key clinicians from the teams and representatives from each major psychiatric unit, as well as a representative from nursing and the Public Affairs division of the Hospital Authority. Members of the steering committee met every month in the first year and then every 2–3 months. They collectively decide on the major aims of the service. Each team then develops its own implementation details according to the local situation. Operational issues are regularly reviewed in the steering committee where experiences can be shared. Core processes (such as evaluation procedures and mass media activities) are shared by all teams. In the pre-launch period ad-hoc workgroups were formed, as described below.

'Naming' workgroup

This workgroup was formed to produce an appropriate translation for the term 'psychosis', which in Chinese translates, inappropriately, as 'serious mental illness'. The group invited suggestions from all levels of mental health workers. It met repeatedly to consider more than 30 suggestions over a series of five meetings, until the current translation, 思覺失調, was agreed. This translation of early onset psychosis literally means a 'dysregulation in thoughts and perception'. Importantly, 'dysregulation' carries the idea of reversibility. The group also decided on the Chinese and English name for the program (EASY) in consultation with the Public Affairs division.

'Education' workgroup

Another workgroup worked extensively on the public health education program. This group was responsible for the design and preparation of media material. The group consists of media experts from the Public Affairs division as well as key clinicians. A painstaking but thorough process of dialog between the professionals from these different disciplines took place until the core message was packaged in an accurate, effective, balanced, and high impact manner. A media skills workshop was also organized for all clinicians by the Hospital Authority personnel department prior to the launch. The information was disseminated in the form of pamphlets, compact disks and radio and television broadcasts.

'Evaluation' workgroup

A third workgroup designed and prepared the evaluation processes. The major domains of outcome were decided and key measures chosen. Major contributions were received from assessment experts in various domains. Prior to launching, a training workshop was held to ensure that clinicians and front line workers would handle the assessments appropriately and competently.

Ongoing EASY operational structure and processes

The operational processes can be divided into five parts: education, assessment, intervention, team building and development, and evaluation. See Figure 13.1 for the structure of EASY.

Education

EASY educational activities consist of mass media and face-to-face activities. Media educational activities are coordinated by the Public Affairs division of the Hospital Authority. A detailed planning process concerning the timing, content, and message ensures that media impact is optimal. The initial wave of media activities aimed at promotion of the service as well as introducing the term 思覺失調 in a high impact manner. This consisted of intensive media exposure (for a period of three weeks) at the launch of the program. This was followed by subsequent news articles that conveyed more detailed information. Subsequent activities included monitoring of media reporting, as well as regular meetings with media representatives in order to ensure correct usage. Face-to-face educational work consists of

meeting with professionals likely to encounter people with early psychosis (social workers, school counselors, psychologists, GPs, and teachers).

Assessment

New to the EASY assessment system is referral by telephone, and this is available to all. Keyworkers conduct a structured assessment by telephone for initial information and to screen inappropriate referrals. This system has enhanced accessibility and the possibility of offering help and advice to the person during the referral process. Following the structured assessment, a diagnostic assessment is arranged in a non-stigmatizing setting. Clinics in general hospitals, as well as community assessment sites, have often been used. This arrangement often decreases the sense of stigmatization.

Intervention

Identified cases receive comprehensive intervention, and following a thorough medical assessment, patients are assigned to a designated keyworker. This keyworker provides in-depth engagement with the patient and also works with the carer. The progress of the patient is reviewed regularly; problems in the recovery process are identified early and managed in an assertive manner, aiming at the best possible outcomes in terms of symptoms, functioning, and subjective recovery. A standardized psychoeducational program is delivered to all patients and their carers. Group therapy has also been offered to patients and their carers. Patients with additional needs (such as residual symptoms, secondary mood and anxiety symptoms) are referred to face-to-face therapy with the clinical psychologist. Psychosocial rehabilitation efforts are also facilitated by collaboration with NGOs and vocational training centers, many of which have organized special programs for recovering early onset psychosis patients.

Team building and development

To enhance a coordinated team effort centralized team building and development activities are

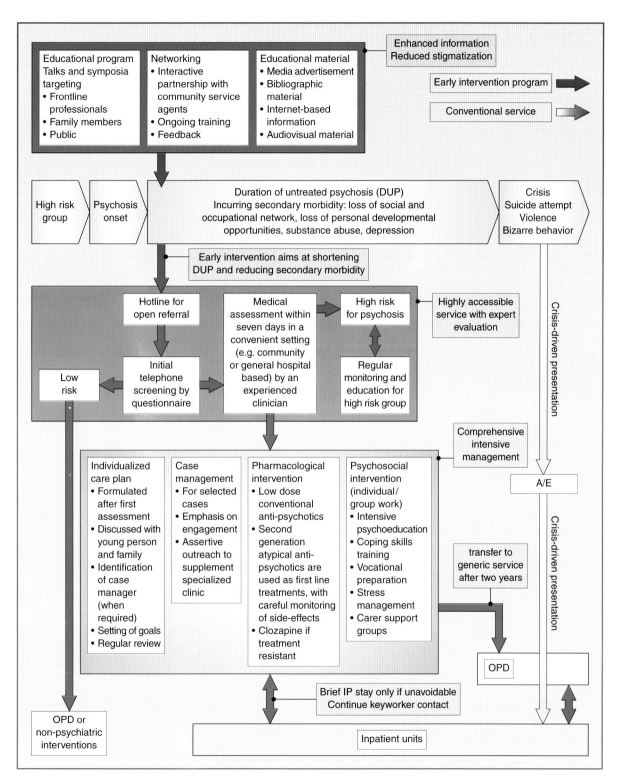

Figure 13.1 The structure of EASY. IP, inpatient unit; OPD, outpatient department

required. Monthly training activities have been organized for EASY clinicians and keyworkers. Training sessions are supported by a variety of local experts and cover a number of relevant areas (e.g. social skills, cognitive therapeutic skills for psychosis, motivational interviewing techniques, advanced medication treatment issues, etc.). All the teams also meet twice yearly for a one day team-building workshop in which key issues of the program can be discussed.

Evaluation

Evaluation of an early intervention service is a complex task. Important decisions need to be made at the beginning to determine the timing and scope of the evaluation. The timing of an evaluative process partly depends on administrative needs. We have found that the first two years of the project largely reflect a transitional state. More representative results probably do not unfold until at least the third or fourth year of the program. It is desirable that the scope of evaluation is fairly broad and includes functioning and subjective outcome parameters as well as symptomatic outcomes. We have included the following domains in the EASY outcome evaluation: presentation including DUP; symptoms; functioning; quality of life; and carer health status. One of the consequences of having such broad outcome categories is that they actually guide the direction of clinical provision. That is, they lead front line practitioners away from the traditional narrow window on symptoms, and facilitate focusing on the wider domains of functioning and quality of life. It would be helpful to have data from a control group for comparison as any results are only of a descriptive nature. Process indicators could also be monitored; these could include response time, screening and diagnostic outcome, and engagement statistics.

Summary

This chapter describes the development of the Hong Kong Early Intervention Program, EASY.

Key processes are outlined from the perspective of project design. We have highlighted how the Hong Kong project has made developmental decisions in the context of the local situation. Many similar issues are likely to arise in other programs and locations. The Hong Kong project is now two years into its operation and can still be considered to be in a stage of development. There are later stage issues that we have not yet faced (e.g. the transition of the patient from the early intervention program to a generic program). This should therefore be considered as an account of the early developmental issues encountered in an Asian urban context.

References

1. Lam LC, Chan CK, Chen EY. Insight and general public attitude on psychotic experiences in Hong Kong. Int J Soc Psychiatry 1996; **42**:10–17.
2. Chen EYH. Early intervention in schizophrenia: rationale and practice. Hong Kong Med J 1998; **5**:57–62.
3. Chen EYH, Dunn ELW, Chen RYL, et al. Duration of untreated psychosis and symptomatic outcome amongst first episode schizophrenic patients in Hong Kong. Schizophr Res 1999; **36**:15.
4. Jarbin H, Ott Y, Von Knorring AL. Adult outcome of social function in adolescent-onset schizophrenia and affective psychosis. J Am Acad Child & Adolesc Psych 2003; **42**:176–83.
5. Werry JS. Child and adolescent (early onset) schizophrenia: a review in light of DSM-III-R. J Autism Dev Disord 1992; **22**:601–24.
6. Carpenter WT, Jr, Strauss JS. The prediction of outcome in schizophrenia: IV. Eleven-year follow-up of the Washington IPSS cohort. J Nerv Ment Dis 1991; **179**:517–25.
7. Harrison G, Croudace T, Mason P, et al. Predicting the long-term outcome of schizophrenia. Psychol Med 1996; **26**:697–705.
8. Mason P, Harrison G, Glazebrook C, et al. Characteristics of outcome in schizophrenia at 13 years. Br J Psychiatry 1995; **167**:596–603.
9. Thara R, Eaton WW. Outcome of schizophrenia: the Madras longitudinal study. Aust N Z J Psychiatry 1996; **30**:516–22.

14

Fraser South Early Psychosis Intervention Program

Karen Tee and Laura Hanson

Introduction

In recent years, the belief in early intervention has inspired reform in mental health practice and the development of specialized early psychosis services. The Early Psychosis Intervention (EPI) Program is an attempt to innovate in a time of systemic and fiscal constraints, while adhering to principles pioneered in the past decade.[1–3] The EPI Program was implemented in 2000 as a collaborative initiative between the government agencies responsible for both adult, and child and youth mental health services in the Fraser South area of British Columbia, Canada. The four communities of Fraser South have a population of 575 000 across about 836 square kilometers. The EPI Program serves young people between the ages of 13 and 35 years with early psychosis (non-affective and affective) and their families. The program bridges youth and adult mental health services, and links community with hospital. Key components include a range of clinical services, community education, research activities, and ongoing evaluation of outcome and service delivery.

The EPI Program aims to improve the mental health and quality of life of young people with psychosis by promoting early identification and providing rapid access to intensive, phase-specific treatment in the critical period of the early years of psychosis. As a community-based, case-finding program, service components include:

- Single entry intake
- Assessment, treatment, and case management for young people with first episode psychosis
- Group intervention
- Family intervention
- Assessment and monitoring/outreach for young people at ultra-high risk for developing psychosis (at-risk mental state).

Hub-and-spoke model

The EPI Program is best described as a hub-and-spoke model for service delivery (see Figure 14.1). There is a multidisciplinary central team (hub), and community teams (spokes). The central team includes a medical director (psychiatrist), program director (psychologist), clinical nurse educator (psychiatric nurse), intake clinician (clinical social worker), and group and family therapist (clinical social worker). A research team, made up of consultant psychologists, a genetic counselor, and research assistants, conducts program evaluation and research studies initiated by the EPI Program and in collaboration with local universities. In total, there are four full-time and one part-time clinical staff,

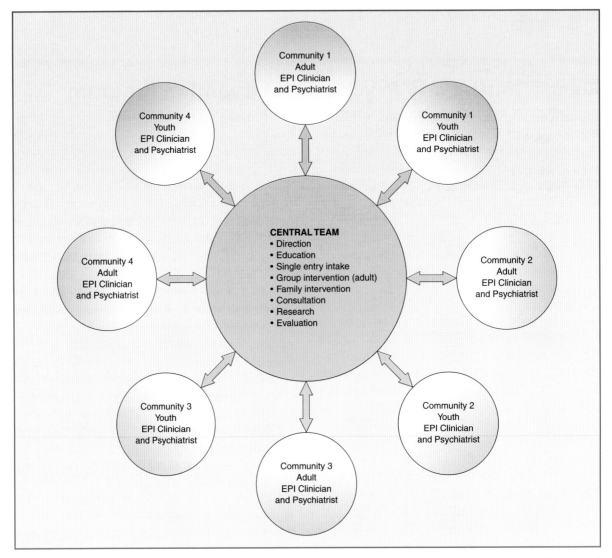

Figure 14.1 The hub-and-spoke model of the Early Psychosis Intervention (EPI) Program. **Hub:** central team provides program direction and regional services, sharing care of clients and families with **Spokes:** community team designated specialists who provide ongoing treatment and case management, according to locality and age.

and five part-time research staff, with dedicated funding through the two ministries and research grants. In addition to providing program direction and coordination, clinical supervision/consultation to the community teams, and delivering/coordinating education for professionals and the public, the central team also provides the pathway into and through care.

The provision of ongoing care is shared with designated early psychosis specialists on the community teams (spokes). The community teams comprise EPI clinicians and EPI psychiatrists in each of the four communities of Fraser South, working in local adult or youth mental health centres. These providers are existing staff on mental health teams who provide general mental health services, with part of their time alloc-ated to providing early psychosis treatment and case management. At this time, there is no dedic-ated funding for these providers. EPI clinicians are psychiatric nurses, psychologists, and master's level counselors. There is at least one EPI clinician on each adult and youth team, with some teams also having a secondary EPI clinician as back up. The central and community teams share the care of clients and families, including some EPI clinicians co-facilitating groups with the central team's group therapist.

Service delivery model

In order to ensure accessibility, community and hospital referrals are made to the EPI Program through a single point of entry (see Figure 14.2). Community referrals indicating a suspected psy-chosis are provided rapid access to screening and psychiatric assessments by the central teams intake clinician and psychiatrist, including out-reach assessments at the young person's school, home, or doctor's office. Upon identification of a first episode psychosis, either through the community assessment or hospital admission, the young person and family members are provided with education and orientation to the program by a central team staff member, either in the community or at the hospital. The central team then facilitates the transition to the adult or youth EPI clinician and psychiatrist in the person's local community. The EPI clinician provides psycho-education, psychosocial treatment, and case man-agement based on the early psychosis care path, a standardized, phase-specific treatment protocol.

Concurrent group and family intervention services are available to clients and their families. Group services include:

- Eight-week psychoeducation and process groups for adolescents
- Eight-week psychoeducation and process group for adults
- Four-week psychoeducation group for family members and significant others

- Psychoeducation group for siblings
- Monthly support group for families and signific-ant others, facilitated in collaboration with community partners (BC Schizophrenia Society and Canadian Mental Health Association).

Family involvement occurs at all stages of assess-ment and treatment. More recently, the EPI Program is developing a family therapy compo-nent as an adjunct to the individual treatment and groups offered. This newly evolving family therapy service will include family assessment, brief intervention with families, and multi-family group intervention for specific issues, such as per-sistent symptoms or drug and alcohol use by their family member.

Young people identified as at risk for develop-ing psychosis are provided with support, educa-tion, monitoring, and outreach by the central team. Ongoing monitoring is provided by the intake clinician for those who do not require mental health treatment. At risk young people, who present with psychiatric symptoms such as depression or anxiety, are treated by their local community mental health service and registered under the EPI Program.

In the 3.5 years since the inception of EPI Program there have been 640 referrals that merited further assessment. A total of 328 cases of first episode psychosis were identified. In the past two years, the incidence rate has remained constant at 19 cases per 100 000. Median age of entry into the program was 20.6 years. Females comprised 30% and males 70%. Almost 55% of referrals were ini-tially hospitalized. Mental health centers provided an additional 22% of referrals, with 9% of referrals from family and friends. General physicians, schools, and community agencies each provided less than 5%. EPI clinicians rated 49% of referrals as having abused substances in the month prior to intake. These ratings have increased over the past three years. Alcohol misuse and violence in the pre-ceding month were present in 12% and 18%, respectively. Suicidal ideation before intake was common (20%) and 6% made a suicide attempt in

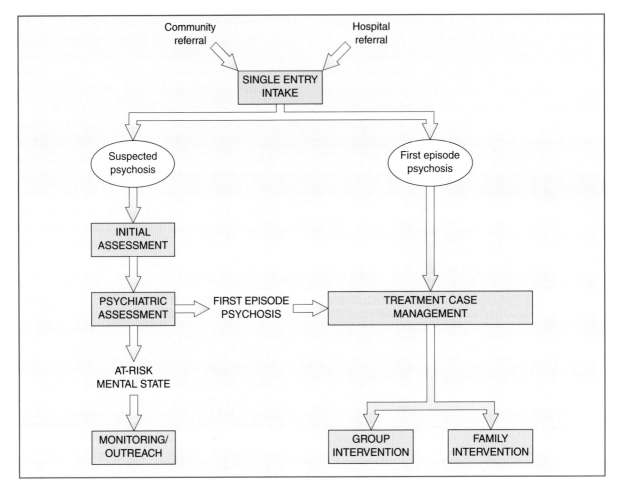

Figure 14.2 The service delivery model

the preceding month. EPI clinicians estimated that the proportions of clients who were psychotic without treatment for less than one month and greater than one year were 42% and 17%, respectively. A total of 116 cases have been discharged; 26% were referred at discharge to continuing services; 29% moved; 14% refused further service; and 24% recovered (64% of these did not require follow-up treatment).

Bridging youth and adult services

A unique aspect of the EPI Program is the bridging of youth and adult services across different ministries, and bringing together their skills, per-

spectives, and experiences into one program serving clients ranging from the age of 13 to 35 years. This bridging is both the greatest strength and challenge of the program in terms of developing strategies for crossing the age division in planning for funding, service delivery, education, and research. The commitment to early intervention in both ministries is most evident in their support of educational strategies. The case finding and early detection approach of the program has sharpened the focus on reaching out to youth. To this end, a public awareness campaign and website (www.psychosissucks.ca) specifically designed for teenagers and young adults were launched early in 2003.

The greatest challenge of the EPI Program model of care has been the joining of community clinicians and psychiatrists on existing mental health teams who have worked either with youth or with older, chronically mentally ill adults, into a program for young, early psychosis clients and their families. The challenges lie in the pursuit of evidence-based practice and crossover of knowledge and skills, against a backdrop of lack of dedicated funding for the community teams and appropriate resources for this age population. Although time is allocated to early psychosis services, EPI psychiatrists, and EPI clinicians especially, struggle with the competing demand of also delivering general mental health services, and an environment that has not yet caught up with practice reform. However, in an attempt to strive for best practices under these conditions and achieve a consistency of care across two ministries, the early psychosis care path was developed.

The early psychosis care path

A care path is a plan that outlines interventions for professional staff caring for a specific client group. While there are many different types of care paths, the vast majority have the following goals:

- Provide a practical 'best practices' guide to care
- Reduce variation in practice
- Provide a method for improving quality of care.

Although there has been a dramatic expansion in care path applications to physical health conditions in the past two decades (e.g. the National Health Service in the UK), relatively few care paths have been developed for use with mental health conditions. Those care paths that have been developed for mental health are primarily for inpatient care,[4–6] and several care paths have now been developed for inpatient care of schizophrenia.[7–10]

For mental health diagnoses including schizophrenia there is often a low rate of adherence to best practices, including both pharmacologic[11] and psychosocial[12] interventions. With increasing fiscal and social pressures to ensure mental health services provide evidence-based interventions, the care path has recently been looked upon as a potential solution to ensure quality care and accountability.[13,14] However, there are numerous challenges facing the use of care paths in outpatient mental health services. These include the fact that longer-term care is often provided, mental health diagnoses tend to be comorbid, and clinicians are often resistant to the notion.[15] This latter fact may be due, in part, to the preference of the clinician to view each client as a unique individual who will not fit into any predetermined treatment plan. While it is true that the experience of each client is unique, it is also true that for any given diagnostic group there will be certain interventions that should be provided to all clients. A care path that details diagnostically specific practices will enable clinicians to spend more time tailoring care to the unique needs of each client.

Development

In summer 2001, the EPI Program took on the challenge of developing a care path, initially limiting the scope to outpatient care provided by EPI clinicians. (The extension to include hospital care is in its preliminary stage and is not discussed here.)

Prior to care path development, current practice was reviewed to allow for identification of gaps between current and best practice:

1. Chart audits: charts were reviewed using an audit tool to assess both treatment process and client outcome.
2. Semistructured interviews: interviews were conducted with all EPI clinicians which covered current practice and obstacles to providing best practices.

The process of carrying out audits made clear the inadequacies of the documentation system.

Charting was narrative and it was very difficult to gauge treatment process and client outcome. Despite these difficulties, a number of areas were identified as problematic: overall levels of family involvement were low and core psychosocial interventions were inconsistently delivered. The interviews suggested that there were other areas wanting improvement including the need for educational curricula. (See Table 14.1 for highlights of the pre-care path review.)

Development of the care path was informed by this review, guided by a task group, and piloted in one community. In an attempt to rectify the issue of poor documentation, key aspects of practice were listed in check-box format. Consistent with recommendations for early psychosis case management,[16] the care path was divided according to stages of recovery. Education materials, assessment templates, and an individualized care plan were developed and included in the care path. (See Table 14.2 for a more detailed breakdown.)

Care path evaluation

The care path was implemented in fall 2002 and evaluated 12 months later with the same audit tool previously used. This evaluation revealed overall compliance with care path use, although progression through the sections was slower than anticipated with only about half of the charts utilizing the recovery section. There may be multiple reasons for this including poor engagement, prolonged recovery, or the care path structure. Individualized care planning was used in only 22% of the charts reviewed. It is hoped that reorganization and streamlining of the care path will ensure better use of individualized care planning and the recovery section.

Evaluation suggested some improvements in practice including increased contact by clinicians working with adults, more individualized family education, and greater use of core psychosocial interventions (see Table 14.2). However, it would be premature to infer that these improvements

Table 14.1 Data highlights from the pre- and post-care path reviews		
Indicator	**Pre-care path**	**Post-care path**
Mean number of in-person visits with client over first three months	Overall = 6.0 ($n = 33$) Child and youth = 6.9 ($n = 15$) Adult = 5.3 ($n = 18$)	Overall = 7.4 ($n =33$) Child and youth = 6.8 ($n = 8$) Adult = 7.6 ($n = 25$)*
Mean number of in-person visits with family over first three months	Overall = 2.2 ($n = 33$) Child and youth = 3.1 ($n = 15$) Adult = 1.2 ($n = 18$)	Overall = 2.7 ($n = 33$) Child and youth = 2.6 ($n = 8$) Adult = 2.8 ($n = 25$)*
Evidence of individualized education provided to family[a]	38% ($n = 26$)	67% ($n = 24$)*
Evidence of relapse prevention provided to clients[a]	46% ($n = 26$)	92% ($n = 24$)*
Evidence of stress management provided to client[a]	34% ($n = 26$)	75% ($n = 24$)*
a Data collected only when there was evidence of adequate engagement. * Significant at $p < .05$		

Table 14.2 Early psychosis care path – description of sections

Section	Description
Referral information and forms	Contains referral and contact information and other forms required by the Mental Health Centre.
Psychiatry	While there is no care path for the EPI psychiatrist, several new forms were developed in the hope that information on medication would be better documented (e.g. medication changes, side effects, compliance). Psychiatry reports and progress notes are included in this section.
Referrals and reports	Referrals made to other services (and follow-through on these) are indicated here. Also contains assessment and treatment reports from service providers other than the EPI clinician and psychiatrist (e.g. hospital reports, vocational assessment reports, etc.)
Initial contact and engagement	Includes the care path starting from when the referral is received and for the initial contacts. The purpose is to establish contact quickly, ensure continuity of care, and actively engage client and family.
Assessment	Includes the care path for the initial assessment. Assessment templates (initial and updates) and termination report are included here and are available as an electronic template as well. The purpose is to assess thoroughly and evaluate progress in treatment.
Individualized care plan	This section is where other treatments (not included in the care path) are planned and documented. The individualized care plan is problem-based and its purpose is to ensure that other client needs (e.g. comorbidity, social problems, etc.) are captured in care.
Recovery	Includes the care path for the period following the initial assessment. The purpose is to facilitate stabilization and reintegration and to provide education and other core psychosocial treatments. Educational handouts and educational session overviews were developed and included for the following topics: what is psychosis, what causes psychosis, early intervention, medications, psychosocial treatments, stress management, relapse prevention, social functioning, lifestyle, goal setting, problem solving, family coping, drugs and alcohol, and coping with persistent symptoms. Additionally, templates are included for the relapse prevention plan, goal setting, and problem solving.
Relapse	Includes the care path for clients who have a relapse (exacerbation of psychosis or psychiatric hospitalization). Not all clients will go onto this part of the care path. The purpose is to ensure safety, minimize disruption, and facilitate stabilization and reintegration.

are a direct result of the care path itself. These improvements may simply be an artifact of improved documentation and/or a reflection of the efforts of the central team to improve practice (e.g. by providing clinician education and peer supervision). The one improvement that is clearly a direct result of the care path is the improvement in documentation. Obtaining standardized process and outcome data is a necessary first step for detection of variations in care, and through this standardization, the care path can now serve as a vehicle for quality improvement. While evaluation revealed some improvements in care, it also has more clearly identified areas needing further improvement (e.g. attention to comorbidity, individualized family education).

The revision of the care path will involve changes to format and content as suggested by evaluation and clinician feedback. Efforts will be made to reduce documentation to the extent possible and improve organization of the care path. In summary, although the implementation of outpatient mental health care paths presents unique challenges, through the EPI Program it has been demonstrated that it is possible to implement such a care path and that this is associated with improvements in clinical practice and documentation.

Future directions

The hub-and-spoke model of care developed by the EPI Program emerged out of fiscal constraint, organization across two ministries, and an expansive geography that necessitates ongoing care within the consumers' own communities. A future direction includes securing funding for the community teams in order to consolidate the program further, and ensure consistency and adherence to the care path. Future program expansion includes developing multicultural service provision, an addictions strategy, and a provincial early psychosis training program for clinicians and physicians.

Acknowledgments

The EPI Program is funded by the Fraser Health Authority (and the previous South Fraser Health Region), and the Ministry for Children and Family Development (Provincial Headquarters and South Fraser Region). The authors would like to acknowledge the dedication of the central team in developing the EPI Program: Bill MacEwan (for leadership), Tom Ehmann, Linda Wowk, Mary McCallum, Walter Lidster, and Dennis Santo. We are especially grateful to Martha Grypma for her invaluable contribution in developing the early psychosis care path. The authors would also like to thank Colleen Meyer, Damon Elgie, Elizabeth Patterson, and the other EPI clinicians for their contributions to the development of the care path.

References

1. McGorry PD, Edwards J, Mihalopoulos C, et al. EPPIC: An evolving system of early detection and optimal management. Schizophr Bull 1996; **22**:305–26.

2. Edwards J, McGorry PD. *Implementing Early Intervention in Psychosis: A Guide to Establishing Early Psychosis Services.* London: Martin Dunitz; 2002.

3. McGlashan M. Early detection and intervention of schizophrenia: rationale and research. Br J Psychiatry Suppl 1998; **172**:3–6.

4. Bultema JK, Mailliard L, Getzfrid MK, et al. Geriatric patients with depression: improving outcomes using a multidisciplinary clinical path model. J Nurs Admin 1996; **26**:31–8.

5. Hassan N, Turner-Stokes L, Pierce K, Clegg F. A completed audit cycle and integrated care pathway for the management of depression following brain injury in a rehabilitation setting, Clin Rehab 2002; **16**:534–40.

6. Andolina K. *Mental Health Critical Path/Care Map Tools and Case Management Systems.* Boston: The Center for Case Management; 1995.

7. Jones A, Kamath PD. Issues for the development of care pathways in mental health services. J Nurs Manag 1998; **6**:87–95.

8. Jones A. Hospital care pathways for patients with schizophrenia. J Clin Nursing 2001; **10**:58–69.

9. Chan SW, Wong K. The use of the critical pathways in caring for schizophrenic patients in a mental hospital. Arch Psychiatr Nurs 1999; **3**:145–53.

10. Baker JA, O'Higgins H, Parkinson J, Tracey N. The construction and implementation of a psychosocial interventions care pathway within a low secure environment: a pilot study. J Psychiatr Ment Health Nurs 2002; **9**:737–9.

11. Owen RR, Fischer EP, Kirchner JE, et al. Clinical practice variations in prescribing antipsychotics for patients with schizophrenia, Am J Med Qual 2003; **18**:140–6.

12. Lehman AF, Steinwachs DM. Patterns of usual care for schizophrenia: initial results from the Schizophrenia Patient Outcomes Research Team (PORT) Client Survey. Schizophr Bull 1998; **24**:11–20.

13. Dunn J, Rodriquez D, Novak JJ. Promoting quality mental health care delivery with critical path care plans. J Psychosocial Nurs Ment Health Serv 1994; **32**:25–9.

14. Smith GB. Critical pathway and patient and family teaching protocol for major depression. Nurs Case Manag 1997; **2**:23–32.

15. Jones A. The development of mental health care pathways: friend or foe? Br J Nursing 1999; **8**:1441–3.

16. Edwards J, Cocks J, Bott J. Preventive case management in first-episode psychosis. In: McGorry PD, Jackson HJ, Perris C (eds). *The Recognition and Management of Early Psychosis.* Cambridge University Press; 1999.

15

Implementing Early Intervention in Switzerland: The Lausanne Early Psychosis Project

Philippe Conus

Introduction

The growing body of evidence linking delay in treatment after the onset of psychosis to clinical and social outcome clearly supports the idea of early intervention.[1] The various programs developed around the world in the last decade have in common the aims of early detection, phase-specific treatment, prevention of secondary psychiatric problems, minimization of family disruption, and best possible level of recovery. The way professionals choose to pursue these goals can, however, vary greatly.

While intervening early is rarely a matter of controversy, some authors have questioned the usefulness of mental health reforms that would implement specialist early intervention services, arguing this would be a waste of valuable resources when generic mental health services could do just as well.[2] The development of intensive case management has faced the same type of criticisms when attempted in Europe, despite its success in the US and Australia. In addition, European research on its efficacy has failed to replicate results of studies conducted in the US. Differences in the structure of mental health systems has been mentioned as one of the explanations for such differences.[3] An assessment of the target population's needs is therefore a necessary preliminary to the implementation of a new program.

The structure of the Swiss mental health system offers a very different context from the one in which the Early Psychosis Prevention and Intervention Centre (EPPIC) was developed in Australia. Switzerland is a country where a high standard of living has until recently allowed the provision of a very wide range of structures that can dispense specialized treatment for psychiatric disorders, regardless of their intensity, in outpatient facilities as well as in a still very high number of inpatient beds. A retrospective file study conducted on first episode psychosis patients hospitalized in 2000 in the Lausanne catchment area (220 000 inhabitants) revealed, however, that despite these dissimilarities in health services and population structures, patients developing a first psychotic episode in Lausanne and their families faced issues similar to those described elsewhere.

In this study, Bonsack et al.[4] found that duration of untreated psychosis (DUP) was usually long and that many family members complained of the complexity of the pathway to care. The effect of DUP appears dramatic in terms of suicide risk (30% with suicide threats before admission, 13% with suicide attempts), rate of comorbidity (50% abuse substances), conflict with family (50% are in conflict with family, 15% have completely lost contact with them), and impact on functional level (44% are unemployed). Admission to hospital is usually compulsory (54%), with frequent need for seclusion (25%) due to violent behavior. Finally, linkage to outpatient treatment is poor, more than 50% of patients failing to attend their first outpatient appointment after discharge.

The Lausanne program

Due to the complexity of the current system and lack of funding, it is neither possible nor necessary to consider the development of an entirely new and specialized treatment structure for early psychosis. The aim is rather to organize appropriately the flux of patients through the existing structure and to combine reallocation of existing resources and new funding (recently secured in the context of project developments in mental health) to develop critical elements of the program (see Table 15.1). The main issues we have to face are:

1. Delay in treatment
2. Lack of community assessment
3. Lack of specialized inpatient treatment
4. Failure to link patients with outpatient care, to ensure continuity of care and to provide specialized outpatient treatment
5. Absence of adequate treatment of comorbidity.

The structure of our program will be composed of three main elements:

1. Assertive treatment team. Even though home-based treatment was relatively common in Lausanne before the 1980s, it almost disappeared during the 1990s. This was because community psychiatry favored office-based treatment on a psychodynamic psychotherapeutic model. Mental health practice emphasized individual choice and responsibility, with strong criticism of the paternalistic aspect of assertive treatment. Although this was useful in preventing some inappropriate treatment, this 'swing of the pendulum' led progressively to the abandonment of difficult-to-engage patients, who were treated only in the context of crisis intervention or compulsory hospitalization. ACT was developed in Lausanne in 2001 in an attempt to address the specific needs of difficult-to-engage patients.[5] *In the context of the early intervention program*, this team will develop a specific focus on early psychosis, promote home-based assessment, and provide intensive support in crisis periods, in order to avoid hospitalization. The team will also facilitate early return to the community by providing intensive support after discharge from hospital.

2. Assertive case management. So far, case management has not developed in Lausanne, and psychiatric treatment is provided by psychiatric registrars supervised by consultants. Nurses and social workers work as members of the multidisciplinary team, but not systematically and specifically in their field of expertise. Due to the rotation of registrars, this model implies an important level of treatment discontinuity and limited availability. *In the context of the early intervention program*, two part-time case manager positions have been created by reallocation of existing resources in the outpatient facility. They will be allocated to patients in the 48 hours following entry into the program and will ensure continuity over the first five years of treatment.

3. Specialized inpatient beds. Seven beds in one of the units servicing psychotic patients (29 beds a total of 97 beds in the hospital) will be reserved for patients going through the first five years of a psychotic disorder (affective and non-affective psychosis). Specific guidelines will be implemented regarding use of atypical antipsychotics, low dose strategy, family support, and involvement of case managers during hospitalization. Group sessions giving information about psychosis already exist and will be adapted to the early phase of the disorder.

Table 15.1 The Lausanne program for early psychosis intervention		
Problem	**Strategy**	
	Available resources	**Development needed**
Treatment delay	Information in the department Information in high schools	Conferences, symposia
Difficulty of access	Community treatment team	
Absence of community assessment	Community treatment team	
Traumatizing admissions	Negotiation before admission with community treatment team	Seven specialized inpatient beds
Lack of treatment continuity, linkage failure	Community treatment team	Two × 0.5 case managers
Medication		Clear guidelines and monitoring tools
Medication	Increase side effects monitoring	Low dose strategy
Information on psychosis	Patient groups	Tools adapted for early psychosis
Family support	Family groups Family associations	Tools adapted for early psychosis
Lack of specific information tools		Translation of international pamphlets
Lack of specific recovery phase therapy	Intensification of collaboration with CBT practitioners	Translation of international tools
Lack of research activity	Competent research teams	Development of specific research projects
CBT, cognitive behavioral therapy		

In addition we will benefit from existing resources, which we will adapt for the needs of young patients:

- To tackle delays in treatment, beside the organization of conferences symposia, and development of personalized contacts with primary care services and providers, information sessions have recently started in high schools and professional schools.

- Early family intervention (debriefing sessions) and family psychoeducation sessions have been proposed for six years for relatives of schizophrenia-spectrum patients. These sessions will be adapted and proposed to families of patients involved in the program.
- Motivational intervention for cannabis abuse: In the framework of a research project, a study will be conducted to assess the efficacy of brief motivational intervention for cannabis abuse.

Research

Finally, research being a strong motor for innovation, motivation, and the development of expertise, various research groups working in the psychiatry department will be involved in the development of projects in the following fields: neurosciences, psychopharmacology, cognitive behavioral therapy, cognitive dysfunction, and evaluative reseach. Funding for research remains however a major hurdle to these developments.

Concluding comments

Despite the availability of a wide range of treatment facilities for psychiatric disorders, first episode psychosis patients face similar difficulties in Switzerland as elsewhere. The limited amount of financial support forced us to develop a simple structure and to rely on reallocation of existing resources in order to start the project. The rapid recruitment of 30 cases in the first three months since implementation of the program in April 2004 will however give momentum to the project and hopefully justify its devclopment in the next few years.

References

1. Norman RMG, Malla AK. Duration of untreated psychosis: a critical examination of the concept and its importance. Psychol Med 2001; **31:**381–400.
2. Pelosi A, Birchwood M. Is early intervention for psychosis a waste of valuable resources? Br J Psychiatry 2003; **182:**196–8.
3. Burns T, Fioritti A, Holloway F, et al. Case management and assertive community treatment in Europe. Psychiatr Serv 2001; **52:**631–6.
4. Bonsack C, Pfister T, Conus P, et al. Predictors of adherence to treatment after first hospitalisation for a psychotic episode. Schizophr Res 2002; **53**(suppl 3):198.
5. Conus P, Bonsack C, Gommeret E, Philippoz R. Le soutien psychiatrique Intensif dans le Milieu (SIM) à Lausanne: un projet pilote. Rev Méd Suisse Romande 2001; **121**(6):475–81.

16

Models of Service Delivery in Early Intervention Teams: UK Variations

Ruth I Ohlsen and Lyn S Pilowsky

Introduction

Research into first episode psychosis has burgeoned over the past few years, and specialized services have become established in many centers worldwide. Early intervention services arise from the 'critical window' hypothesis.[1] The early period after the onset of psychotic illness presents significant opportunities for secondary prevention, stabilizing developing disabilities, reducing treatment resistance, and influencing the way people view and treat their illness. There is evidence that 66% of all suicides in this group occur in the first six years.[2,3] Relapse risk is as high as 80%.[4] Optimal management of first episode psychosis is thought to maximize chances of full recovery, and minimize the likelihood of relapse and comorbidity.[5] Interventions should, ideally, be intense and multimodal[6] and sustained over at least two years.[7] Several service models for managing first episode psychosis have been developed.[6,8,9] These services are in the early stages of development, however, and a definitive treatment model has yet to be established.[10]

The UK government has called for all National Health Service (NHS) Trusts to provide specialized early intervention teams by the end of 2004, and has developed commissioning guidelines for their establishment with the National Service Framework (NSF).[11] The proposed and existing care models, while still being decided on and varying between localities, span a range of logistical, economic, and philosophical constructs.

What are the requirements for a specialized early intervention service? How can such services be constructed and implemented to provide the most clinically and socially effective care? This chapter will examine some different early intervention care models, from a logistical and a philosophical viewpoint.

Requirements of an early episode psychosis service

According to the NSF, several vital qualities should set apart an effective early episode psychosis service from its standardized mental health delivery model counterpart. These are:

- Acceptability for young people
- Accessibility/reduced waiting time for assessment
- Non-stigmatizing environment
- Collaborative treatment planning
- Willingness to initiate early, appropriate treatment,[12] involving identification of treatment resistance and assertive provision of appropriate interventions, such as clozapine treatment and cognitive therapy
- Holistic approach: not solely focused on

symptom reduction, but committed to improving functional, social, and vocational outcome

- Engagement with and involvement of carers/significant others[13]
- Addresses the specific needs of people with first episode psychosis
- Assertive vocational rehabilitation and de-stigmatization
- Risk assessment and prevention of suicide
- Identification and treatment of comorbidity[14]
- Prevention of physical morbidity and healthy lifestyle promotion[15,16]
- Relapse prevention and crisis planning.

While these remain the abiding principles of care provision for this group, other factors will necessarily come into play when planning care delivery and organization. These include:

- Size of the population catchment area
- Inclusion criteria, such as lower and upper age limits, diagnosis
- Cultural and ethnic composition of the catchment area
- Mode of referral to service
- Research remit of the service.

Table 16.1 amplifies the factors affecting planning and delivery.

Logistically, services may be placed within the existing mental healthcare structure in three main ways. The adoption of any of these models may be based on economic considerations more than clinical or philosophical credos.

Model 1

A 'stand-alone', independent specialist first episode team that manages care wholly from initial presentation up to two to three years later (the NSF recommends three years). This model has been adopted in and around several locations in London and throughout the UK. Examples of this are Lambeth early onset team (LEO), St. Georges' Team.

Model 2

A specialist service 'embedded' in the existing structure, which may consist of one or more specially trained members of staff who work within the team and provide key-worker input to first episode patients. To our knowledge, there are no working examples of this model in the UK at present.

Model 3

A 'hub-and-spokes' model, where primary care and care program approach (CPA) responsibility is held by the mainstream mental health service (the 'spokes'), but specialist input is provided by a team of dedicated first episode experts (the 'hub'). The specialist team may provide advice, consultancy, and therapy in such areas as medication review and management, cognitive behavioral interventions, compliance therapy, diet, exercise and lifestyle, vocational rehabilitation, and family work. Examples of this are the Southwark First Onset Psychosis Service (FIRST Team) and Birmingham Early Onset Team.

All three models have advantages and disadvantages in the level and quality of care they can provide. The advantages and disadvantages of these care models are detailed in Tables 16.2–16.4

Table 16.1 Factors affecting service planning and delivery

Size of catchment area (geographical)	Geographically large catchment areas may benefit from several specialist sites, and decentralized referral points staffed by personnel trained in first episode issues.
Population of catchment area	Large populations will naturally require more staff, but during the planning process, a 'needs assessment' should be undertaken to ascertain how many new cases of psychosis might be expected to present during a given time period (e.g. a year). The incidence and prevalence of psychosis will be higher in areas with high rates of unemployment, homelessness, deprivation, immigration, asylum seekers, and ethnic minorities than in more affluent, homogenous areas, and will require higher staffing levels and more intensive input from staff in the absence of family or other community support.
Composition of catchment area	As stated above, demographics will dictate specific needs. Areas with diverse ethnic composition should take account of the special needs of ethnic populations and ensure that appropriate support is available, and that staff have a working knowledge of cultural issues affecting and relating to mental healthcare delivery.
Service inclusion criteria (age)	Upper and lower age limits need to be defined. Consultation and liaison with Child and Adolescent Mental Health Services should occur at an early stage of planning to ensure seamless transition between services. Defining lower and upper age entry to services may depend on the amount of money available. Age limits into services in the UK range from 14–18 yrs (lower) and 27–65 yrs (upper).
Service inclusion criteria (diagnostic)	This will depend on the nature of the service (i.e. is it a prodromal service, in which entry criteria will be defined according to symptomatology and family history?). Early psychosis services will require a diagnosis of psychosis, but some services may restrict this to people presenting with schizophreniform psychoses and exclude affective psychoses. Comorbid conditions, such as organic illness, learning disability, or substance misuse, may be grounds for exclusion, although substance misuse remains a significant correlate of early episode psychosis, and excluding this group from a specialist service would involve denying a large proportion of patients urgently needed treatment. As diagnosis at a very early stage of illness may not be particularly relevant or accurate, many clinicians prefer symptom-based treatment.

continues

Table 16.1 continued	
Mode of referral to the service	Again, the service remit will dictate this. Prodromal services may outreach directly to and accept referrals directly from non-health related social/community organs, such as schools, churches, and youth clubs. Many referrals will also come from primary care. An early psychosis service will accept referrals from secondary care, most will accept referrals from primary care, and there may be referrals directly from the community facilities listed above. Individuals who are floridly psychotic may come to the attention of mental health services via the police/legal system. Both services will probably accept self-referrals.
Research remit	Whether a service intends to carry out research, or act purely as a clinical care model, will have financial implications. More funding will probably be available if research is ongoing. This will increase the number of staff available, and possibly improve the quality and intensity of care offered.

Table 16.2 The 'stand-alone' model	
Advantages	**Disadvantages**
Acquisition of expert, skilled staff	Potential problems in 'poaching' staff from existing mainstream services[17]
Ability to focus skills on one specific area	Staff from mainstream services feel 'deskilled'
Opportunity for development of specialist skills and expertise	More expensive to set up and run
Single point of contact for patients and carers	Money involved in setting up such a service could be perhaps better spent on the improvement and development of existing services, rather than leaching funds from them into a service, the efficacy and value of which has not been conclusively/systematically proven[17]
Continuity of care at critical stage[1,7]	
Provision of holistic, first episode specific service incorporating clinical, vocational, and functional outcome expectations	
Allows flexibility of care	
Where inpatient care is necessary, provides a more appropriate, user-friendly, less 'toxic' environment on a specialist first episode ward	
Care can be individually tailored and 'user friendly'	

Table 16.3 The 'embedded' model

Advantages	Disadvantages
Inexpensive to run	Fewer specialized staff members – potential staffing problems during periods of sickness, annual leave, etc.
	Potential for specialist staff roles to be subsumed into mainstream work and ethos
Potential for mainstream staff to develop skills and expertise in dealing with first episode patients	Little opportunity for the development of expertise on site
	Potential problems with supervision and access to expert opinion and help
	Potential safety issues – lack of staff to perform paired domiciliary visits if needed
	No identified geographic center or point of contact

Table 16.4 The 'hub-and-spokes' model (see also Figure 16.1)

Advantages	Disadvantages
Inexpensive to run	Potential for confusion about clinical/treatment boundaries between specialist service and mainstream service, on the part of clinicians, patients, and carers
Centralized area of expertise	May compromise continuity of care – 'too many cooks'
Provides an opportunity to train mainstream staff in specialized areas of expertise	May allow quiet, or less severely ill patients to 'fall through the net' and not receive specialist intervention
Allows individualization and flexibility of care	Effectiveness depends on mainstream staff not versed in specific first episode issues to identify needs and refer for specialist input
Allows continuity of care	

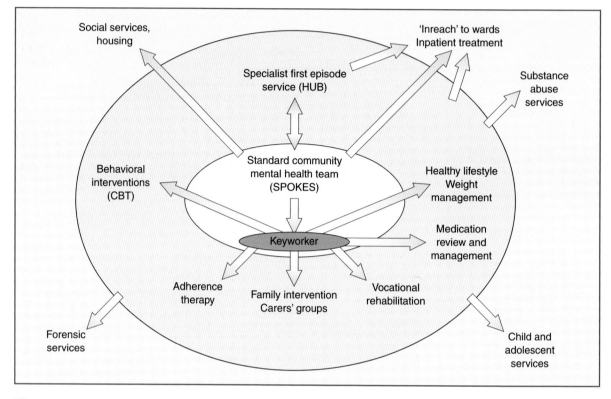

Figure 16.1 A schematic of the 'hub-and-spokes' model: CBT, cognitive behavioral therapy

Specific requirements of first episode teams may be met by some of these models, whereas without a dedicated service, some may be difficult to implement (see Table 16.5)

Early intervention

When to intervene, or 'How early is too early?'

The clinical basis for early intervention is still a matter of much debate.[17] At what stage clinical intervention ought to occur is controversial, and has political as well as clinical implications (Table 16.6). While some early intervention services focus on identifying high risk groups in the pro-dromal stage, most intervene only when psychotic features are already clearly present.

A working example of the 'hub-and-spokes' model

The Southwark First Onset Psychosis Service (FIRST Team) was a specialist community-based mental health team in the London Borough of Southwark caring for individuals in the first or early stages of a psychotic illness. The service was set up in January 2001 and initially funded by a charitable research grant with a view to further expansion of the service and funding from main-stream sources should this approach prove effect-ive. The FIRST Team worked in conjunction with existing resources as a 'hub-and-spokes' model. The level of funding required for a stand-alone service was prohibitive, and the potential value of merging and co-working with existing services (community mental health teams [CMHTs]), rather than developing a discrete service, lay in

Table 16.5 Requirements of the three models

Requirement	'Stand-alone'	'Embedded'	'Hub-and-spokes'
Addresses the specific needs of people with first episode psychosis	Yes	No	Yes
Acceptability for young people	Yes	No	Yes
Accessibility/ reduced waiting time for assessment	Yes	Probably not	Yes
Non-stigmatizing environment	Yes	No	Yes
Collaborative treatment planning	Yes	Maybe	Yes
Initiation of early, appropriate treatment, identification of treatment resistance, and assertive provision of appropriate interventions, such as clozapine and cognitive therapy	Yes	Maybe—staffing shortages may mitigate against this, requiring outside referral	Yes
Holistic approach: not solely focused on symptom reduction, but committed to improving functional, social, and vocational outcome	Yes	As above	Yes
Engagement with and involvement of carers/significant others	Yes	Maybe	Yes
Assertive vocational rehabilitation and destigmatization	Yes	Maybe—may need outside referral	Yes
Risk assessment and prevention of suicide	Yes	Yes	Yes
Identification and treatment of comorbidity	Yes	Maybe	Yes
Prevention of physical morbidity and healthy lifestyle promotion	Yes	Maybe	Yes
Relapse prevention and crisis planning	Yes	Yes	Yes

ensuring continuity of care was maintained, and the opportunity for CMHT personnel to be trained. This facilitated subsequent dissemination of expertise within mainstream psychiatric services. The co-working 'hub-and-spokes' model also addressed the controversial issue of diverting funding from existing services to specialist teams, the value of which had not yet been systematically audited.

All aspects of the service were comprehensively evaluated for both research and audit purposes. Specialist services such as these are a major cost to the health service, and we were required to demonstrate whether this type of service was effective before Health Authority funding could be invested.

Quantitative outcome measures indicated significant improvements in symptoms, cognition,

Table 16.6 The case for and against early intervention at the prodromal stage	
For intervention	**Against intervention**
Prevention of neurotoxicity caused by psychosis[7]	Misidentification—'false positives' receiving potentially harmful medications
Prevention of neurodegeneration occurring at the onset of psychosis[18]	Potential for stigmatization at a vulnerable stage because of misidentification
Prevention of functional, academic, and social decline at a critical stage	Not cost effective
Prevention of a long prodrome and subsequent poor prognosis	Leaches money from resources that could otherwise be channelled into improving care for people with established illness
Opportunity to engage with user-specific, user-friendly services at a critical stage	'Need to treat'—40% go on to develop psychosis within 1–2 yrs
Research	
Prevention of the onset of frank psychotic symptoms by means of cognitive behavioral intervention may be possible at an early stage[12]	

functioning, and quality of life. The FIRST Team also wanted to explore the experiences of service users to establish the specific elements of the service that users did or did not find helpful and beneficial. Their views were considered essential for informing future service provision.

Referrals

Referrals were accepted from CMHTs, early detection services, and psychiatric emergency services. Primary care referrals were diverted to the appropriate CMHT for assessment, with the expectation of rapid referral to FIRST. Flexible service provision ensured that patients who needed to be seen in their homes on a daily basis were accommodated, or that patients who worked could be seen before or after their working day. Early intervention and rapid response were a priority—patients were seen where possible, within hours of presenting to psychiatric services, or when presentation occurred after hours or on weekends, within 48 hours.

Intervention

The interventions offered by FIRST were based on the standards set out in the NSF Commissioning Guidelines. All patients were offered care 'modules' according to their individual needs. We adopted a collaborative approach to care, and regarded continuing engagement with the service as a vital prevention strategy. A keyworker was identified at an early stage to stay with the patient throughout the first two years. The keyworker was either part of the sector CMHT, or a FIRST Team member. CPA responsibility for patients was allocated on an ad-hoc basis.

Medication management

A thorough psychiatric and physical review was undertaken. Quantitative outcomes were assessed by means of standardized psychiatric symptom and side effect rating scales at baseline and regular intervals thereafter. This approach was integral to assessing treatment response and identifying treatment resistance. Patients requiring a change in their medication regime were switched, and the switching process managed by the specialist service in collaboration with the referring CMHT. FIRST acted in accordance with the National Institute for Clinical Excellence (NICE) guidelines, by recommending first line treatment with an atypical antipsychotic and adopting a collaborative approach to treatment. Where appropriate, and with the patient's permission, family and carers were involved in treatment planning.

Where treatment response remained incomplete, or residual symptoms remained, FIRST initiated clozapine treatment or suggested referral for psychosocial intervention.

Additional interventions
Assertive vocational rehabilitation and job coaching

This module addressed destigmatization by re-establishing and reintegrating first episode patients into their vocational and social milieu at the earliest possible opportunity. Data from the FIRST service suggested that high level support was necessary to enhance motivation and ensure continuing attendance at retraining schemes. A dedicated job coach, with well established links to work retraining schemes, mainstream employers willing to employ people with mental health problems, local colleges and voluntary work organizations, was available to work alongside patients wishing to go back to work, training, or to continue education. Neuropsychological testing proved a valuable tool in assessing patients' premorbid functioning, which was taken into account when planning vocational rehabilitation.

Healthy lifestyle program

Schizophrenia per se appears to be a risk factor for poor physical health.[15,16] Given this pre-existing vulnerability, it is incumbent on clinicians to monitor and take active steps to enhance the physical health of patients in the early stages of schizophrenia.

FIRST provided a weight management intervention comprising dietary planning, exercise (weekly exercise classes and individualized training programs), and motivational interviewing. This approach successfully mitigated against significant antipsychotic-induced weight gain, provided structured healthy activity, and raised awareness of health, fitness, and lifestyle issues at an early stage in the illness.

In order to confirm psychiatric diagnosis, monitor physical health, and prevent or recognize early signs of iatrogenic disease,[19] some physical measures were taken including regular weight, body mass index (BMI), and blood tests (urea and electrolytes, liver function test, glucose, triglycerides, prolactin).

Assessment and treatment of comorbidity (substance misuse)

The most significant predictor of non-compliance is comorbid substance misuse.[14] Identifying and treating substance misuse in this population is integral to diagnosis, effective treatment, and prevention of relapse.

Patients with a dual diagnosis were referred to specialist substance misuse services.

Assessment of risk

This was undertaken and discussed with the team. Suicide risk was monitored on an ongoing basis, by means of a standardized risk assessment instrument and other standardized, internationally validated measures (Calgary Depression Scale in Schizophrenia, Beck Hopelessness Scale).

Carer workshops and education groups

The FIRST Team provided education and support for families and carers on both an individual and a group basis. Where necessary, families were referred to specialist family intervention services for assessment and ongoing therapy. The FIRST team package:

- Provided up to date information about mental illness, treatments, and side effect management

- Promoted awareness of the role carers can play in relapse prevention, by briefly discussing issues such as expressed emotion
- Enabled recognition of early signs of relapse, and appropriate responses
- Taught simple problem-solving techniques, using examples from participants' personal experience
- Provided a milieu whereby families and friends can support each other, and share their experiences
- Alleviated guilt felt by families and carers, and encouraged them to pay attention to their own needs
- Promoted awareness of community facilities, such as community mental health teams, support organizations, retraining facilities, and other services, such as befrienders and user groups.

A user evaluation of the service in which patients were asked to feed back their experiences of and 'journey' through the service was conducted using the focus group interview technique.

The data analysis revealed several emergent themes that highlighted the aspects of the service deemed to be most helpful:

- Collaborative approach to treatment: vital in terms of gaining trust and allowing the patient to assume responsibility for their treatment
- Ease of access to and flexibility of the service
- Structured interventions centred on vocational rehabilitation
- Healthy lifestyle package.

Conclusions

The holistic approach offered by the FIRST Team appears to have been beneficial in terms of promoting recovery, effecting good functional outcome, and preventing relapse. In terms of clinical outcome, the interventions offered were effective, and served also to enhance social and vocational functioning. Perhaps even more significantly, feedback from the service users indicated

that the treatment package was accessible, non-stigmatizing, and provided a safe environment that promoted continuing engagement and a positive experience of mental health services at an early and vulnerable stage.

Acknowledgments

The authors would like to thank AstraZeneca for funding the FIRST study through an unrestricted charitable grant, and also the Medical Research Council who funded Dr Lyn Pilowsky.

References

1. Birchwood M, Todd P, Jackson C. Early intervention in psychosis: the critical period hypothesis. Br J Psychiatry 1998; **172**(Suppl 33):53–9.
2. Westermeyer JF, Harrow M, Marengo JT. Risk for suicide in schizophrenia and other psychotic and non-psychotic disorders. J Nerv Ment Dis 1991; **179**:259–66.
3. Mortensen PB, Juel K. Mortality and the causes of death in first admitted schizophrenic patients. Br J Psychiatry 1993; **163**:183–9.
4. Shepherd M, Watt D, Falloon I. The natural history of schizophrenia: a five-year follow-up in a representative sample of schizophrenics. Psychol Med 1989; **15**(Monograph Suppl):53–9.
5. Power P, Elkins K, Adlard S, et al. Analysis of the initial treatment phase in first-episode psychosis. Br J Psychiatry 1998; **172**(Suppl 33):71–6.
6. Preston NJ. Predicting community survival in early psychosis and schizophrenia populations after receiving intensive case management. Aust N Z J Psychiatry 2000; **34**:122–6.
7. Birchwood M. The critical period for early intervention. In Birchwood M, Fowler D, Jackson C (eds). *Early Intervention in Psychosis.* Chichester: Wiley, 2000; 28–63.
8. Jackson C, Farmer A. Early intervention in psychosis. J Ment Health 1998; **7**(2):157–64.
9. McGorry PD, Edwards J, Mihalopoulos C, et al. EPPIC: An evolving system of early detection and optimal management. Schizophr Bull 1996; **22**(2): 305–25.
10. Verdoux H. Have the times come for early inter-

vention in psychosis? Acta Psychiatr Scand 2001; **103**:321–2.

11. National Services Framework (UK) at: http://www. iris-initiative.org.uk (accessed January 2004).

12. Gleeson J, Larsen TK, McGorry P. Psychological treatment in pre- and early psychosis. J Am Acad Psychoanal Dyn Psychiatry 2003; **31**(1):229–45.

13. Tennakoon L, Fannon D, Doku V, et al. Experience of caregiving: relatives of people experiencing a first episode psychosis. Br J Psychiatry 2001; **178**:575.

14. Bebbington PE. The content and context of compliance. Int Clin Psychopharmacology 1995; **9**(Suppl 5):41–50.

15. Brown S, Birtwhistle J, Roe L, Thompson C. The unhealthy lifestyle of people with schizophrenia. Psychol Med 1999; **29**(3):697–701.

16. Ryan M, Thakore J. Physical consequences of schizophrenia and its treatment. The metabolic syndrome. Life Sci 2002; **71**(3):239–57.

17. Pelosi AJ, Birchwood M. Is early intervention for psychosis a waste of valuable resources? Br J Psychiatry 2003; **182**:196–8.

18. Pantellis C, Velakoulis D, McGorry PD, et al. Neuroroanatomical abnormalities before and after onset of psychosis: a cross-sectional and longitudinal MRI comparison. Lancet 2003; **361**(9354): 281–8.

19. Nasrallah HA, Mulvihill T. Iatrogenic disorders associated with conventional vs atypical antipsychotics. Ann Clin Psychiatry 2001; **13**:215–37.

17

Implementing Early Detection and Intervention in Psychosis: The German Approach

Thomas Wobrock, Peter Falkai, and Wolfgang Gaebel

Introduction

Approximately 1% of the population worldwide will develop schizophrenia in their lifetime. Despite modern treatment techniques, schizophrenia still presents an enormous burden to the patients and their relatives and reduces quality of life especially due to chronic impairment in two thirds of cases. Of people suffering from schizophrenia, 10–15% commit suicide. Schizophrenia is the most expensive psychiatric disorder, with direct and indirect treatment in Germany costing a total of approximately €3.5 billion annually.

Many efforts have been made to influence the disabling course of the disease. Shortening the period of untreated psychosis has now become a primary goal. Mental health services, primary care, and individual clinicians have searched for strategies to reduce delays in accessing treatment. Strategies to reduce duration of untreated psychosis (DUP) include improving recognition through education and awareness, increasing referrals through providing a responsive user friendly service, and reducing fear and stigma associated with psychiatric services. Psychiatric services have to provide easy access, rapid response on demand, a flexible approach, and assertive outreach.

Retrospective assessment of patients with first episode schizophrenia showed that social functioning is already impaired before the first psychotic symptoms appear. Focusing on the initial prodromal stage allowed the development of instruments to predict transition into full-blown psychosis and to characterize subgroups of patients and young people in a high risk state.

Reducing the duration of untreated psychotic illness (DUI) recently entered into the scope of clinicians worldwide. Programs for early recognition and early intervention have been initiated and the first results of controlled studies evaluating the influence of psychotherapeutic and pharmacotherapeutic strategies are encouraging. A range of ethical and conceptual issues needs to be considered in relation to this emerging field. The concept of indicated prevention supports this approach from an ethical point of view, especially as patients suffer from significant disability and are seeking help.

This chapter highlights the German approach to diagnosing and treating early psychosis. Many of the ideas of German psychiatrists at the beginning of the last century dealing with the prodromal phases of schizophrenia (e.g. Bleuler, Schneider, Huber, Conrad) were adopted from other countries and included in more pragmatic approaches to research as well as inpatient and outpatient care. Implementation of psychiatric services aiming at early intervention was successful in Scandinavia (e.g. TIPS, 1997), Australia (e.g. EPPIC, 1992), Canada (e.g. EPP, PEPP, 1996), the UK (e.g. EIS, 1995), and Germany (e.g. FETZ, 1997). Even if today's literature is full of interesting results and recommendations of Australian and North American centers, this article summarizes German activities in this area, which are closely linked to the roots of early prodromal research in Germany.

Development of early detection: historical background

In 1896, the German psychiatrist Emil Kraepelin developed his concept of dementia praecox from the poor outcome of the psychotic patients he observed. He has been accused of being the architect of an entrenched pessimism due to the former nihilistic treatment possibilities in the pre-neuroleptic era. Nevertheless, he pointed out that it may be of the greatest practical importance to diagnose cases of dementia praecox at an early stage. The German psychiatrist Eugen Bleuler, introducing the term 'schizophrenia' to psychiatry, noted in 1908 that the sooner the patients remit to their former level of functioning and the less they are allowed to withdraw into a world of their own, the better will be their prognosis.

Further research on the course of schizophrenia demonstrated that a considerable proportion of patients recover or display only very mild deficits. In a review of 44 long-term follow-up studies (mean follow-up more than 10 years), in 17 studies the proportion of fully recovered patients was between 21% and 30%.[1] An early occurrence of negative symptoms and a prolonged onset of illness predicted a poor outcome in these studies.

One of the early German follow-up studies (Bonn study) demonstrated that most schizophrenics are not continuously experiencing psychotic symptoms, but suffer from more-or-less uncharacteristic 'basic deficiencies'.[2] Therefore, the 'basic symptom' concept was developed stepwise from the beginning of the 1950s. Basic symptoms are considered to be nearer to the 'somatic substrate' than the psychotic end-phenomena and comprise subtle, often only self-experienced deficiencies in several domains. They can occur in prepsychotic outpost syndromes, prodromes, and postpsychotic reversible and irreversible basic stages.[3] For standardized assessment and documentation, the Bonn Schedule for the Assessment of Basic Symptoms (BSABS) was introduced, a rating scale reliable for demonstrating self-reported impairments of the patients. In the Bonn study it was observed that complete remissions were more seldom the longer the (untreated) prodromes last, or in other words, the duration of untreated illness (DUI) was associated with poor outcome. In 1970, a prospective study was initiated to investigate basic symptoms as early signs of a developing psychosis. The rate of transition into schizophrenic psychosis with first rank symptoms after a mean follow-up of 7.5 years was 31.2%. In this sample, cognitive basic symptoms like thought interference, thought blockade, disturbances of receptive speech in reading and listening were seen most frequently. Based on this data it was possible to differentiate from a sample of patients with neurotic or psychopathic personality disorders a subgroup with a highly significant increased risk of developing schizophrenia at a later stage.

At the same time as Huber et al. conceptualized the basic symptom approach, K Conrad, later the head of the University Clinic of Saarland, systematically investigated recruits admitted for unspecific or psychotic signs to a military hospital. From the description of subjective, self-reported changes in mood, thoughts, and behavior, and observed objective psychopathological phenomena of mostly first episode psychosis, he developed a stage-specific model of beginning schizophrenia. This stepwise model of understanding the progressive deterioration and disintegration of psychic functions was particularly influential in German psychiatry. Nearly 40 years later the ABC Schizophrenia Study (Age, Beginning, Course) confirmed his hypothesized first stage 'Trema' occurring with high frequency, but not the presumed order of the two following phases (Apophänie, then Apokalypse).[4]

To study the assumed later onset of illness in women with schizophrenia and therefore to investigate further for the pathogenetic issues of the disease, a reliable instrument for the retrospective assessment of the onset of schizophrenia (IRAOS) was developed. This semistructured interview became the basis of the Mannheimer ABC Study, an investigation of 232 patients aged 12–59 years with first illness episodes of broadly defined schizophrenia. This sample comprised 84% of all patients admitted for the first time with a diagnosis of schizophrenia to 10 hospitals, representing a catchment area of nearly 1.5 million people. Much of our knowledge about the initial prodrome, and the later rationale on early detection and intervention, came from the results of this study. The prodromal stage with a mean duration of five years and the psychotic pre-stage, from the first positive symptoms to the full-blown psychosis, with an average duration of 1.3 years, characterizes the window for early treatment.[5]

Framework of early detection and intervention

The Cologne Early Recognition (CER) study prospectively investigated the predictive accuracy of basic symptoms in 160 of 338 patients. Almost half of the patients developed schizophrenia during the follow-up period of 9.6 years. The absence of prodromal symptoms excluded a subsequent schizophrenia with a probability of 96%, whereas their presence predicted schizophrenia with a probability of 70%, certain disturbances even up to 91%.[6]

Contributing to basic symptoms, and as a result of the cited studies, the Early Recognition Inventory (ERI) was developed. For further investigations, items from the ERI and the IRAOS of the Mannheimer group were taken to construct a new valid instrument (ERIraos), a structured interview of 110 items. This inventory includes modules to

estimate the risk due to pre- and/or perinatal complications, substance abuse, and genetic risks (family history), and also documents social functioning, forensic problems, relatives' reports of changes in behavior, and subtle self-experienced impairments. Ten basic symptoms precisely described in ERIraos showing high prognostic accuracy were selected to create inclusion criteria for diagnosing the early initial prodromal state (EIPS). The presence of additional risk factors (first degree relative with schizophrenia/schizophrenia spectrum disorder or pre- and/or perinatal complications) and evidence for a decline in functioning were further items added to the EIPS (see Table 17.1).

The late initial prodromal state (LIPS), which is assumed to have a higher probability of transition to schizophrenia than EIPS, is defined analogously to the Australian ultra-high risk criteria (see Table 17.2). Trait risk factors are not part of the definition of LIPS. The definitions of EIPS and LIPS presented here serve as inclusion criteria for different stage-specific treatment strategies in the early detection and intervention programs, being part of the German Research Network on Schizophrenia. The network collates information from several German centers which deal with the problem of early detection of psychosis and develops effective treatment strategies.

Early detection and intervention

The German Network on Schizophrenia (KNS: Kompetenz Netzwerk Schizophrenie) is one of 14 competence networks in the field of medicine in Germany.[12] It is supported by the Federal Ministry for Research and Education to bring together the leading research institutes (horizontal network) and qualified routine care facilities (vertical network) to provide better care for patients suffering from schizophrenia. Approximately 20 psychiatric university clinics, including child and adolescent psychiatry, 14 state, district, and specialized hospitals, and six psychiatric and general practice networks are integrated in this

Table 17.1 The early initial prodromal state (EIPS)

Self-experienced neuropsychological deficits (basic symptoms)

Presence of at least one of the following symptoms:

- Thought interference
- Compulsive perseverance of thoughts
- Thought pressure
- Thought blockade
- Disturbances of receptive language, either heard or read
- Decreased ability to discriminate between ideas and perception, fantasy and true memories
- Unstable ideas of reference (subject-centrism)
- Derealization
- Visual perceptual disturbances (blurred vision, transitory blindness, partial seeing, hypersensitivity to light, etc.)
- Acoustic perceptual disturbances (hypersensitivity to sound or noise, etc.)

Occurrence in the last 3 months prior to the study for several times a week

AND/OR

Reduction in the Global Assessment of Functioning Score (GAF)
According to DSM-IV of at least 30 points within the past year

AND

At least one of the following risk factors:

- First degree relative with a lifetime diagnosis of schizophrenia or a schizophrenia spectrum disorder
- Pre- or perinatal complications

Table 17.2 The late initial prodromal state (LIPS)

Attenuated positive symptoms

Presence of at least one of the following symptoms:

- Ideas of reference
- Odd belief or magical thinking
- Unusual perceptual experience
- Odd thinking and speech
- Suspiciousness and paranoid ideation

Symptoms have to appear several times per week for a period of at least one week during the three months prior to the study

AND/OR

Brief limited intermittent psychotic symptoms (BLIPS)

- Duration of episode less than one week, interval between episodes at least one week
- Symptoms resolve spontaneously
- Presence of at least one of the following symptoms during the three months prior to the study:
  - Hallucinations
  - Delusions
  - Formal thought disorder
  - Gross disorganized or catatonic behavior

institution. The KNS has an orientation towards the vulnerability-stress-coping-illness model in scientific and routine clinical care projects. One of the main goals is the use of basic research results for the development of course and therapy predictors, and the development and evaluation of strategies for early recognition and early intervention at all stages of the illness. Furthermore, a stage-specific integration of strategies of primary, secondary, and tertiary prevention into clinical practice will be developed. The aims of the KNS are to:

- Advance early discovery and recognition of people at risk of developing schizophrenia through the development and evaluation of an early recognition inventory
- Optimize prevention of first episode psychosis through psychological and pharmacological early treatment in people identified to be at risk
- Optimize acute and long-term treatment of first episodes of schizophrenia
- Improve relapse prevention through relapse prediction and early intervention guided by a prodrome based early intervention algorithm
- Improve treatment quality through the use of guidelines in inpatient and outpatient settings
- Prevent the illness from becoming chronic through specific rehabilitation
- Proceed in research into the biological and genetic foundations of the disorder
- Apply the findings of basic research to treatment practice
- Analyse the benefit and cost of innovative treatment procedures
- Improve education and information for lay people, relatives, and experts through specific application of knowledge.

To improve awareness of early psychosis, several options for educating the public or distributing specific information were developed. The network provides educational materials for primary medical care as well as for advisory

---

Table 17.3 Checklist for early signs of psychotic illness

Do you agree with the following statements, describing your current life?	Yes	No

1. You keep silent and avoid social activities.
2. You become shy in contact with others.
3. You have felt sad over several weeks.
4. You have developed sleep disturbance and less appetite.
5. Your way of moving, thinking, and talking has slowed down.
6. Your engagement and motivation in school, education, job, and leisure time has diminished.
7. You have neglected personal care, health, and hygiene.
8. You are often nervous and tense and cannot relax.
9. You frequently enter into discussion, conflicts, and struggle with others.
10. Thoughts are intrusive.
11. You often have the impression that you are let down and misused by other people.
12. Some events in your daily routine get a special meaning for you and serve as hidden hints to change your former behavior.
13. Your usual environment changes in an unreal, bizarre manner.

Have you had the following experiences at any time in your life?

14. You perceived noises or colors in your environment in an intense, unrealistic, and extraordinary manner. Or people and objects changed in shape, volume, or color and you could not explain why this happened.
15. Your own way of thinking is disturbed by other, alien thoughts.
16. You sometimes feel watched, threatened, and persecuted.
17. You saw, heard, tasted, or smelled something that other people could not detect or perceive.

Table 17.4 Psychological intervention in the early initial prodromal state (EIPS): components and main topics of the cognitive behavioral program

Individual therapy (30 sessions) focuses on:
- A therapeutic partnership/alliance with the patient
- Psychoeducation (information about the nature of the illness, treatment possibilities, personnel involved in the treatment, and future prospects)
- Analysing and managing the individual's symptoms, distress, and crisis
- Working on coping strategies
- Developing a crisis management plan including the definition of key persons for help

Group therapy (15 sessions, 4–8 participants) focuses on:
- Encouraging communication and discussion of their problems with others
- Reducing emotional distress and negative self-evaluations through group feedback
- Leaning how to build up positive activities
- Learning how to deal with close relationships and increasing social competence
- Training problem-solving strategies

Cognitive training (12 sessions, individual setting) focuses on:
- Improving concentration, attention, and memory
- Computer-based approach including daily living components

Family intervention (3 sessions) focuses on:
- Family psychoeducation
- Providing information about being at risk for early psychosis
- Giving practical advice to deal with the clients' attitudes and behavior
- Managing feelings of loss, grief, and guilt

centers and schools. Young people with an increased possible risk may be referred to early recognition centers by consultative teachers, education advice centers, and family doctors/general practitioners. To provide access to the early detection and intervention centres for the general population, a screening checklist with several self-maintained symptoms (17 items) was introduced. Using a cut-off score of positively identified items, contacting the center by phone, e-mail, or personal consultation is recommended (see the checklist in Table 17.3).

Nonetheless, after transition to first episode in schizophrenia, it is very difficult to keep these patients in treatment, which emphasizes the need for a special support program.[7] Therefore, further efforts of the KNS include the optimization of

acute and long-term treatment in schizophrenia, the development of treatment guidelines, their implementation in standard care, and the support of programs against stigma in schizophrenia. Additionally, concerted instruments for prodrome assessment enable the comparison of initial and relapse prodromes.

In addition to the focus on early detection there is the second target of early intervention. Two treatment studies were initiated for people at risk for early psychosis with the aim of improving diagnosis of prodromal syndromes, preventing social decline, and delaying progression into full-blown psychotic illness.

The treatment of prodromal schizophrenia was assisted by the development of a multimodal cognitive behavioral treatment program on the early initial prodromal state (see Table 17.4). A controlled randomized study is comparing this program with clinical management. Preliminary outcome data suggest that multimodal psychological treatment improves self-perceived neuropsychological deficits, depression, anxiety, and social decline.[8]

For those in late initial prodromal states, a pharmacological treatment with amisulpride (50–800 mg per day) or a psychologically advanced clinical management including crisis intervention and family counseling in a supportive manner is offered. These two treatment conditions are being compared in a randomized controlled parallel group design. The first preliminary results have been published. Despite the small sample size, significantly decreased psychopathology and improved general level of functioning were observed in the neuroleptic-treated group.[9]

As well as the activities of the German KNS, an increasing number of local centers for early detection and intervention are developing.

Table 17.5 German centers of early detection and intervention		
Name of the center	**Department**	**City**
Early Detection and Intervention Center (FETZ)	Psychiatry and Psychotherapy, University of Cologne (Head: Prof Dr J Klosterkötter)	Cologne
Early Detection and Intervention Center (FEZ)	Psychiatry and Psychotherapy, Heinrich-Heine-University (Head: Prof Dr W Gaebel)	Düsseldorf
Early Detection and Intervention Center (ZEBB)	Psychiatry and Psychotherapy, Rheinische Friedrich-Wilhelm-University of Bonn (Head: Prof Dr W Maier)	Bonn
Schizophrenia Research Unit Central Institute of Mental Health (ZI)	Schizophrenia Research Unit Central Institute of Mental Health (Head: Prof Dr H Häfner)	Mannheim
Early Detection and Intervention Center (FETZ)	Psychiatry and Psychotherapy, Ludwig-Maximilians-University (Head: Prof Dr HJ Möller)	Munich
Early Detection and Intervention Center (FETZ)	Psychiatry and Psychotherapy, Charité (Head: Prof Dr A Heinz)	Berlin
Heidelberg Early Adolescent and Adult Recognition and Therapy Center for Psychosis (HEART) (Frühbehandlungs-zentrum für junge Menschen in Krisen)	Psychiatry and Psychotherapy, University of Heidelberg (Heads: Prof Dr Ch Mundt, Adult Psychiatry; Prof Dr F Resch, Child and Adolescent Psychiatry)	Heidelberg
Early Detection and Intervention Center Saarland (FETS)	Psychiatry and Psychotherapy, University of Saarland (Head: Prof Dr P Falkai)	Homburg/Saar

However, work on early psychosis is in most cases still restricted to university clinics or similar institutions.

Early psychosis services in local centers

A variety of research and routine care approaches characterize work on early psychosis. For example, different centers may focus on initial prodromal states, first episode schizophrenia, or early warning signs of relapse. Table 17.5 lists most of the German centers.

Many centers involve cooperation between departments of child/adolescent psychiatry and adult psychiatry because the target group of young people aged 15–18 is at higher risk for developing psychosis. Joint facilities for treatment of early psychosis have been established in several locations (e.g. the Heidelberg Early Adolescent and Adult Recognition and Therapy Centre for Psychosis, HEART), because child psychiatry services often provide excellent psychotherapeutic interventions. However, these centers frequently lack experience with acute psychosis while adult services often lack skills in youth-oriented psychotherapeutic approaches. To lower the threshold of care access and because of the often non-specific symptoms in most help seekers, the focus lies on crisis evaluation and treatment. Staff

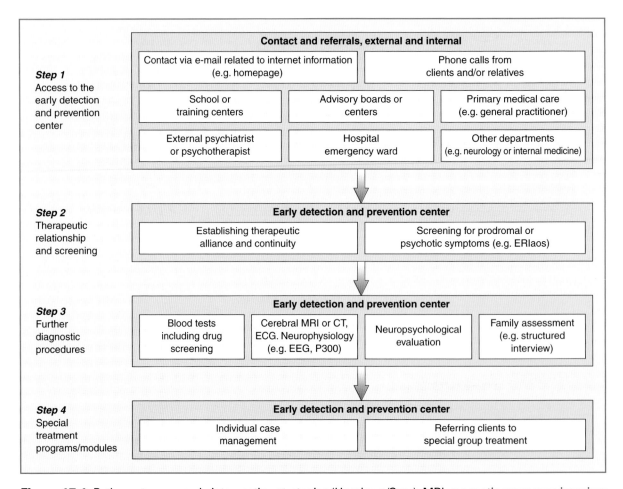

Figure 17.1 Pathway to care: early intervention strategies (Homburg/Saar). MRI, magnetic resonance imaging; CT, computed tomography; ECG, electrocardiogram; EEG, electroencephalogram; P300, event-related potential.

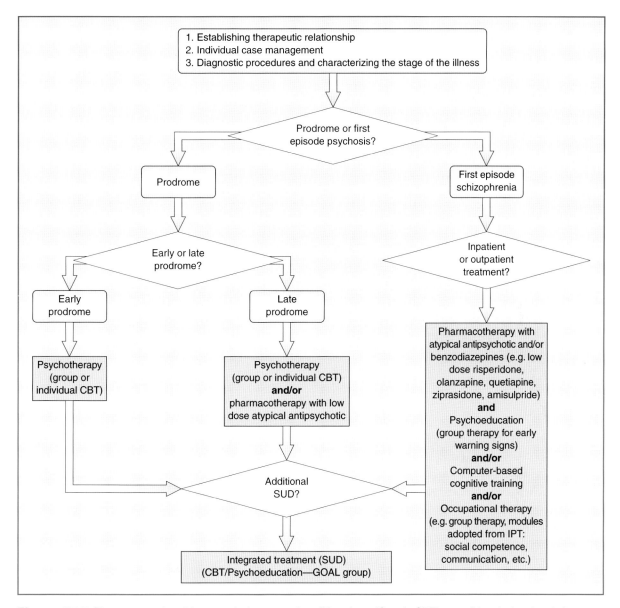

Figure 17.2 Treatment algorithm: early intervention (Homburg/Saar). CBT, cognitive behavioral therapy; SUD, substance abuse disorder; IPT, Integrated Psychological Therapy Program.

members for inpatient and outpatient care are provided by both departments and belong to the same treatment team to ensure therapeutic continuity.

Other departments of psychiatry and psychotherapy focus on the early recognition of first episode schizophrenia and the detection of early warning signs of relapse (e.g. the inpatient and outpatient service of the Homburg department of

psychiatry and psychotherapy, University of Saarland). This has led to the study of indications of relapse in schizophrenic patients.[10] In addition, an integrated treatment service for patients with schizophrenia and comorbid substance abuse has been developed. High rates of comorbidity with substance abuse occur in first episode schizophrenia. The self-medication hypothesis has been studied,[11] and substance abuse in schizophrenic patients has been found to be associated with poorer prognosis, more admissions to hospital, and medication non-adherence, if the abuse persists. As a consequence, special programs for dual diagnosis patients are going to be established in Homburg as in other centers.

Figures 17.1 and 17.2 show the pathway to care and early intervention strategies in Homburg/Saar, Germany.

Planning the therapeutic regimen in advance via a multimodular treatment setting gives more flexibility and takes the limited personnel resources into account. Working with modules allows tailoring treatment strategy to the individual needs of the client if a constant key person coordinates the therapeutic process. In Germany, this is usually a psychiatrist (physician). The key coordinator must establish a trusting relationship, provide continuity of care, and be accessible in emergency situations (psychotic or suicidal crisis).

Conclusions

The German approach to early detection and intervention does not differ substantially from other countries'. It takes a long time from the conception of the need for early treatment strategies and actual implementation in psychiatric services. Perhaps the German structure of medical care with local independent psychiatrists not being attached to a local mental heath center, together with a discouraging bureaucracy, may be responsible for the delays in translating research findings into practice. Nevertheless, the German Network on Schizophrenia is integrated into European and worldwide early detection and treatment programs and young scientists and clinicians are finally engaged in the development of better care for people with prodromal signs of psychosis.

References

1. Häfner H, an der Heiden W. Course and outcome of schizophrenia. In: Hirsch SR, Weinberger DR (eds). *Schizophrenia*, Oxford: Blackwell Science; 2003:101–41.
2. Huber G, Gross G, Schüttler R, Linz M. Longitudinal studies of schizophrenic patients. Schizophr Bull 1980; **6**:592–605.
3. Gross G, Huber H, Klosterkötter J. Early diagnosis of schizophrenia. Neurol, Psychiatry Brain Res 1992; **1**:17–22.
4. Hambrecht M, Häfner H. 'Trema, Apophänie, Apokalypse'—Ist Conrads Phasenmodell empirisch begründbar? Fortschr Neurol Psychiatr 1993; **61**:418–23.
5. Häfner H, Maurer K, Löffler W, Riecher-Rössler A. The influence of age and sex on the onset and early course of schizophrenia, Br J Psychiatry 1993; **162**:80–6.
6. Klosterkötter J, Hellmich M, Steinmeyer EM, Schultze-Lutter F. Diagnosing schizophrenia in the initial prodromal phase. Arch Gen Psychiatry 2001; **58**:158–64.
7. Gaebel W, Möller HJ, Buchkremer G, et al. Pharmacological long-term treatment strategies in first episode schizophrenia. Study design and preliminary results of an ongoing RCT within the German Research Network on Schizophrenia. Eur Arch Psychiatry Clin Neurosci 2004; **254**:129–40.
8. Bechdolf A, Wagner M, Hambrecht M. Psychological intervention in the pre-psychotic phase: preliminary results of a multicentre trial. Acta Psychiatr Scand 2002; **106**(Suppl 413):41.
9. Ruhrmann S, Schultze-Lutter F, Klosterkötter J. Early detection and intervention in the initial prodromal phase. Pharmacopsychiatry 2003; **36**(Suppl 3):S162–7.
10. Behrendt B, Sittinger H, Wobrock T. Personal relapse signature in the relapse prevention of schizophrenic patients. Paper presented at the *WAPR, 8th World Congress for Psychosocial Rehabilitation*, 3–5 August 2003, New York.
11. Wobrock T, Caspari D, Behrendt B, Sittinger H. Cannabis and psychopathology in first-episode schizophrenia. Eur Arch Psychiatr Clin Neurosci 2000; **250**(Suppl 1):I35.
12. Wölwer W, Buchremer G, Häfner H, et al. German Research Network on Schizophrenia – bridging the gap between research and care. Eur Arch Psychiatry Clin Neurosci 2003; **253**:321–9.

18

Evaluating Treatment Integrity in First Episode Psychosis Programs: Comparing What is Promised With What is Delivered

Meredith G Harris, Jane Edwards, Deepika Ratnaike, Lisa Wong, Darryl Wade, and Warrick Brewer

Introduction

The experimental evaluation of multicomponent or 'complex' treatment models, such as first episode psychosis (FEP) intervention programs, presents numerous methodological challenges.[1] There are presently few well designed studies, completed or underway, evaluating whether specialized biopsychosocial treatment of FEP, delivered at initiation of treatment for FEP, is associated with better outcomes.[2] An important study design issue is the measurement of treatment integrity. Measurement of treatment integrity is essential for demonstrating the program's capacity to provide good quality, specific treatment for FEP, and for ensuring that valid conclusions can be drawn about the effectiveness of the intervention under study.[3] Program evaluation activities, such as clinical audits and measurement of performance indicators, conducted as part of routine program operation, may help to ensure treatment integrity in routine practice. This chapter discusses the importance of treatment integrity in the evaluation of FEP programs, from both research and service delivery perspectives.

Treatment integrity in mental health services research

Treatment integrity (or treatment fidelity) is the extent to which interventions are delivered according to a defined program model.[4] In mental health services research, fidelity measures have been developed to assess the critical 'ingredients of care' of service models, particularly in assertive case management[5,6] and supported employment programs.[7,8]

The evaluation of treatment integrity addresses two key questions: What is the intervention? To what extent did the individual patient receive it? This is similar to the concept of compliance in medication trials. Inadequate description and measurement of treatment integrity may undermine the validity of an evaluation. Appraisal and replication is problematic if the intervention, including key treatment elements and constraining or enabling factors in the program environment, is not precisely described. It is then difficult to judge whether what is described is actually implemented,[1] and it may not be possible to relate client outcomes to the treatments provided.[9]

Importance of treatment integrity in evaluations of first episode psychosis programs

The evaluation of treatment integrity is of particular importance for FEP programs, for several reasons. First, there has been enormous growth and investment in early intervention in psychosis worldwide.[10,11] Evidence from controlled experimental studies, particularly randomized controlled trials, is likely to have significant impact on the scientific evidence base as well as on policymakers and funders.

Second, there is increasing support for the view that early intervention constitutes more than reducing delays into treatment. Malla and Norman argue that the impact of FEP programs is also likely to depend on the content of treatment provided during the critical period of the first five years following the onset of psychosis.[12] Treatment content should be tailored to the early phases of psychotic illness and specific to the needs and circumstances of young people, to optimize effectiveness and engagement.[12,13] Evaluative studies must be conducted in programs that can demonstrate capacity to provide good quality care that is specific to FEP, and based on up-to-date thinking and best available evidence. The results of studies conducted in services where this is not the case may underestimate the value of FEP programs.

Third, there is significant variation between intervention programs for FEP, reflecting differences in underlying philosophies, service foci, degree of specialization of the service model, and local context factors. The details of the intervention must be well described to enable judgments about whether it can be exported and implemented faithfully in another context, and can be expected to achieve the same results.[14]

The effectiveness of complex FEP intervention programs, initiated after the onset of psychosis, has been evaluated using a range of study designs.[15–23] Results from more recent studies are emerging. The following questions regarding treatment integrity may be useful in appraising the results of FEP intervention studies:

1. Are the treatments and services provided: (a) well articulated in detailed treatment manuals and service description documents; (b) replicable; and (c) reflective of best practice treatment for FEP?[2]
2. Are the treatments specific to FEP wherever possible? For example, are the psychosocial components of treatment tailored to the needs of first episode psychosis patients, or is the FEP intervention standard care supplemented by generic psychosocial interventions?
3. Are the treatments and services well tested and established in the program? It is preferable that a process of developing, documenting and piloting component treatments and services,[24] training and clinical skill development, and an adequate period of evaluation precede the conduct of trials of complex interventions.[21]
4. Are the experimental and comparison treatments sufficiently different? Do medication doses and regimens differ? Does the standard care condition reflect the deficiencies of standard care in real world practice?[11]
5. Has treatment integrity been measured reliably? Are data presented describing: (a) the treatments received on an individual patients basis during the study period; and (b) the extent of adherence to best practice, or practice as otherwise defined by the underlying service model?

Ensuring treatment integrity in the real world clinical setting

Comprehensive program evaluation may help to ensure treatment integrity in routine clinical practice. The Early Psychosis Prevention and Intervention Centre (EPPIC) in Melbourne, Australia, has developed a five-phase approach to program description and evaluation, described in full elsewhere.[25] The five phases are:

1. Program description
2. Clarification
3. Program monitoring
4. Process evaluation
5. Outcome evaluation.

The approach focuses on developing and maintaining treatment integrity within day-to-day clinical practice. Examples of recent service-based efforts to ensure and examine treatment integrity, from the EPPIC program and elsewhere, are discussed.

Developments in program description

FEP programs around the world are increasingly providing published descriptions of their clinical programs, developing manuals and articulating clinical guidelines.[25] Descriptive accounts reflect the evolutionary stage of the program. For example, the focus of program description documents published by EPPIC has shifted over time

from broad service model description,[26–28] to specific detailing of case management,[29] psychological interventions based on randomized controlled trials,[30–33] and supportive psychoeducational materials.[34] This shift reflects the need for detailed information about specific psychological therapies provided by FEP programs, and recent efforts to address service gaps for specific patient groups, highlighted via internal clinical reviews. These developments have been incorporated into the revised *EPPIC Clinical Guidelines* (see Box 18.1), which provide a basis for many of the program monitoring and process evaluation activities undertaken at EPPIC. An extract from the guidelines is provided in Table 18.1.

Process evaluation

Techniques for process evaluation include: measuring performance indicators derived from practice guidelines and standards; benchmarking against agreed targets and thresholds; and clinical auditing (see Box 18.2). Process evaluations can highlight real world problems in maintaining adherence to clinical guidelines and standards, and provide opportunities for examining the impact of variability in practice on patient outcomes.

The use of clinical audit to assess treatment integrity

Published audits have examined the treatment of early psychosis delivered within the context of specialist programs[35–37] and generic mental health services.[38–42] Further FEP audits are in progress in Melbourne, the United Kingdom, Vienna, and Sydney. Audits have been used to: describe the patients treated within a particular service for planning and service development purposes (see Box 18.3: audit example 1);[40] compare service delivery against clinical guidelines or standards,[35] and between services[41] (see Box 18.4: audit example 2); and support a continuous quality improvement cycle.[38,43]

Audit designs are attractive for a number of reasons. For example, they are relatively efficient

---

Box 18.1 *EPPIC Clinical Guidelines, 2003*©

The *EPPIC Clinical Guidelines* are tailored to the EPPIC service setting, providing guidance to clinicians regarding the optimal timing and/or intensity of clinical interventions and activities. Developed in 1996 and most recently updated in April 2003, the guidelines reflect the guiding philosophies of the EPPIC model of care (e.g. providing treatment in the least restrictive environment possible, and reducing trauma related to hospital admission). Key features have been maintained from previous versions (e.g. grouping standards of care according to phase of illness). The current version adds procedures for elevated suicide risk, persisting positive and negative symptoms, poor service engagement, and individual psychological interventions for appropriate patient subgroups. There are quantifiable indicators for key standards, and a range of formats for clinicians and consumers are under development.

Table 18.1 Extract from the *EPPIC Clinical Guidelines*, 2003©

Guideline   Standard
EPPIC will offer an accessible and responsive service
> Delays in treatment should be minimized: all clients suspected of experiencing a first episode psychosis should be considered a priority and be assessed within 24 hours of EPPIC receiving a referral.

Gain a thorough understanding of the person and their situation as quickly as possible
> All clients should have a comprehensive biopsychosocial assessment undertaken by the acute treating team within 48 hours after entry to the service. This should include a mental state examination (MSE), physical examination including body weight, neurological examination, risk assessment, drug and alcohol use, personal history and family history, formulation, and management plan.

Provide regular review of client's progress with treatment
> All clients should be seen at least twice weekly during the acute phase by the acute treating team and/or outpatient case manager (OCM), and a doctor.

> All clients with persisting positive or negative symptoms, or high suicide risk, should be referred by the treating team to TREAT[a] for review and consultation within three months after entry to service, and then at any point during treatment at EPPIC.

Regular risk assessments are undertaken with each client to inform treatment planning
> An immediate risk management plan should be developed and documented in conjunction with the client, carers, consultant psychiatrist, and other members of the treating team (e.g. OCM or doctor, youth access team (YAT),[b] inpatient unit) for all clients identified at high suicide risk.

Individual psychological interventions are provided by the OCM (when training has been provided) and specialist workers as a means of enhancing the individual's ability to cope with early psychosis
> All clients with comorbid psychological disorders (e.g. adjustment difficulties, anxiety, or depression) should be offered COPE[c] as part of standard case management.

> All clients with persisting suicidality should be offered LifeSPAN[d] as part of standard case management.

> All clients with problematic cannabis use should be offered CAP[e] as part of standard case management.

EPPIC treatment should be in the least restrictive environment and manner
> Involvement of police to enforce treatment should be kept to a minimum.

> The use of seclusion and intensive care area (ICA) should be kept to the minimum frequency and duration to meet treatment aims of managing high risk patients.

[a] TREAT is a panel of senior clinicians that meets weekly to provide consultation to EPPIC clinicians whose clients are experiencing problematic recovery 12 weeks into treatment.
[b] YAT is a multidisciplinary mobile assessment, crisis intervention, and community treatment team which is the first point of contact with EPPIC.
[c] COPE (cognitively oriented psychotherapy for early psychosis) focuses on promoting recovery from the first episode of psychosis.
[d] LifeSPAN is a cognitive behavioral therapy addressing feelings of hopelessness, suicidal ideation, and depression.
[e] CAP (cannabis and psychosis) is a brief intervention for individuals with problematic cannabis use.

Box 18.2 Process evaluation example: EPPIC clinical practice reviews

EPPIC has implemented a schedule of 'clinical practice reviews', in which small teams of clinician 'reviewers' evaluate aspects of care against existing best practice standards, such as the *EPPIC Clinical Guidelines*. The aim is to encourage staff to reflect critically on clinical practice and identify possible areas for improvement in service delivery. Data are collected via clinical file audit or, on occasion, patient and carer surveys or focus groups.

Topics have included adherence to guidelines for low dose medication strategy, the provision of psychoeducation to carers, minimizing delays to assessment, and police involvement in referral and inpatient admission. Resulting improvements in service delivery include: the establishment of an intensive case management team for clients aged 18–24 years experiencing difficulty engaging with the service or requiring intensive support; and strategies to improve the identification and monitoring of clients at risk of suicide.

Box 18.3 Audit example 1: the Vienna FEP File Audit Survey (V-FFAS)

The V-FFAS is being undertaken to inform planning for the provision of specialist services for young people with FEP at the Department of Child and Adolescent Neuropsychiatry, Vienna (population approximately 1.6 million). All individuals with FEP who commenced treatment between January 2001 and March 2003 were identified from the inpatient medical record database, outpatient case lists, and discussions with clinic staff. A total of 43 cases were identified comprising 25 males and 18 females, aged 13–18 years.

Existing FEP audit tools were identified from published studies and knowledge of unpublished audits and audits in progress. A 'best fit' audit tool was selected and modified for the Vienna context. Pilot testing revealed limitations to the information that could be gained from the clinical files. The most reliable data items were medication details and inpatient length of stay. Duration of untreated psychosis and pathways to care will require prospective data collection.[48, 49] Consumer satisfaction surveys may also be necessary.

The audit will review the first six months of treatment. Each file will take approximately two hours to review. Audits will be undertaken in pairs by two trainee psychiatrists and a doctoral level research assistant, with input from a consultant psychiatrist, and will be completed during 2004.

---

to conduct, and offer flexibility in terms of sampling and defining the period of assessment. However, these benefits need to be balanced against the limitations of routine clinical information, some of which are discussed here.

Pharmacological treatments and inpatient treatment for FEP have been explored using file audit.[35,44] Assessing the content of psychological treatments provided in mental health services is considerably more difficult, due to challenges in operationalizing and coding these treatments, and the possibility that detailed information regarding the content of each treatment occasion may not have been documented. As a consequence, attempts to develop precise criteria to measure adherence to treatment recommendations may be hampered by the specificity and range of information required.[45]

This problem is illustrated by two US studies which evaluated the quality of routine care provided to individuals with schizophrenia, using indicators derived from practice guidelines. Goldman et al. were unable to obtain sufficient data from medical records adequately to assesses adherence to the selected guidelines.[46] Young et al. obtained data from patient interviews and medical record abstraction.[47] They found that

> **Box 18.4 Audit example 2: the St Vincents Mental Health Service (SVMHS) audit**
>
> The SVMHS audit examined the management of patients with early psychosis at a generic mental health service in Melbourne, Australia. The sample comprised 62 patients currently in treatment, experiencing a first episode of psychosis or within the first 2 years following an initial episode. A standardized audit tool was used to collect data from clinical files.
>
> The study reported longer DUP, a higher proportion of inpatient admissions, longer length of stay, greater use of seclusion, and more police involvement in admissions compared to published data from a specialized first episode psychosis service (EPPIC). The authors suggested that current practice in generic services is not optimal. Treatment is focused on the needs of the clients with more established and severe mental illnesses, who comprise the majority of the patient population. Areas of practice requiring improvement included: lack of assertive assessment and follow-up and long delays to treatment; lengthy hospitalization; high use of seclusion; high rates of police involvement. Results suggested that clinical staff may benefit from interventions to increase awareness of the special needs of early psychosis patients and improve confidence in providing treatment to these patients.

using data from both sources resulted in the identification of twice as many cases of poor quality pharmacological care than using medical record data only. However, they were not able to determine whether this was due to poor file documentation or inadequate detection of symptoms and side effects.

Summary and conclusions

The evaluation of treatment integrity requires the measurement and comparison of what is prom-ised with what is delivered. Failure to evaluate treatment integrity has been acknowledged as a problem in interpreting the results of effectiveness studies in mental health.[50,51] Articulation of treatment components and services is essential to ensure that the intervention can be appraised and replicated. From a research perspective, the assessment of treatment integrity is a necessary component of good quality research design, ensuring that conclusions about the effectiveness of the FEP intervention under study are valid. In the clinical setting, process evaluation activities, such as audits and performance indicators, can help to focus quality improvement efforts by showing variance between actual practice and standards of care.

References

1. Wolff N. Randomised trials of socially complex interventions: promise or peril? J Health Serv Res Policy 2001; **6**:123–6.
2. Edwards J. Developing first-episode psychosis services. Br J Psychiatry (Suppl): (in press).
3. Bickman L. The most dangerous and difficult question in mental health services research [Editorial]. Ment Health Serv Res 2000; **2**:71–2.
4. Bond G, Evans L, Salyers M, et al. Measurement of fidelity in psychiatric rehabilitation. Ment Health Serv Res 2000; **2**:75–87.
5. McGrew J, Bond G, Dietzen L, Salyers M. Measuring the fidelity of implementation of a mental health program model. J Consult Clin Psychol 1994; **62**:670–8.
6. Fiander M, Burns T, McHugo G, Drake R. Assertive community treatment across the Atlantic: comparison of model fidelity in the UK and USA. Br J Psychiatry 2003; **182**:248–54.
7. Becker D, Smith J, Tanzman B, et al. Fidelity of supported employment programs and employment outcomes. Psychiatr Serv 2001; **52**:834–6.
8. Resnick S, Neale M, Rosenheck R. Impact of public support payments, intensive psychiatric community care, and program fidelity on employment outcomes for people with severe mental illness. J Nerv Ment Dis 2003; **191**:139–44.
9. Mechanic D. Emerging issues in international

mental health services research. Psychiatr Serv 1996; **47:**371–5.

10. Lewis S. The European First-Episode Schizophrenia Network [Editorial]. Br J Psychiatry 2002; **181**(Suppl):S1–S2.

11. McGorry P. Early psychosis reform: too fast or too slow? [Editorial]. Acta Psychiatr Scand 2002; **106**:249–51.

12. Malla A, Norman R. Early intervention in schizophrenia and related disorders: advantages and pitfalls. Curr Opin Psychiatry 2002; **15:**17–23.

13. Edwards J, McGorry P. *Implementing Early Intervention in Psychosis. A Guide to Establishing Early Psychosis Services.* London: Martin Dunitz; 2002: 145–55.

14. Paulson R, Post R, Herinckx H, Risser P. Beyond components: using fidelity scales to measure and assure choice in program implementation and quality assurance. Community Ment Health J 2002; **38:**119–28.

15. McGorry P, Edwards J, Mihalopoulos C, et al. EPPIC: An evolving system of early detection and optimal management. Schizophr Bull 1996; **22:**305–26.

16. Mihalopoulos C, McGorry P, Carter R. Is phase-specific, community-oriented treatment of early psychosis an economically viable method of improving outcome? Acta Psychiatr Scand 1999; **54:**1–9.

17. Addington J, Leriger E, Addington D. Symptom outcome 1 year after admission to an early psychosis program. Can J Psychiatry 2003; **48:**204–7.

18. Malla A, Norman R, McLean T, McIntosh E. Impact of phase-specific treatment of first episode of psychosis on Wisconsin Quality of Life Index (client version). Acta Psychiatr Scand 2001; **103:**355–61.

19. Malla A, Norman R, Manchanda R, et al. Status of patients with first-episode psychosis after one year of phase specific community-oriented treatment. Psychiatr Serv 2002; **53:**458–63.

20. Cullberg J, Levander S, Holmqvist R, et al. One-year outcome in first episode psychosis patients in the Swedish Parachute project. Acta Psychiatr Scand 2002; **106:**276–85.

21. Catts S, O'Donnell M, Spencer E, et al. Early psychosis intervention in routine service environments: implications for case management and service evaluation. In: Kashima H, Falloon I, Mizuno M, Asai M (eds). *Comprehensive Treatment of Schizophrenia: Linking Neurobehavioral Findings to Psychosocial Approaches.* Berlin: Springer; 2002: 309–30.

22. Nordentoft M, Jeppesen P, Abel M, et al. OPUS Study: suicidal behaviour, suicidal ideation and hopelessness among patients with first-episode psychosis. One year follow-up of a randomised controlled trial. Br J Psychiatry 2002; **181**(Suppl): S98–S106.

23. Jorgensen P, Nordentoft M, Abel M, et al. Early detection and assertive community treatment of young psychotics: the OPUS study. Soc Psychiatry Psychiatr Epidemiol 2000; **35:**283–7.

24. Campbell M, Fitzpatrick R, Haines A, et al, Framework for design and evaluation of complex interventions to improve health. BMJ 2000; **321:**694–6.

25. Edwards J, McGorry P. *Implementing Early Intervention in Psychosis. A Guide to Establishing Early Psychosis Services.* London: Martin Dunitz; 2002: 107–26.

26. Edwards J, Francey S, McGorry P, Jackson H. Early psychosis prevention and intervention: evolution of a comprehensive community-based specialised service. Behav Change 1994; **11:**223–33.

27. McGorry P. The Centre for Young People's Mental Health: blending epidemiology and developmental psychiatry. Australas Psychiatry 1996; **4:**243–7.

28. Edwards J, McGorry P. Early intervention in psychotic disorders: a critical step in the prevention of psychological morbidity. In: Perris C, McGorry P (eds). *Cognitive Psychotherapy of Psychotic and Personality Disorders.* Chichester: Wiley; 1998: 168–95.

29. EPPIC. *Case Management in Early Psychosis: A Handbook.* Melbourne: Early Psychosis Prevention and Intervention Centre; 2001.

30. Herrmann-Doig T, Maude D, Edwards J. *Systematic Treatment of Persistent Psychosis (STOPP): A Psychological Approach to Facilitating Recovery in Young People With First-Episode Psychosis.* London: Martin Dunitz; 2003.

31. Power P, Bell R, Mills R, et al. Suicide prevention in first episode psychosis: the development of a randomised controlled trial of cognitive therapy for acutely suicidal patients with early psychosis. Aust N Z J Psychiatry 2003; **37:**414–20.

32. Jackson H, McGorry P, Edwards J. Cognitively oriented psychotherapy for early psychosis (COPE):

theory, praxis, outcome and challenges. In: Corrigan P, Penn D (eds). *Social Cognition and Schizophrenia.* Washington DC: APA Press; 2001: 249–84.

33. Edwards J, Hinton M, Elkins K, et al. Cannabis and first-episode psychosis: the CAP project. In: Graham H, Copello A, Birchwood M, et al (eds). *Substance Misuse in Psychosis: Approaches to Treatment and Service Delivery.* Chichester: Wiley; 2003: 283–304.

34. EPPIC. *Prolonged Recovery in Early Psychosis: A Treatment Manual and Video.* Melbourne: Early Psychosis Prevention and Intervention Centre; 2002.

35. Power P, Elkins K, Adlard S, et al. Analysis of the initial treatment phase in first-episode psychosis. Br J Psychiatry 1998; **172**(Suppl):71–6.

36. Edwards J, Harris M, Herman A. The Early Psychosis Prevention and Intervention Centre, Melbourne, Australia: an overview, November 2001. In: Ogura C (ed). *Recent Advances in Early Intervention and Prevention in Psychiatric Disorders.* Tokyo: Seiwa Shoten Publishers; 2002: 26–33.

37. Svedberg B, Mesterton A, Cullberg J. First-episode non-affective psychosis in a total urban population: a 5-year follow-up. Soc Psychiatry Psychiatr Epidemiol 2001; **36**:332–7.

38. Tobin M. Initiation of quality improvement activities in mental health services. J Quality Clin Pract 1999; **19**:111–6.

39. Tobin M, Hickie I, Yeo F, Chen L. Discussing the impact of first onset psychosis programs on public sector health services. Australas Psychiatry 1998; **6**:181–3.

40. Rowlands R. Auditing first episode psychosis: giving meaning to clinical governance. Int J Clin Pract 2001; **55**:669–72.

41. Yung A, Organ B, Harris M. Management of early psychosis in a generic adult mental health service. Aust N Z J Psychiatry 2003; **37**:429–36.

42. Milner E, Rowlands P, Gardner B, Ashby F. First episode of psychosis—an audit of service engagement and management at 1–2 year follow-up. Med Sci Monit 2001; **7**:1299–302.

43. Gorrell J, Cornish A, Rosen A, et al. What are we doing differently? The process and outcome of a medical record audit [abstract]. Acta Psychiatr Scand 2002; **413**(Suppl):63.

44. Lambert M, Conus P, McGorry P. FEPOS study: methodology, diagnostic distribution and stability over the 18–month treatment period [abstract]. Acta Psychiatr Scand 2002; **106**(Suppl):45.

45. Young A. Evaluating and improving the appropriateness of treatment for schizophrenia. Harv Rev Psychiatry 1999; **7**:114–8.

46. Goldman M, Healy D, Florence T, et al. Assessing conformance to medication treatment guidelines for schizophrenia in a Community Mental Health Center (CMHC). Community Ment Health J 2003; **39**:549–55.

47. Young A, Sullivan G, Burnam M, Brook R. Measuring the quality of outpatient treatment for schizophrenia. Arch Gen Psychiatry 1998; **55**:611–7.

48. Addington J, van Mastrigt S, Hutchinson J, et al. Pathways to care: help seeking behaviour in first episode psychosis. Acta Psychiatr Scand 2002; **106**:358–64.

49. Norman R, Malla A, Verdi M, Hassall L, Fazekas C. Understanding delay in treatment for first-epsiode psychosis. Psychol Med 2004; **34**:255–66.

50. Mueser K, Bond G, Drake R, Resnick S. Models of community care for severe mental illness: a review of research on case management. Schizophr Bull 1998; **24**:37–74.

51. Rosen A, Teesson M. Does case management work? The evidence and the abuse of evidence-based medicine. Aust N Z J Psychiatry 2001; **35**:731–46.

19

The Benefits of Incorporating Research into Clinical Programs

Kimberley P Good, Warrick J Brewer, and Lili C Kopala

Introduction

The main aim of this chapter is to promote improved clinical care as a result of incorporating research into a first episode clinical treatment program. We will begin by outlining the advantages of clinical research for patients, family members, and staff. The second section presents a prototype research model to illustrate the simplicity of a research question that spurred almost two decades of research.

Direct and indirect benefits of participating in research

Clinical trials

Clinical trials frequently allow treatment with the new generation of antipsychotic medications. This is particularly important for those patients without subsidized healthcare plans as the cost of these agents can limit their use. As significant deleterious effects are likely to occur early in the course of illness,[1] access to the second generation antipsychotics (SGA), with potentially fewer problematic side effects, is beneficial. Evolving data suggest that the earlier a patient is optimally treated with an effective and well tolerated agent, the faster and more complete is the recovery.[2] Involvement in a clinical trial is one way to maximize exposure of patients to effective medications, enhance adherence, and also to improve therapeutic alliance. Many clinical trials include specialized nurses who are not only familiar with the medication, but more importantly, with the patient and possibly his or her family. This resource acts to structure and motivate closely monitored intervention. In turn, clinical trials provide patients with access to not yet approved, but potentially useful medications.

Research MRI scans

Canadian Best Practice Guidelines for the Treatment of Early Psychosis (November 1998) advocate the use of neuroimaging procedures in order to rule out other neurological conditions. Cost constraints normally dictate a less expensive computed tomographic (CT) scan but this technology is not sufficiently sensitive to uncover the subtle and non-specific neuropathology demonstrated by many patients with psychotic disorders. Although the early morphometric studies of patients with psychotic disorders used CT scan technology,[3] the ubiquitous availability of magnetic resonance imaging (MRI) scanners currently allows for this latter technology to be exploited. However, the cost of an MRI scan coupled with the clinical backlog may make it generally unavailable to a patient with a psychotic disorder.

Involving patients in research projects using MRI (or functional MRI) may have distinct advantages. Although no pathognomonic features have been discerned in patients in this group, there is imaging evidence of subtle brain abnormalities.[4] Such studies can contribute valuable information for patients and family members in that these conditions are brain disorders (see Figures 19.1). Consequently, these data are more convincing educational material regarding the biological aspects of the illness. Alternatively, a lack of palpable anatomical abnormalities may help provide peace of mind in that neurological causes have been ruled out.

Psychological counseling, neuropsychological testing, occupational therapy

At many centers, a lack of skilled and trained psychologists represents challenges for front line clinicians. Information that could potentially improve prognostic ability (i.e. a detailed assessment of cognitive function) or give an indication of current functional capacity (occupational therapy) is desirable. As with functional neuroimaging, objective neuropsychological evidence of impaired cognitive functioning may also allow patients and their families to come to appreciate the fact that psychosis frequently involves difficulties in attention, memory, and sensory processing. Assessment of the cognitive measures that are often impaired in psychotic disorders would allow for appropriate rehabilitation measures. This is particularly pertinent as many domains of cognitive function, such as verbal working memory, attention, and executive function are predictors of social and vocational adaptability.[5]

Psychological counseling, as well as rehabilitation programs, may be made available as a consequence of participating in research protocols. These aspects of clinical care are essential for maximizing the individual's potential for recovery. As the translation of cognitive improvement after treatment with the SGA into distinct positive changes in social and vocational outcome has not yet been demonstrated,[6] enhancing adaptive functioning is dependent on other, established methods (e.g. psychosocial programming, methods to augment independence).

Extended supportive environment

Often, a psychotic disorder emerges insidiously without family members being aware of the developing dysfunction. Having patients/family members recollect (often difficult) scenarios and memories may be distressing. Recall and articulation of complex emotions may be facilitated in a supportive and structured environment that is characteristic of the course of a clinical trial or investigation.[7] As structured clinical interviews are mandatory for most clinical research, missing important information is less likely to occur. Full

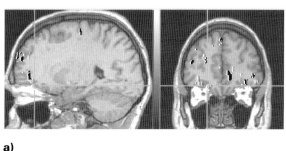
a)

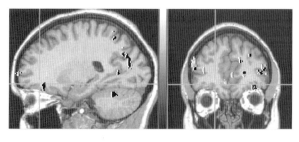
b)

Figure 19.1 Functional magnetic resonance imaging (fMRI) scan during presentation of a pleasant odor in (a) healthy controls, showing activation in orbitofrontal regions, and (b) patients with psychotic disorders, showing a lack of activation in orbitofrontal regions. (Good et al. 2003, unpublished data.)

and accurate disclosure may not only aid in the diagnostic process, but also guide appropriate rehabilitation programs.

Education for patients and family members

A further advantage of incorporating research into clinical programs includes the provision of formal or informal education sessions for patients and their families. Education is a key component of any clinical program involving patients who are likely to have to adhere to medication for extended periods of time. If the family are aware of the importance of various aspects of the treatment, then they can advocate on behalf of their relative. Adherence to treatment is crucial to recovery and education of all members of the team is essential. Various modules, focusing on a variety of learner-driven topics, can incorporate up-to-date information on how to get well, stay well, and reduce the likelihood of relapse. Finally, patients and families can take ownership and experience pride in being involved in activities that benefit themselves and others with similar conditions.

Benefits for trainees and staff

The development of integrated clinical research models encourages the scientist-practitioner model for staff, which in turn is more likely to result in real world practical research findings. Extra resources are inevitably attracted to often-struggling clinical programs. These include staff, information technology upgrades, conference attendance, training seminars for clinical staff, and psychometric evaluation to supplement clinical judgment. A professional work ethos amongst clinicians that encourages rigorous testing of working hypotheses in diagnoses also reflects a progressive and structured treatment approach to patients, which enhances therapeutic response. In addition, the inclusion of clinical staff in research and authorship of consequent publications is a valuable motivation reinforcing the elements of successful research activities. These include optimizing recruitment rates and enhancing team spirit and morale which, again, reflects back to patients and their families for therapeutic benefit.

Development of a clinical research framework reflects more clearly the structured progress of a research agenda, and promotes the development of focused and integrated research hypotheses. These often 'contained' projects can be metamorphosed into a larger research endeavor. As some students and clinicians can be initially intimidated by the plethora of mandatory and time-consuming elements of research (e.g. diagnostic and IQ assessment, and the sometimes arduous preparation of multiple research funding and ethics applications), these preliminary undertakings are attractive. A working model that expands this point is found at the ORYGEN Research Centre, Melbourne, Australia where one of the authors (WJB) regularly provides the under- and postgraduate programs with mini research projects in the form of abstract proposals that are attractive to students as they kick-start their careers and study. Furthermore, such a framework allows for the rationalization and matching of student interests and clinical placements during their training. Moreover, it is often the interesting projects that involve clinical populations that are more likely to attract potential trainees. The ORYGEN Research Centre model supports a more formalized research supervision/mentoring framework, whereby selected honors level (final year undergraduate) students are offered structured projects and potentially casual employment in a clinical setting via closer collaboration with site clinical directors. This provides the opportunity for students to network and to evaluate the real possibility of extending their undergraduate interests to a postgraduate level, along with offering them more immediate access to associated further employment opportunities within their developing area of expertise. This process also expands student access to regions of study that are not solely restricted to the interests and expertise of more purely academic supervisors.

Evidence-based practice is the goal

This point is discussed and expanded in Chapter 18. The importance of measuring treatment integrity has been reinforced by recent studies demonstrating that when mental health programs attempt to implement evidence-based practices, programs with higher fidelity to the defined practice tend to attain better outcomes.[6] Successful working models, such as EPPIC in Australia, as described elsewhere in this book, reflect the benefits of not only incorporating rigorous evidence-based practice and evaluation into the clinical program,[9] but of co-siting a clinical program with structured research activities. This allows for an active and immediate synergy of ideas regarding research foci from clinical observations, and in turn ready access for researchers to significant clinical populations.

Consensus diagnosis

Despite the limitations of the current diagnostic system, accurate diagnosis is paramount to providing appropriate treatment and for the initiation of social supports. Inaccurate diagnosis can lead to much frustration and anxiety as different (and probably ineffective) treatments are applied. The resources required in a busy inpatient setting rarely allow psychometric confirmation/clarification of diagnosis to supplement clinical judgment and information gathering. In contrast, patients who are involved in research studies tend to be more highly scrutinized and are subject to a multidisciplinary team for diagnosis, treatment, education, and rehabilitation. At times, a consensus diagnosis is required and this stimulates discussion and consideration of all available information.

Olfaction as a prototype research protocol

Case study

A 20-year-old male college student, Adam, is accompanied to your office by his parents. This young man appears to be guarded, admits to suspiciousness, but denies that he has any problems apart from difficulty concentrating in class. Despite the presence of positive psychotic symptoms, he has been doing reasonably well in university (B average). However, he was always an A student in high school and one might expect him to be performing at an even higher level given that all his siblings are now professionals. Structured neuropsychological assessment was not available, but olfactory testing revealed olfactory identification to be in the normal range (normosmic). There is a positive family history of psychotic illness in a maternal grandparent. Although never having been treated with any antipsychotic medications, Adam demonstrates mild extrapyramidal motor dysfunction. Upon reflection, the parents estimate that Adam has 'not been himself' for at least two years. He admits to occasional use of cannabis and alcohol.

What advice can you reliably give to this family regarding the most likely course of illness or response to medication? What of time to recovery or the potential for subsequent functional recovery?

The amount of information available to the practitioner at first episode can be considerable, particularly if reliable collateral information is obtained. However, one's capacity for predicting ultimate outcome remains limited. In the clinical vignette, there are conflicting risks and strengths. On one hand, male sex, relatively early age of onset, significant duration of untreated psychosis (DUP), pre-existing extrapyramidal motor dysfunction, use of substances, and a positive family history of psychosis all mitigate against a favorable response to treatment.[10–12] On the other hand, cognitive functioning appears to be intact, which bodes well for his subsequent functioning. Without a formal neuropsychological evaluation, however, it is impossible to determine whether a decline in cognitive abilities has occurred and whether remaining relative cognitive strengths can be usefully employed in vocational and educational endeavors. It may be assumed that cognitive efficiency has been compromised in this individual as evidenced by comparisons with family members or with premorbid levels. In any case, as Adam is continuing to perform at above average levels academically, prior research would predict a more favorable functional outcome for this individual,[5] as long as his positive symptoms can be well controlled. Intact olfactory identification ability would also support this prediction,[11] as it implies that specific brain circuits are intact. If he had exhibited significant deficits, then closer monitoring and allocation of resources would be warranted to buffer him from increased risk for development of negative symptoms and potential treatment resistance, along with a higher chance of receiving a diagnosis of schizophrenia.[14–17] (For further information, see below.)

Additionally, a limited awareness of psychotic symptoms at this point could interfere with adherence and, as such, targeted education is indicated in order to improve his awareness of his condition. If Adam is willing to engage with the treatment team and participate in education sessions about the deleterious effects of substances, his prospects for recovery are enhanced. Adherence to medications will be essential.

The next section describes a model outlining the advantages of having accessible research resources allocated to clinical programs. Specific principles reflect the three authors' collaborative experience of clinical olfactory research.

Olfactory connections and the pathology of psychotic disorders

In the mid 1980s, while training as a psychiatry resident, one of the current authors (LCK) was struck by a statement made to her by a young psychotic patient. He said simply: 'I can't smell anything'. Intrigued, but unable to find any pertinent literature on the subject, Dr Kopala immersed herself in this area of research. The central question was the relationship between olfactory deficits and the underlying brain dysfunction producing the psychotic symptoms. At that time, major impairments in olfactory function in patients with Alzheimer's disease had been demonstrated while anecdotal evidence existed pointing to a defect in the perception of specific steroidal odors in patients with schizophrenia. The literature was devoid of any reference to objective olfactory assessment in patients with schizophrenia.

Dr Kopala's pioneering work spawned a surge of interest that has persisted for almost 20 years. Other notable laboratories worldwide (e.g. Melbourne, New York, Lyon, Philadelphia) have furthered our understanding of this topic. In fact, in the most recent International Congress on Schizophrenia Research (2003, Colorado Springs), a symposium was devoted to the complexities of olfactory dysfunction in patients with psychotic disorders.

> Clinicians are in a unique position to observe phenomena which inevitably raise questions. The answers to these questions lead one down a systematic path of enquiry.

What Dr Kopala discovered was that many of the brain regions identified as being abnormal in schizophrenia have direct or indirect olfactory connections. This neuroanatomical correlate provided the rationale for olfactory assessment in patients with psychoses. In the earliest report of olfactory identification deficits,[18] patients with schizophrenia were shown to be impaired relative to a bipolar disorder or normal control group. Neither the use of medications, duration of illness, effects of smoking, task complexity, nor positive symptoms could account for the olfactory deficits observed.[19] Patients with schizophrenia and olfactory identification deficits (OID) had intact olfactory acuity suggesting that they had an olfactory agnosia, similar to that reported in Korsakoff's amnestic syndrome and in patients with focal lesions of the orbitofrontal cortex or temporal lobe.[20–22]

Impaired olfactory function as an biological marker of pathology

Emerging evidence suggests that employing olfactory function as a neurobehavioral probe is a useful way to identify distinct subtypes of patients with psychotic disorders.[13,16,23,24] Furthermore, patient subgroups have been identified who have relative one-sided (unirhinal) microsmia.[23,24] Preliminary data suggest that first episode patients with unirhinal OID are more likely than those whose olfactory function is intact to have difficulties with social and occupational functioning.[13] Biologically, these subgroups may also be distinct and represent discrete neuropathological substrates.

Because not all patients with psychotic disorders demonstrate olfactory abnormalities, it is possible that those who do represent a distinct subtype of patients with abnormal neurogenesis or development. Their brain development may well be distinct from non-psychotic controls, and from psychotic patients without olfactory dysfunction.[25] Several lines of evidence support this hypothesis. Patients with left or right nostril unirhinal OID show unique patterns of neuropsychological abnormalities.[24] Structural brain abnormalities in the temporal lobe, as measured by magnetic resonance imaging (MRI), also differentiated patients with unirhinal OID from normosmic patients (Good et al., in prep). Finally, using positron emission tomography (PET), it has been demonstrated that right-sided basal ganglia and thalamic metabolism was reduced in patients who had OID when compared to those patients with normal olfactory function.[26]

The development of intact olfactory function progresses throughout childhood and adolescence and stabilises in early adulthood.[27] This process is consistent with parallel maturation of the prefrontal cortex. Therefore, early detection of potential neurodevelopmental arrest of limbic-prefrontal pathways, that may be reflected by OIDs, appears to be a promising approach to screening at-risk youth. Indeed, these early deficits may become an exciting and important early marker for later diagnostic specificity,[16] not only in the early detection of first episode psychosis and for schizophrenia specifically, but in other disorders of development that are mediated by these same prefrontal pathways. Certainly, early detection of *neurodegenerative* processes, such as Alzheimer, Huntington, and Parkinsons diseases utilizing olfactory identification has been described.[28]

Impaired olfactory function as a indicator of risk and prognosticator of outcome

There is potential utility in finding olfactory deficits in subjects deemed to be at ultra-high risk for psychosis, where initial results suggest that those individuals with olfactory deficits are more likely to develop schizophrenia.[16] This finding, along with the association of olfactory deficits and more pronounced negative symptoms,[14,15,17,29] has important implications for the earlier detection of those subjects. They are more likely to require greater service resources as their response to treatment is less robust. The finding of impaired olfactory function as a predictor of poor functional adaptation is also consistent with this point.[13] Here, strategic investment of resources in those patients who are likely to be more vulnerable in their responses to optimal treatment may be facilitated. For example, the early implementation of a vocational or social structure may provide important buffering for these apparently more vulnerable patients from earlier on during the course of their psychosis, thereby enhancing the probability of higher levels of recovery.

Conclusions

A simple approach to a complex problem

As outlined earlier, the ability to predict functional recovery or outcome for a particular patient with a first episode of psychosis continues to be problematic. From clinical observations, many important discoveries have occurred. Henri Laborit noted that psychotic patients were calm after receiving the anesthetic agent chlorpromazine.[30] It took many years to convince psychiatrists that this might be a useful agent. History is replete with other examples of enquiring minds seeking answers to their questions. The question: 'Is olfactory function impaired in patients with psychotic disorders?' raised a series of other questions and serves as a example of how such a marker of abnormal brain development might enhance our ability to predict risk for the expression of psychosis. Furthermore, does the presence of olfactory dysfunction indicate and predict a poorer response to treatment with subsequent lower levels of function? Finally, impaired olfactory function may provide information regarding specific underlying neuropathology in distinct brain regions.

Our proposal is consistent with ideas put forward by Tsuang et al.[31] wherein the behavioral aspects of the disorder (i.e. cognition—and our specific example of the cognitive process of olfaction identification) and not symptoms may be used to categorize patients uniquely. This approach has been successfully incorporated into an amalgamated clinical/research program and continues to provide a structured direction for theoretical exploration.

References

1. McGlashan T. Duration of untreated psychosis in first-episode schizophrenia: marker or determinant of course. Biol Psychiatry 1999; **46**:899–907.
2. Miller T, McGlashan T, Woods S, et al. Symptom assessment in schizophrenic prodromal states. Psychiatr Q 1999; **70**(4):273–87.
3. Johnstone E, Crow T, Frith C, et al. Cerebral ventricular size and cognitive impairment in chronic schizophrenia. Lancet 1976; **2**:924–6.
4. Pantelis C, Velakoulis D, McGorry P, et al. Neuroanatomical abnormalities before and after onset of psychosis: a cross-sectional and longitudinal MRI comparison. Lancet 2003; **361**:281–8.
5. Green M, Kern R, Braff D, Mint J. Neurocognitive deficits and functional outcome in schizophrenia: are we measuring the 'right stuff'? Schizophr Bull 2000; **26**(1):119–36.
6. Velligan D, Prihoda T, Sui D, et al. The effectiveness of quetiapine versus conventional antipsychotics in improving cognitive and functional outcomes in standard treatment settings. J Clin Psychiatry 2003; **64**:524–31.
7. Scott D, Valery P, Boyle F, Bain C. Does research into sensitive areas do harm? Experiences of research participation after a child's diagnosis with Ewing's sarcoma. Med J Aust 2002; **177**(9):507–10.
8. Drake R, Goldman H, Leff H. Implementing evidence-based practices in routine mental health service settings. Psychiatr Serv 2001; **52**:179–82.
9. Edwards J, McGorry P. *Implementing Early Intervention in Psychosis: A Guide to Establishing Early Psychosis Services.* London: Martin Dunitz Ltd; 2002.
10. Drake R, Haley C, Akhtar S, Lewis S. Causes and consequences of duration of untreated psychosis in schizophrenia. Br J Psychiatry 2000; **177**:511–15.
11. Hafner H. Gender differences in schizophrenia. Psychoneuroendocrinology 2003; **28**(Suppl 2): 17–54.
12. Jarbin H, Ott Y, Von Knorring A. Adult outcome of social function in adolescent-onset schizophrenia and affective psychosis. J Am Acad Child Adolesc Psychiatry 2003; **42**(2):176–83.
13. Good K, Kopala L, Kiss I, et al. Predicting future social and occupational adaptation based on olfactory identification performance at a first episode psychosis. International Early Psychosis Association Syllabus; 2000.
14. Brewer W, Edwards J, Anderson V, et al. Neuropsychological, olfactory hygiene deficits in men with negative symptom schiozphrenia. Biol Psychiatry 1996; **40**:1021–31.
15. Brewer W, Pantelis C, Anderson V, et al. Stability of olfactory identification deficits in neuroleptic-naive patients with first-episode psychosis. Am J Psychiatry 2001; **158**:107–15.
16. Brewer W, Wood S, McGorry P, et al. Impairment of olfactory identification ability in individuals at ultra-high risk for psychosis who later develop schizophrenia. Am J Psychiatry 2003; **160**:1790–4.
17. Malaspina D, Coleman E. Olfaction and social drive in schizophrenia. Arch Gen Psychiatry 2003; **60**(6):578–84.

18. Hurwitz T, Kopala L, Clark C, Jones B. Olfactory deficits in schizophrenia. Biol Psychiatry 1988; **23**:123–8.

19. Martzke J, Kopala L, Good K. Olfactory dysfunction in neuropsychiatric disorders: review and methodological considerations. Biol Psychiatry 1997; **42**:231–7.

20. Potter H, Butters N. An assessment of olfactory deficits in patients with damage to prefrontal cortex. Neuropsychologia 1980; **18**:621–8.

21. Jones B, Moskowitz H, Butters N. Olfactory discrimination in alcoholic Korsakoff patients. Neuropsychologia 1975; **13**:173–9.

22. Jones-Gotman M, Zatorre R. Contribution of the right temporal lobe to odor memory. Epilepsia 1988; **29**:661.

23. Good K, Martzke J, Honer W, Kopala L. Left nostril olfactory identification impairment in a subgroup of male patients with schizophrenia. Schizophr Res 1998; **33**:45–53.

24. Good K, Martzke J, Milliken H, et al. Unirhinal olfactory identification deficits in young male patients with schizophrenia and related disorders: association with impaired memory. Schizophr Res 2002; **56**:211–23.

25. Kopala L, Clark C. Implications of olfactory agnosia for understanding sex differences in schizophrenia. Schizophr Bull 1990; **16**(2):255–61.

26. Clark C. Kopala L, Hurwitz T, Li D. Regional metabolism in microsmic patients with schizophrenia. Can J Psychiatry 1991; **36**:645–50.

27. Doty R, Shaman P, Dann M. Development of the University of Pennsylvania Smell Test: standardized microencapsulated test for olfactory function. Physiol Behav 1984; **32**:489–502.

28. Murphy C. Loss of olfactory function in dementing disease. Physiol Behav 1999; **66**(2):177–82.

29. Geddes J, Huws R, Pratt P. Olfactory acuity in the positive and negative syndromes of schizophrenia. Biol Psychiatry 1991; **29**(8):774–8.

30. Rosenbloom, M. Chlorpromazine and the psychopharmacologic revolution. JAMA 2002; **287**: 1860–1.

31. Tsuang M, Stone W, Faraone S. Toward reformulating the diagnosis of schizophrenia. Am J Psychiatry 2000; **157**(7):1041–50.

20

First Episode Schizophrenia in British Columbia between 1896 and 1950

Geoffrey N Smith, Kathryn McKay, and William G Honer

Introduction

The study of the past provides invaluable insights into the present. With regard to schizophrenia, the explanatory potential of history is largely unrealized. An abundant literature has described the lifetime course of schizophrenia in the pre-neuroleptic era.[1–6] Historical studies suggest that the majority of cases of schizophrenia deteriorated within the first two to five years of illness and the course of illness was marked by a predominantly negative state or repeated episodes.[7] Only 10–15% of patients recovered.[7–9] However, the results of these studies are often contradictory. The extent to which this variability results from sampling differences and the degree to which it is a consequence of the limitations of the studies is unclear. The conclusions of many historical studies are diminished by unrepresentative or poorly described samples, inadequate prognostic, course, and outcome measures, and poorly defined diagnostic criteria. These and other limitations have been discussed in several reviews of the historical literature.[1,6,10] In addition to observing the natural course of schizophrenia, several research groups have compared pre- and post-neuroleptic era samples. Most of these 'mirror-image' studies compared patients admitted between the late 1930s and the early 1950s with patients from the late 1950s and early 1960s.[6] Most pre-neuroleptic patient groups were from the era when insulin coma and electroconvulsive therapy (ECT) were available and course of illness may be influenced by these treatments.[6,11,12] In addition, antipsychotic treatment groups were taken from the first years these medications were used when the value of maintenance therapy had not been realized and atypical neuroleptics were not available.

Kraepelin (1919) observed almost a century ago that the outcome of schizophrenia might be improved by prompt treatment. The current availability of effective antipsychotic medications and psychosocial therapies has resulted in renewed interest in early identification and treatment. Nevertheless, there remains considerable debate about early intervention and which patients are most likely to benefit from early treatment. In order to assess accurately the long-term efficacy of early intervention, we need to determine the natural course of illness in the absence of any treatment. Clearly, it is neither desirable nor ethically permissible to withhold treatment. In the absence of a contemporary sample, historical records may provide valuable information about the course of illness in the absence of neuroleptics.

The purpose of the present study was to

determine whether historical records could provide accurate information about the course of schizophrenia in patients who received no neuroleptic medication. In order to achieve this goal, the data set must provide detailed information about a large representative sample of patients. Information in the records should provide an adequate description of prognostic and outcome measures and sufficient clinical detail reliably to make contemporary diagnoses. The level of detail should be consistent across records and any ratings that are based on information from the records should be reliable. The specific purposes are as follows, to:

1. Describe the pre-neuroleptic psychiatric population in British Columbia and assess the consistency and detail of available clinical and demographic information
2. Determine the feasibility of re-diagnosing patients using DSM-IV criteria
3. Describe changes in the incidence, course, and phenomenology of schizophrenia and the factors associated with any changes.

British Columbia and psychiatric populations

The British Columbia population

This short history describes events that affected British Columbians during the years covered by this study. British Columbia (BC) joined the confederation of Canada in 1871 and, in the first four decades, was settled primarily by single men from Europe and Asia who came to work in fishing, mining, logging, and railway construction. The first decade of the 20th century saw a rapid expansion in both population (Table 20.1) and economy and a substantial expansion of the transportation system. The completion of the Trans-Canada railway in 1886 and the opening of the Panama Canal in 1914 allowed increased travel and the shipment of goods between BC and both Eastern North America and Europe. The prosperity of the early years ended during the first decade

of the 20th century. By 1910, the province was in an economic depression and jobs were scarce. Not until the early 1920s did BC see better times. This era saw the rise of socialist movements, considerable labor unrest, and racial tension. Asians faced legalized discrimination, anti-oriental riots and, in 1921, the Oriental Exclusion Act. The declining economy also resulted in increased aggression directed at other immigrants.[13] Europeans and working-class Britons were particularly unwelcome.[14] Immigration laws of 1906 and 1910 resulted in a substantial increase in deportations.[15]

Approximately 39 000 men enlisted in the First World War of which half were killed or wounded. Many non-Canadian-born men returned to Europe to fight for their home country or moved to the United States to avoid conscription or detention. This exodus resulted in a substantial decline in the proportion of males between the 1911 and 1921 censuses (Table 20.1). The BC population became more stable and prosperous during the 1920s but the depression of the 1930s changed the face of the province. Many unemployed men moved to the mild climate of the West Coast and by 1931, BC had the largest unemployed population in Canada. With over 20% unemployment, relief camps were established in remote areas of the province to move unemployed men away from the cities. In response to the economic crisis, immigration was restricted and a third of those who arrived in Canada were deported.[15] The economic situation finally improved during the Second World War and BC achieved full employment. Prosperity continued after the war and large numbers of people arrived from other parts of Canada and from abroad.

Psychiatric hospital population

The rapidly expanding provincial population was mirrored in the psychiatric admission rate (Table 20.1). The total number of admissions and the average number of inpatients increased each year and the psychiatric hospitals were expanded on

Table 20.1 British Columbian and psychiatric hospital populations: 1896–1950

British Columbian statistics for each census year

	1901	1911	1921	1931	1941	1951
Population	178 657	392 480	524 582	694 263	817 861	1 165 210
% male	71%	70%	59%	57%	54%	51%
% 10–59 yrs	70%	79%	74%	75%	72%	65%

Hospital statistics for each decade[a]

	1896–1905	1906–15	1916–25	1926–35	1936–45	1946–50
Admissions	933	2697	3814	5119	6935	4865
% 15–59 yrs	90%	91%	83%	77%	66%	63%
% male	77%	73%	68%	65%	59%	56%

Hospital statistics for patients with a functional psychosis[b]

Admissions	623	1935	2320	2879	3334	2151
(% of total)	67%	72%	61%	56%	48%	44%
% male	73%	71%	65%	61%	54%	48%

[a]Each decade from 1896 to 1945 and the quinquennial 1946 to 1950.
[b]Dementia praecox, schizophrenia, paranoia, terminal dementia, adolescent insanity, manic depression, depression, psychosis not otherwise specified.

average every five years. Overcrowding was a constant problem but there is no indication of changes in admission policies based on bed availability. Hospital expansions tended to follow rather than precede an increased hospital population. Periods of economic depression, when hospital budgets were likely to be restricted, were associated with an increase rather than a decrease in admissions. The hospital population reached a maximum of 6327 in 1956 and then declined steadily. This reduction followed the opening of general hospital psychiatric wards, the introduction of antipsychotic medication, and the development of community psychiatry. None of these alternatives were available before 1950. The provincial mental hospitals provided virtually all psychiatric care between 1872 and 1950. Before the 1950s, close to 100% of those with schizophrenia received hospital care at some time during their illness.[16] This finding suggests that historical hospital samples can accurately reflect the population of those with schizophrenia.[17,18]

Between 1872 and 1950, 24 983 patients accounted for 29 268 hospital admissions. The proportion of the patient population with either dementia or mental retardation increased steadily with increases in the proportion of older and younger British Columbians (Table 20.1). Men were over-represented in the hospital population relative to the provincial population. This difference was due in large part to the high percentage of men relative to women with a primary diagnosis of syphilis (85%) or alcohol abuse (80%).

Before 1936, patients were treated with hydrotherapy (warm baths, steam baths, and needle showers), bed rest, and a nutritious diet. This was followed by a period of work, fresh air, and exercise. When necessary, sedating medication was used (e.g. veronal, hyoscine, chloral hydrate). The era of somatic therapies began in 1937 with insulin coma therapy. Chemically (metrazol) induced seizures were used between 1937 and 1944 but this treatment was replaced by electroconvulsive therapy (ECT) in 1943. Psychosurgery was first used in 1944 and its use continued for nearly two decades. Up until 1950, 197 lobotomies were performed. Neuroleptic medications were not used in BC until 1954.

Method

Information obtained from admission and discharge registers was reviewed for all patients who were admitted to a provincial hospital between 1896 and 1950. This information was used to exclude patients over 59 years of age, those with no psychotic symptoms (e.g. mental retardation, anxiety disorders) and those for whom psychosis resulted from a general medical condition (e.g. dementia, epilepsy, brain injury, syphilis). Patients with multiple admissions were included if the diagnosis during at least one admission suggested a psychotic or mood disorder that was not the result of a medical condition. All cases with an ambiguous diagnosis (e.g. masturbatory insanity, primary dementia, psychopathic deviate with psychosis), mental retardation with psychosis, or a substance-induced psychosis were assessed. If there was evidence of psychosis or mood symptoms not due to the direct physiological effects of a substance or a general medical condition, the file was reviewed in detail (see the next main section).

Results

Over 98% of the hospital files have been located and these show increasing clinical detail over time. Virtually all files contain an application for hospitalization, two medical certificates, a brief life history, clinical progress notes, and a medical examination report. Records after 1932 included detailed social service notes. The medical certificates describe functioning immediately before admission and the application for hospitalization provides demographic information and specific items concerned with current and past illnesses. Basic demographic data were obtained from admission and discharge registers for all 24 364 patients admitted between 1896 and 1950 (Figure 20.1). These registers provided name, gender, date of admission, number of admissions, and diagnosis for every patient admitted after 1896. The results of this initial review indicated that 12 524 patients were under 60 years of age and presented with psychotic symptoms that were unlikely to be a consequence of a general medical condition. Most files contain sufficient detail to allow a rating of severity of illness at admission and degree of improvement by the time of discharge. Level of functioning after discharge was reported only after 1932 when social service notes became available.

Diagnosis in first episode psychosis

Psychiatric diagnoses underwent substantial changes during the latter part of the 19th century and the first half of the 20th century. The BC files reveal two major periods. Early diagnoses reflect the nosological confusion of the times and followed no single diagnostic scheme. Diagnoses commonly made during this era include hebephrenia, adolescent insanity, terminal dementia, delusional insanity, and masturbatory insanity. Hebephrenia, masturbatory insanity, and adolescent insanity were not used after 1902. Terminal dementia continued to be used until 1923 and delusional insanity or paranoia became less common but were used until after 1950. Kraepelin's influence on diagnosis was evident in BC by the mid 1890s and his diagnosis of dementia praecox was only replaced by Bleuler's schizophrenia toward the middle of the century. The early use of the term 'dementia' was ambiguous. Dementia in young patients was used in the Kraepelinian sense to denote predominant negative symptoms.[8] Memory in these young 'demented' patients was normally unimpaired but behavior was frequently described as demented, dull, withdrawn or stupid. Dementia in older patients was used in the modern sense to denote impairments in memory. A diagnosis of manic-depression in BC appears to be synonymous with agitation, irritability or 'behavioral excitement'. Included in

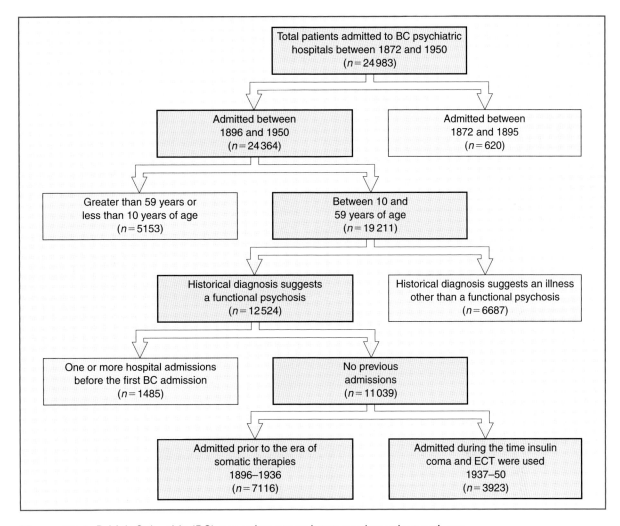

Figure 20.1 British Columbia (BC) screening procedures used to select patients

this diagnostic category are delirium, dementia with agitation, alcohol withdrawal, and agitated patients with schizophrenia. This diagnosis also included many depressed patients whether or not they presented with agitation. All diagnoses in the present study preceded the first edition of the *Diagnostic and Statistical Manual* (DSM).[19] It is clear from the historical literature and from a review of the BC files that there is likely to be disagreement between historical and contemporary diagnoses. One goal of this study was to determine the feasibility of making DSM-IV diagnoses from historical records.[20]

Method

The following screening procedures were used to identify cases that met DSM-IV criteria for schizophrenia or a related disorder or for a mood disorder (Figure 20.1).

Initial screening

The files of all patients between 10 and 60 years of age with a diagnosis that suggested schizophrenia or a related disorder or a mood disorder were assessed in order to identify previous psychiatric hospitalizations. Patients with an admission before their first BC admission were excluded and the files of those with no previous admissions were reviewed in detail (see the next main section).

Review diagnosis

Database entries were reviewed for patients who passed the initial screening in order to assign a DSM-IV diagnosis. All information on a database page was considered when making the review diagnosis. This included DSM-IV inclusion criteria (the presence, duration, and co-occurrence of psychotic and mood symptoms, and changes to level of functioning) and exclusion criteria (the presence of a general medical condition or substance abuse disorder that probably accounts for the mood or psychotic symptoms).

DSM-IV Diagnostic Evaluation After Death

The complete clinical files of 20% of first episode patients were reviewed in detail in order to obtain a DSM-IV diagnosis. A structured symptom checklist was developed from the Diagnostic Evaluation After Death scale (DEAD).[21] The DEAD is used to make post-mortem DSM-III-R diagnoses,[22] and has high inter-rater reliability and excellent correspondence between ante-mortem and post-mortem diagnoses.[23] The modified version used in the present study included items needed to make DSM-IV diagnoses. Clinicians were blind to historical and review diagnoses.

Results

The first screening procedure was completed for all 12 524 patients with a diagnosis suggesting a functional psychosis. The majority (88%) had no psychiatric admissions before their first BC admission. Of these first episode patients, 7116 were admitted before any somatic treatment was available and 3923 were admitted when insulin coma therapy or ECT were in use. A DSM-IV-Review diagnosis was made for 1425 patients and a detailed DSM-IV-DEAD diagnosis was completed for 457 patients. The concordance between Review and DEAD diagnoses is shown in Table 20.2. Agreement between the two diagnostic pro-

cedures was achieved in 86% of the cases. In most cases of schizophrenia (236/257, 92%) and of other disorders (organic, substance-related, or non-psychotic, 49/53, 92%), the DSM-IV-DEAD diagnosis was confirmed by the DSM-IV-Review diagnosis. When making a DSM-IV-Review diagnosis, separating mood disorders from schizoaffective disorder using only the summarized clinical notes was difficult in some cases. However, if these two diagnoses were combined, the Review diagnosis agreed with the DEAD diagnosis in 95% (140/147) of the cases. The level of agreement between historical and DSM-IV diagnoses are shown in Table 20.2. In most cases, an ambiguous historical diagnosis was equivalent to DSM-IV schizophrenia. If ambiguous diagnoses were included with schizophrenia and dementia praecox, the correspondence with DSM-IV schizophrenia was relatively high (214/257, 83%). A DSM-IV diagnosed mood disorder was equivalent to a historical diagnosis of manic-depression or depression in 72% of cases. However, only 24% of patients who were diagnosed with manic-depression met DSM-IV criteria for bipolar disorder. It is noteworthy that 12% of patients with a historical diagnosis suggesting a functional psychosis would today receive a diagnosis of psychosis due to a general medical condition, or substance-induced psychosis.

Historical changes in schizophrenia

Historical evidence suggests that the course, phenomenology, and incidence of schizophrenia have changed over the past two centuries.[24–30] The decline of catastrophic and catatonic schizophrenia are well documented,[2,25] although other changes are not widely acknowledged.[26,31] In addition, the causes of any observed changes remain obscure but recent evidence suggests the influence of environmental factors.[32–35] A detailed analysis of a large DSM-IV diagnosed representative sample that extends over a long period of time would be an invaluable means of examining these issues.

Table 20.2 Correspondence between DSM-IV-Diagnostic Evaluation After Death (DEAD) diagnoses and both DSM-IV-Review diagnoses and historical diagnoses

DSM IV Review diagnosis	DSM-IV-DEAD diagnosis				
	Schizophrenia[a]	Schizo-affective	Mood disorder	Other diagnosis[b]	Total
Schizophrenia[a]	**236 (92%)[e]**	5	2	2	245
Schizoaffective	16	**6 (46%)[e]**	**31 (23%)[e]**	0	53
Mood disorder	3	**2 (15%)[e]**	**101 (75%)[e]**	2	108
Other diagnoses[b]	2	0	0	**49 (92%)[e]**	51
Historical diagnosis					
Schizophrenia[c]	**197 (76%)[5]**	8	31	31	267
Manic depression	33	2	**61 (45%)[e]**	17	113
Depression	10	2	**36 (27%)[e]**	3	51
Ambiguous diagnoses[d]	**17 (7%)[e]**	1	4	4	26
Total	257	13	134	53	457

[a]Schizophrenia, schizophreniform disorder, brief psychotic disorder, psychosis not otherwise specified.
[b]Psychosis due to a general medical condition, dementia, substance-induced psychosis, non-psychotic disorder.
[c]Dementia praecox, delusional insanity, schizophrenia.
[d]Adolescent insanity, hebephrenia, terminal dementia, primary dementia, psychopathic deviant with psychosis, substance-induced psychosis.
[e]Percent of cases in which the detailed DSM-IV-DEAD diagnosis was confirmed.

Method

The file of every patient who met the inclusion criteria (Figure 20.1) was reviewed. Demographic, life history, and clinical information was entered in a database. This included a narrative of each patient's life history before admission and clinical notes describing the onset of illness, hospitalization, and treatment. The following preliminary results are based on information obtained from those patients for whom a DSM-IV diagnosis has been made. Of the 1425 patients for whom a DSM-IV-Review diagnosis was made, 1266 had first episode schizophrenia or a related disorder or a mood disorder (Table 20.3).

Results

Males were over-represented in the hospital population although the proportion of males decreased from 70% in the first half of the study to 57% during the last half. The decline in the proportion of males occurred for each DSM-IV diagnosis (Figure 20.2) and reflects the change in gender distribution in the BC population (Table 20.1). Patients with schizophrenia or a related disorder tended to be younger than those with a mood disorder (Table 20.3) and age at admission increased in mood disorder patients (Figure 20.3). Males were more likely to be single than females and this was more often the case for schizophrenia than for schizoaffective disorder or mood disorder (Table 20.3). As the gender ratio of the BC population became more equal, the likelihood for males to be single declined (Table 20.1, Figure 20.4). There was a minority of women in the BC population before the 1950s and no change in the proportion of single female patients over time. Canadian-born patients accounted for 36% of admissions and those born outside Canada came from Britain (30%), Europe (19%), the USA (8%), or Asia (7%). Relative to the population of BC, there were fewer than expected Canadian-born patients. British immigrants were

Table 20.3 Demographic characteristics of patients with a DSM-IV-Review diagnosis

	DSM-IV-Review diagnosis			
	Non-affective psychosis	Schizoaffective	Mood disorder	Total
Number of patients	798	149	319	1266
Gender (% male)	73%	57%	51%	65%
Marital status (% single, M:F)	74%:33%	64%:19%	58%:18%	70%:25%
Age at admission (SD)	35.5 (10.5)	36.2 (11.1)	37.7 (11.8)	36.1 (10.9)
Outcome of first admission				
• Died[a]	28%	13%	20%	25%
• Transferred[b]	29%	23%	17%	25%
• Discharged	43%	64%	63%	50%
% discharged patients readmitted	29%	37%	27%	31%

[a]Died or discharged to a home for the aged.
[b]Deported, transferred to another Canadian province, or escaped. SD, standard deviation.

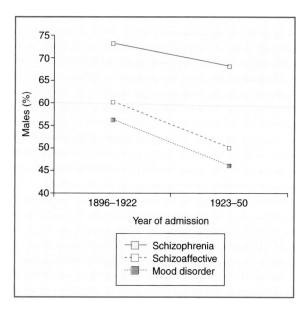

Figure 20.2 Percentage of males in each diagnostic group for the first and last half of the study period

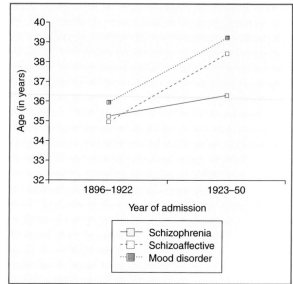

Figure 20.3 Mean age at admission for each diagnostic group in the first and second half of the study period

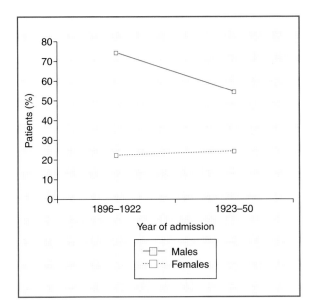

Figure 20.4 Percentage of male and female patients who were single

over-represented in the hospital population early in the 20th century and Europeans were over-represented throughout the study period (Figure 20.5).

Duration of the first hospital admission ranged from one day to 61 years with a median of 30 weeks. Length of hospitalization remained relatively stable in mood disorder patients but declined markedly in those with schizophrenia who were admitted from the 1920s to 1950 (Figure 20.6). It is noteworthy that this change occurred more than a decade before somatic therapies became available. Of patients with schizophrenia, 43% were discharged after their first admission and the remaining 57% died in hospital, were deported, transferred to another Canadian province, or escaped. The rate of discharge was higher for mood disorder patients (63%). The probability of being discharged after the first three years of hospitalization was very low and

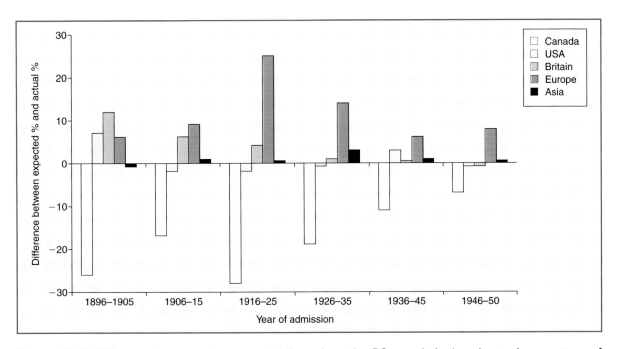

Figure 20.5 Difference between the expected (based on the BC population) and actual percentage of DSM-IV diagnosed patients for each place of birth

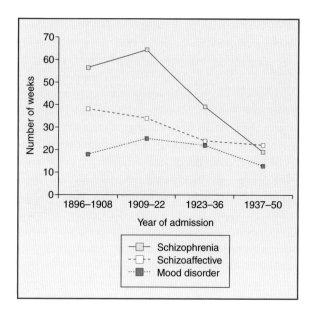

Figure 20.6 Median duration of hospitalization in weeks for patients with each DSM-IV diagnosis

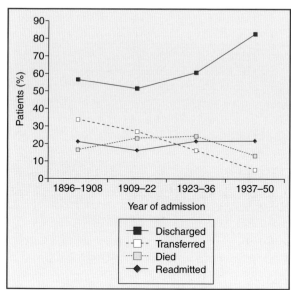

Figure 20.8 Outcome for DSM-IV diagnosed patients with schizoaffective disorder or mood disorder

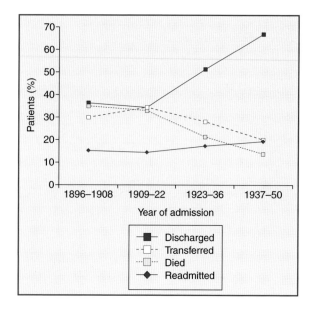

Figure 20.7 Outcome for patients with DSM-IV schizophrenia who were admitted between 1896 and 1950

only 12% of those with schizophrenia and 8% of mood disorder patients were discharged after two years of hospitalization. This finding supports the observations of Kraepelin in 1919, who indicated that irreversible deterioration tends to occur within the first three years of illness. The likelihood of being discharged increased in patients admitted during the last two decades of the study for both schizophrenia and mood disorder patients (Figures 20.7 and 20.8). The readmission rate tended to remain stable throughout this time suggesting improved prognosis.

Discussion

The first goal of the present study was achieved. Historical case files can provide useful information about the natural course of DSM-IV diagnosed schizophrenia. British Columbia retains a comprehensive record of all psychiatric admissions between 1896 and 1950. The provincial hospitals provided virtually all psychiatric care in BC and over 98% of the clinical records have been preserved. Prior to the introduction of antipsychotic medication, almost all individuals with schizophrenia received hospital care.[16] This suggests that hospital records provide a relatively complete record of schizophrenia in BC. Detailed demographic and clinical information is available on almost all patients. Of the patients with a first episode functional psychosis, 64% were admitted before somatic therapies were introduced (1896–1936) and 36% were admitted when insulin coma, metrazol or electroconvulsive therapies (ECT) were available (1937–50). Preliminary results suggest the second goal of this study was achievable. In virtually all cases, clinical notes were sufficiently detailed to allow an accurate DSM-IV diagnosis to be made. As predicted, historical diagnoses do not correspond to DSM-IV diagnoses in many cases. The correspondence for manic-depression was particularly poor.

With regard to the third goal, the present study provides intriguing albeit preliminary findings. Results suggest that societal factors influenced the incidence and course of psychiatric illness. This finding is consistent with recent studies that suggest urbanization, migration, and childhood environment increase the level of risk for schizophrenia.[32–35] British Columbia underwent dramatic changes between 1896 and 1950. Population growth, urbanization, immigration, war, and economic depressions all affected the lives of those who lived through this era. The degree to which these stresses were psychopathogenic is uncertain. However, the impact of these factors is suggested by increasing patient populations, changes in gender distribution, and age at illness onset. In addition, the incidence of schizophrenia in British and European immigrants was greater than in those who were Canadian-born. The excess of British and European patients was greatest during periods of high immigration and when these groups were most marginalized in the BC population.[13,14] The course of illness also appeared to change in BC. The present results and those from previous investigations suggest that treatment innovations, such as insulin coma, metrazol therapy, and ECT, may have an ameliorating effect on the course of illness.[11,12] However, it appears from the present results that the prognosis for schizophrenia was improving for more than a decade before these treatment innovations. The degree to which sociocultural and treatment-related factors affected the incidence and course of illness awaits a more complete investigation of the historical records.

Well defined first episode historical samples can provide useful descriptions of the natural course of illness in schizophrenia. Such samples could be matched with contemporary first episode groups in order to assess the efficacy of early intervention. Comparisons could be weighted according to a number of potentially useful variables, such as gender, age at onset, socioeconomic status, and place of birth. Historical samples can also be used to predict the probability of developing schizophrenia and the natural outcome of illness based on a range of variables. These prediction models could be applied to contemporary populations in order to compare probable with actual outcome.

References

1. an der Heiden W, Hafner H. The epidemiology of onset and course of schizophrenia. Eur Arch Psychiatry Clin Neurosci 2000; **250**:292–303.
2. Bleuler M. A 23-year longitudinal study of 208 schizophrenics and impressions in regard to the nature of schizophrenia. In: Rosenthal D, Kety SS (eds). *Transmission of Schizophrenia.* New York: Pergamon Press; 1968: 3–12.
3. Landis C, Farwell JE. Trend analysis of age at first-admission, age at death, and years of residence for state mental hospitals: 1913–1941. J Abnorm Soc Psychology 1944; **39**:3–23.
4. Langfeldt G. Schizophrenia: diagnosis and prognosis. Behav Sci 1969; **14**:173–82.
5. Valliant GE. Prospective prediction of schizophrenic remission. Arch Gen Psychiatry 1964; **11**:509–18.
6. Wyatt RJ. Neuroleptics and the natural course of schizophrenia. Schizophr Bull 1991; **17**:235–80.

7. Bleuler M. *The Schizophrenic Disorders: Long-term Patient and Family Studies.* New Haven, CT: Yale University Press; 1978.

8. Kraepelin E. *Dementia Praecox and Paraphrenia.* New York: Robert E Krieger Publishing; 1919.

9. Modestin J, Huber A, Satirli E, et al. Long-term course of schizophrenic illness: Bleuler's study reconsidered. Am J Psychiatry 2003; **160**:2202–8.

10. Hegarty JD, Baldessarini RJ, Tohen M, et al. One hundred years of schizophrenia: a meta-analysis of the outcome literature. Am J Psychiatry 1994; **151**:1409–16.

11. May PRA, Tuma AH, Yale C, et al. Schizophrenia – a follow-up study of the results of treatment: II. Hospital stay over two to five years. Arch Gen Psychiatry 1976; **33**:481–6.

12. Staudt VM, Zubin J. A biometric evaluation of somatotherapies in schizophrenia. Psychol Bull 1957; **54**:171–96.

13. Kelley N, Trebilcock M. *The Making of the Mosaic: A History of Canadian Immigration Policy.* Toronto: University of Toronto Press; 1998.

14. Barman J. *The West Beyond the West: A History of British Columbia.* Toronto: University of Toronto Press; 1996.

15. Roberts B. *Whence they Came: Deportation from Canada.* Ottawa: University of Ottowa Press; 1988.

16. Odegard O. Pattern of discharge from Norwegian psychiatric hospitals before and after the introduction of psychotropic drugs. Am J Psychiatry 1964; **120**:772–8.

17. Dilling H, Wayerer S. Prevalence of mental disorders in the small-town rural region of Traunstein (Upper Bavaria). Acta Psychiatr Scandi 1984; **69**:60–79.

18. Maurer K, Hafner H. Methodological assessment of onset of illness in schizophrenia. Schizophr Bull 1995; **15**:265–76.

19. American Psychiatric Association. *Diagnostic and Statistical Manual of Mental Disorders.* Washington, DC: American Psychiatric Association; 1952.

20. American Psychiatric Association. *Diagnostic and Statistical Manual of Mental Disorders* (4th edn). Washington, DC: American Psychiatric Association; 1994.

21. Zalcman S, Endicott J. *Diagnostic Evaluation After Death.* New York: Developed for NIMH Neurosciences Research Branch, Department of Research Assessment and Training; 1983.

22. American Psychiatric Association. *Diagnostic and Statistical Manual of Mental Disorders* (3rd edn, rev). Washington, DC: American Psychiatric Association; 1987.

23. Keilp JG, Waniek C, Goldman RG, et al. Reliability of post-mortem chart diagnoses of schizophrenia and dementia. Schizophr Res 1995; **17**:221–8.

24. Goldner EM, Hsu L, Waraich P, Somers JM. Prevalence and incidence studies of schizophrenic disorders: a systematic review of the literature. Can J Psychiatry 2002; **47**:833–43.

25. Hare EH. The changing content of psychiatric illness. J Psychosom Res 1974; **18**:283–9.

26. Hare EH. Was insanity on the increase? Br J Psychiatry 1983; **142**:439–55.

27. Israel RH, Johnson NA. Discharge and readmission rates in 4254 consecutive first admissions of schizophrenia. Am J Psychiatry 1956; **112**:903–9.

28. Page JD, Landis C. Trends in mental disease. J Abnorm Soc Psychol 1943; **38**:518–24.

29. Stephens JH, Richard P, McHugh PR. Long-term follow-up of patients hospitalized for schizophrenia, 1913 to 1940. J Ner Ment Dis 1997; **185**:715–21.

30. Torrey EF. Prevalence studies in schizophrenia. Br J Psychiatry 1987; **150**:598–608.

31. Torrey EF, Miller J. *The Invisible Plague: The Rise of Mental Illness from 1750 to the Present.* London: Rutgers University Press; 2001.

32. Boydell J, van Os J, Allardyce J, et al. Incidence of schizophrenia in ethnic minorities in London: ecological study into interactions with environment. BMJ 2001; **323**:1336–8.

33. Sharpley M, Hutchinson G, McKenzie K, Murray RM. Understanding the excess of psychosis among African-Caribbean population in England. Br J Psychiatry 2001; **178**(Suppl 40):60–8.

34. van Os J, Hanssen M, Bak M, et al. Do urbanicity and familial liability coparticipate in causing psychosis? Am J Psychiatry 2003; **160**:477–82.

35. Wahlbeck K, Osmond C, Forsen T, et al. Associations between childhood living circumstances and schizophrenia: a population-based cohort study. Acta Psychiatr Scand 2001; **104**:356–60.

Section III State-of-the-Art Applications

21

Prodromal Research and Interventions

G Paul Amminger and Claudia Klier

Introduction

Schizophrenia is often preceded by a prodromal phase. There is a suggestion that the earlier the treatment of schizophrenia begins the more rapid the immediate recovery and the better the overall outcome.[1] However, intervention in the pre-psychotic phase has been questioned as, using current criteria, only 20–50% of individuals classified as prodromal develop a psychotic disorder within a 1–2 year period.[2] Treatment agents investigated in the pre-psychotic phase of schizophrenia and other psychotic disorders should, therefore, not have major side effects. Nevertheless, as it is generally acknowledged that most psychosocial impairment develops in the prodromal and onset phase,[3] the question of whether treatment of subthreshold symptoms should be initiated before a psychotic disorder as currently defined by DSM-IV or ICD-10 can be diagnosed remains controversial. Also, it is unclear whether treatments that are effective for schizophrenia (e.g. neuroleptics) are optimal for the prodromal phase to prevent the onset of schizophrenia and minimize or reverse processes of neurodegeneration and cell death, which potentially occur during a first psychotic episode.

Research on the prodrome has a long tradition in Germany but most of this research has been retrospective and was mainly driven by psychopathological interests.[4,5] More recently, prospective research in the emerging phase of psychotic disorders has aimed to build an evidence base to guide therapeutic intervention and tries to clarify biological and psychological factors and mechanisms that are involved in the psychotic breakdown. The goal of this research is to be able to prevent or at least ameliorate psychotic disorder. This chapter:

1. Describes the rationale for (pre-psychotic) intervention in the onset phase of schizophrenia
2. Reviews prediction and intervention studies conducted in individuals with subthreshold psychotic symptoms
3. Proposes omega-3 essential fatty acids (EFAs) as beneficial and potentially preventative therapeutic agents in young people at immediate risk for psychosis.

Prodrome definitions

Psychosis usually develops gradually. The boundary between 'different but not psychotic' ('pre-psychotic') and 'frankly psychotic' is often blurred. Prodromal symptoms and behaviors may include attenuated positive symptoms (e.g. illusions, ideas of reference, and magical thinking), mood symptoms (e.g. anxiety, dysphoria, mood lability, and irritability), cognitive symptoms (e.g. distractibility and difficulty concentrating), social withdrawal, and obsessive behaviors.[6] Because these prodromal phenomena extensively overlap with the mental experiences and behaviors of persons in the age group at risk for schizophrenia who do not subsequently develop the disorder, they cannot be considered diagnostic.[7] Accordingly, such disturbances in individuals who have not yet experienced a psychotic episode can be viewed as indicators of an elevated risk of becoming psychotic, rather than signs inevitably associated with progression to a psychotic disorder. The term 'at-risk mental state' has been suggested for this phase of illness. 'At-risk mental state' can be applied prospectively, in contrast to a 'prodrome' which can only be defined retrospectively once a disorder has been diagnosed.[8]

Crucial for research in the period of emerging psychosis is the certainty with which individuals truly at risk for imminent psychosis can be identified. McGorry and colleagues from the PACE (Personal Assessment Crises Evaluation) clinic in Melbourne, Australia, developed prodromal criteria to identify individuals at risk of developing psychosis in the near future using the Comprehensive Assessment of At-Risk Mental States (CAARMS; Yung et al., 1998).[9] In brief, CAARMS defines three subgroups characterized by a recent functional decline plus genetic risk (Group 1), the recent onset of subthreshold psychotic symptoms (Group 2), or the onset of brief transient psychotic symptoms (Group 3). Diagnoses of Groups 2–3 are based on the experience of positive symptoms as rated on a checklist including disorders of thought content, perceptual abnormalities, and disorganized speech. Each item is rated by severity, frequency, and duration. Additional ratings record the relation of symptoms to stressful experience and/or substance use. The assessment of severity, frequency, and duration of prodromal experiences is an important advance from earlier approaches that focused solely on the quality of symptoms. In studies conducted in the PACE clinic between 30% and 40% of individuals who fulfilled the CAARMS at-risk criteria developed psychosis within 6–12 months.[9,10] The theory behind this strategy is based on the observation that the emergence of some subthreshold symptoms greatly increases the risk of transition to a fully fledged disorder, which has been articulated in the concept of 'indicated prevention'.[11] Indicated prevention is aimed at individuals who have symptoms of a mental disorder but do not meet diagnostic criteria. While the incidence of mental disorders is never higher than 10–15% in asymptomatic genetic high risk groups (with usual follow-up periods of many years), the incidence in subjects who already have some symptoms of the disorder can be much higher and transition more immediate. McGlashan and colleagues developed a diagnostic semistructured interview (Structured Interview for Prodromal Symptoms: SIPS), and a severity scale (Scale of Prodromal Symptoms: SOPS) closely modeled on the CAARMS to diagnose and measure psychopathological symptoms in individuals who may be in a pre-psychotic state.[12] Prodrome classification using SIPS and SOPS yielded acceptable inter-rater reliability (kappa = 0.81).[13]

Other currently employed prodrome definitions in schizophrenia include:

1. The concept of basic symptoms:[14] subjectively experienced neuropsychological deficits particularly in cognition, attention, perception, and movement
2. An approach by Tsuang et al. (2002),[15] who propose that non-psychotic forms of schizophrenia exist, which are characterized by neurocognitive deficits and negative symptoms[15]
3. An approach by Cornblatt et al. (2002),[16] which includes a subgroup with attenuated negative symptoms (in particular, social withdrawal/isolation and school withdrawal/ difficulties) or attenuated disorganized symptoms (such as poor grooming and hygiene).[16]

Prediction studies

Klosterkötter and colleagues prospectively investigated 160 individuals of whom 110 met the description of prodromal state according to BSABS (Bonn Scale Assessment Basic Symptoms) criteria.[17] At follow-up after a mean of 9.6 years, 49% (79 of 160) had developed DSM-IV schizophrenia.[18] Of those, 98% (77 of 79) met BSABS prodromal criteria at the first assessment. Only two of 50 individuals who were not considered prodromal at baseline developed schizophrenia. The absence of prodromal symptoms excluded subsequent schizophrenia with a probability of 96% (sensitivity: 0.98; false-negative predictions: 1.3%). Presence of prodromal symptoms predicted schizophrenia with a probability of 70% (specificity: 0.59; false-positive predictions: 20%). Among the 66 BSABS symptoms, those most predictive of schizophrenia were thought interference, disturbances of receptive language, and visual distortions. Transition to psychosis was observed after a mean duration of follow-up of 6.7 years in males and 4.3 years in females after the onset of the prodromal symptoms.

To enhance predictive accuracy, additional variables as well as the CAARMS intake criteria[9] have been under investigation by McGorry and colleagues from the PACE clinic. Significant clinical predictors of progression to psychosis were: long duration of prodromal symptoms, poor functioning, cannabis dependence, and high thresholds of attenuated psychotic symptoms, depression, and disorganization at baseline.[19,20] Among neuroanatomical parameters, larger left hippocampal volume,[21] less grey matter in the right medial temporal, lateral temporal, and inferior frontal cortex, and in the cingulate cortex bilaterally were found to be associated with progression to psychosis.[22] There is also the suggestion that olfactory identification impairment is specifically associated with the development of schizophrenia.[23]

Clinical setting and transition rate

Carr et al. reported that when they applied the PACE prodrome criteria in a clinical setting with fewer severely ill individuals than in previous studies the transition rate was substantially lower than 30–40%, at about 9%.[24] This finding indicates that the recruitment environment might have a strong influence on the transition rate. Screening and recruitment of potentially prodromal individuals for participation in intervention studies might therefore concentrate on psychiatric clinics rather than primary care settings to yield a low number of false positives (those who do not develop a psychotic disorder). On the other hand, a recent analysis from the PACE clinic (mean duration of follow-up 759 days) revealed that there might be certain subgroups among individuals classified as prodromal with an even higher risk for transition than the overall rate observed in previous samples; for example, 50% of 14- to 19-year-old individuals developed a psychotic disorder, whereas the transition rate for individuals in the third life decade was significantly lower (20%).[25] The high transition rate among teenagers might be associated with a peak incidence of schizophrenia during the late teens and first half of the third life decade.[26] Taking into account that a prodrome can precede the onset of schizophrenia by years,[3] it is not surprising that significantly more true positives were found before the age of 20. If this finding can be replicated, future intervention studies in the onset phase of psychosis might consider focusing in particular on adolescents.

Intervention studies

A pioneering study introducing the concept of pre-psychotic intervention in everyday clinical practice has been conducted by Falloon (1992),[27] demonstrating the feasibility of engaging patients with subthreshold psychotic symptoms in treatment.[27] The study also illustrated the need for new criteria for subthreshold forms of psychosis, which were subsequently developed. The first generation of intervention studies investigated neuroleptics and/or cognitive behavioral therapy (CBT) as potentially helpful tools in the pre-psychotic phase with two intervention targets in comparison with standard care: to reduce current prodromal symptoms and improve functioning; and to prevent a progression to psychotic disorder.

From 1996 to 1999 the first randomized controlled trial (RCT) was conducted in the PACE clinic which examined the efficacy of low dose risperidone plus CBT compared to standard treatment in 59 individuals with subthreshold symptoms.[19] By the end of treatment after six months, 35.7% of those receiving standard care developed psychosis compared to only 9.7% of those who received low dose risperidone (mean dose 1.3 mg/day) and CBT (the difference was statistically significant). Treatment was initiated with 0.5 mg risperidone daily and increased by 0.5 mg weekly to 2.0 mg per day if well tolerated. The most common side effects were akathisia, sedation, and weight gain. This study showed that more specific pharmacotherapy and psychotherapy reduces the risk of early transition to psychosis in individuals experiencing prodromal symptoms.

The statistic 'number needed to treat' (NNT) is a clinically appealing way of summarizing the effect of treatment in terms of the number of individuals a clinician needs to treat with a particular therapy to expect to prevent an adverse event. In the PACE study, McGorry et al. (2002)[19] NNT would be defined as the number of individuals who would need to be treated with risperidone and CBT in addition to unspecific interventions to prevent one making the transition to psychosis. The NNT was four for the end of treatment and five for 12 month follow-up. This contrasts with NNT of 13 for the treatment of moderate hypertension in the prevention of stroke.

Another intervention study focused on short-term medication effects—whether the atypical antipsychotic olanzapine could reduce prodromal symptoms, compared with placebo.[28] The olanzapine–placebo difference was statistically signific-

ant at week eight ($p < .05$). Ratings of extrapyramidal symptoms remained low in each group and were not significantly different. However, over the eight week study period individuals who received olanzapine gained 4.5 kg (9.9 lb) versus 0.32 kg (0.7 lb) for placebo patients ($p < .001$). The authors concluded that olanzapine is associated with significantly greater immediate symptomatic improvement but significantly greater weight gain than is placebo in prodromal patients and that future research over the longer term with more patients will be needed before recommendations can be made regarding routine treatment.

A third study, a randomized treatment trial of early detection and investigation of a cognitive behavioral intervention for preventing transition to psychosis in individuals with prodromal symptoms is underway in the UK.[29] In an interim analysis the authors reported that their findings confirm that the indicated prevention approach is a viable procedure for detecting individuals who are likely to develop a psychotic illness in the very near future. Of 23 prodromal patients monitored for 6–12 months 22% developed a psychotic disorder. These authors also assessed psychological measures of psychosis proneness, such as schizotypy, metacognitive beliefs, and dysfunctional self-schemas (sociotropy); the prodromal individuals in general scored significantly higher than a non-patient group. The elevated scores are consistent with the view that these psychological dimensions may play a significant role in the development of hallucinations and delusions.

Psychotherapeutic intervention in the prodromal phase

Francey and colleagues from the PACE clinic have designed an integrated cognitive therapy specifically tailored for young people at high risk of developing a psychotic disorder (Francey et al. in prep.). The principle objective of the intervention is to use cognitive strategies to strengthen the individual's coping resources. Environmental stressors, such as relationship problems, societal commitments, and lifestyle factors, appear to increase vulnerability to psychotic and other psychiatric symptoms. Cognitive behavioral therapy (CBT) involves the client and therapist working together on an agreed problem list which may prioritize problems unrelated to psychosis, such as family relationships, occupational concerns, social anxiety, and depression. Therefore, CBT would pose little risk to the false-positive group; indeed the problem-oriented nature of this intervention would mean that it is likely to be of benefit to these individuals.[29]

Novel treatments

Together, the intervention studies described above suggest that individuals with subthreshold psychotic manifestations can receive preventive benefit as well as treatment benefit from intervention. Taking into account that treatment benefit is generally accepted to justify exposure to treatment risks the results strengthen the argument that carefully designed intervention studies can be ethical with prodromal patients. Safety concerns, however, must be balanced with efficacy considerations. The main ethical criticism against specific treatment in the prodromal phase is that only about one third of individuals with prodromal symptoms develop psychosis, so the majority of individuals are exposed to potentially harmful interventions for no reason (e.g. the effects of antipsychotics on the developing brain are unknown). Although atypical antipsychotics are associated with fewer extrapyramidal side effects, other side effects such as weight gain, hyperglycemia, and hyperlipidemia are not uncommon.[30] In addition, neuroleptic medication might be compensatory rather than curative in the treatment of schizophrenia. Therefore, the investigation of safer and potentially more effective pharmacological treatment strategies needs to be pursued for the prodromal phase.

Neuroprotective substances

There is a suggestion that N-methyl-D-aspartic acid (NMDA) receptor hypofunction state plays a pathogenic role in neurodegenerative disorders (e.g. Alzheimer's disease) and psychotic disorders. The NMDA subtype of the glutamate receptor may be particularly important for schizophrenia, as blockade by substances such as phencyclidine (PCP) or ketamine increases dopamine release in the mesolimbic system and causes schizophrenia-like psychosis.[31] NMDA receptor hypofunction might be linked with glutamate-mediated neurotoxicity involving calcium release from nerve cells and subsequent release of nucleases and proteases which might lead to excessive pruning of nerve cells.[32] Substances that influence the process of neurodegeneration and cell death may be therapeutic or curative in the onset phase of psychosis, even those substances are not helpful in later stages of the disorder. For instance, lithium or lamotrigine, which have been shown to be neuroprotective in animal models, are candidates for further investigation in prodromal schizophrenia. Furthermore, vitamins C and E, which are effective antioxidants and scavenge neurotoxic hydrogen peroxide (H_2O_2) and nitric oxide (NO), warrant further investigation in the initial onset phase of psychosis.

Bioactive lipids

Bioactive lipids are molecules that have both intra- and intercellular roles, including mediation, modulation, and control of neurobiological processes, such as ion channel and receptor activity, neurotransmitter release, synaptic plasticity, second messenger pathways, and neuronal gene expression. Abnormal membrane glycerol-phospholipids (GPL) essential fatty acid (EFA) metabolism has been suggested to contribute to the etiopathophysiology of schizophrenia. A recent review of 15 studies confirmed a depletion of bioactive lipids in cell membranes of patients with schizophrenia.[33] The most consistent findings were reductions in arachidonic acid (AA) and its precursors, and these were independent of drug treatment (Yao et al., 1996). Khan et al. reported on erythrocyte membrane EFA levels and levels of plasma lipid peroxides, products of damaged EFAs, in drug-naïve patients within a few days of onset of psychosis.[34] The levels of EFAs, particularly AA and docosahexaenoic acid (DHA) were significantly lower in drug-naïve patients at the onset of psychosis compared to matched normal controls. These lower EFA levels were associated with significantly higher levels of lipid peroxides in individuals with schizophrenia. Interestingly, EFA levels were higher in chronic medicated patients than drug-naïve first episode patients. Khan et al. concluded that these findings could indicate that lower membrane AA and DHA predate the illness and probably contribute to the onset of illness.[34] Increased lipid peroxidation in never-medicated individuals with schizophrenia suggests that possible oxidative stress may be one of the mechanisms of reduced membrane EFAs.[34] These findings imply that supplementation of EFAs and/or antioxidants might provide effective treatments for early psychosis. This view is supported by Horrobin et al. who showed that increase in red cell AA levels resulted from treatment with the optimal levels of eicosapentaenoic acid (EPA), and that clinical improvement was highly significantly positively correlated with rises in red cell membrane AA in individuals with schizophrenia.[35]

Three randomized controlled treatment studies in individuals with schizophrenia found 2 g EPA/day significantly more effective than placebo in reducing psychopathological symptoms.[36,37] Symptom improvements in those studies were both clinically relevant and statistically significant. A dose-ranging exploratory study of the effects of EPA in individuals with schizophrenia who experienced persistent symptoms found 2 g EPA/day significantly more effective in reducing symptom scores on psychiatric rating scales than 1 g and 4 g EPA/day.[38]

Fenton et al. investigated augmentation of neuroleptics with 3 g EPA/day on symptoms and cognition in patients with schizophrenia or schizoaffective disorder and reported a negative finding.[39] The patients in Fenton et al.'s study had, however, been ill for two decades and had substantial symptoms, despite treatment with newer neuroleptics, including clozapine. The patients described as benefiting from EPA in the other studies were younger and had a shorter duration of illness.[37]

It must be emphasized that in all EPA treatment studies, no treatment-related side effects or adverse biochemical or hematological effects have been observed. EPA did not cause side effects other than mild gastrointestinal symptoms by itself, nor did it enhance the side effects of existing drugs. Patients reported EPA highly tolerable. The proportion of patients who completed 12 weeks (89%) compares favorably with mean withdrawal rates of 54% in the novel neuroleptic groups and 67% in the placebo groups in trials in the Federal Drug Administration (FDA) database.[38] Acceptance of a substance which is normally found in the human body without significant side effects, with a potency potentially similar to the antipsychotic drugs in the emerging phase of psychotic disorders, could contribute to reduce the duration of untreated psychosis and to increase compliance.

Summary

There is consistent evidence that there are now reliable ways to identify individuals who appear to stand a 30–40% risk of a psychotic disorder within a year. This degree of increased incidence (3000–4000 per 10 000 person-years) is about 200–300 times that of the general population at this age (Amminger et al. in prep.). Studies in the PACE clinic and other centers have provided encouraging preliminary information on treatments to reduce current symptoms and the risk of transition to psychosis. To bring the focus of intervention to current symptom reduction rather than future syndrome prevention might reduce stigmatization, clarify the question of how long to continue treatment,[40] and make obvious that indicated prevention in emerging psychosis is not an 'all or nothing phenomenon' as might be emphasized by terms such as 'transition to psychosis' or the labeling of individuals who recover in this phase of illness as 'false positives'. However, more data are needed and the risk: benefit ratio of various interventions must be determined. Antipsychotic medications are only indicated in RCTs or if a person meets diagnostic criteria for a psychotic disorder, except possibly: when rapid deterioration is occurring; where the risk of suicide is very high and treatment of any depression had proved ineffective; and when aggression or hostility is increasing and poses a risk to others.[41]

The extent to which the onset of schizophrenia follows a typical course from non-specific, negative symptoms to positive-like symptoms that gradually increase in severity requires further clarification. It is possible that the various symptom clusters (i.e. attenuated negative vs attenuated positive) represent etiologically different clinical entities. This raises the question as to whether the same type of (preventive) intervention should be given, regardless of the specific characteristics of the prodrome, or whether the different subgroups require different interventions (i.e. antidepressant vs antipsychotic medication).[16] Essential fatty acids (e.g. EPA) and CBT are effective treatments for both mood and psychotic symptoms. When considered, together with the controversy concerned with the extent to which an intervention is intrusive or may produce harm that outweighs the benefits, EPA and CBT are prime candidates for immediate further evaluation in RCTs in individuals with prodromal symptoms. Treatment research means RCTs, which are the only secure way of showing if a potential treatment is beneficial or not. As emphasized by McGorry et al.: 'this type of research is the best antidote to risky off-label atypical antipsychotic drug use among clinicians'.[42]

References

1. Norman RM, Malla AK. Duration of untreated psychosis: a critical examination of the concept and its importance. Psychol Med 2001; **31**(3):381–400.
2. McGlashan TH, Miller TJ, Woods SW. Pre-onset detection and intervention research in schizophrenia psychoses: current estimates of benefit and risk. Schizophr Bull 2001; **27**(4):563–70.
3. Häfner H, Nowotny B, Loffler W, et al. When and how does schizophrenia produce social deficits? Eur Arch Psychiatry Clin Neurosci 1995; **246**(1):17–28.
4. Huber G, Gross G, Schuttler R, Linz M. Longitudinal studies of schizophrenic patients. Schizophr Bull 1980; **6**(4):592–605.
5. Klosterkötter J. Basic symptoms and end phenomena of schizophrenia. An empirical study of psychopathologic transitional signs between deficit and productive symptoms of schizophrenia. Monogr Gesamtgeb Psychiatr Psychiatry Ser 1988; **52**:1–267.
6. Yung AR, McGorry PD. The prodromal phase of first-episode psychosis: past and current conceptualizations. Schizophr Bull 1996; **22**(2):353–70.
7. McGorry PD, McFarlane C, Patton GC, et al. The prevalence of prodromal features of schizophrenia in adolescence: a preliminary survey. Acta Psychiatr Scand 1995; **92**(4):241–9.
8. McGorry PD, Singh BS. Schizophrenia: risk and possibility. In: Raphael B, Burrows GD (eds). *Handbook of Studies on Preventative Psychiatry*. Amsterdam: Elsevier; 1995: 491–514.
9. Yung AR, Phillips LJ, McGorry PD, et al. Prediction of psychosis. A step towards indicated prevention of schizophrenia. Br J Psychiatry Suppl 1998; **172**(33):14–20.
10. Phillips LJ, Yung AR, McGorry PD. Identification of young people at risk of psychosis: validation of Personal Assessment and Crisis Evaluation Clinic intake criteria. Aust N Z J Psychiatry 2000; **34**(Suppl):S164–9.
11. Mrazek PJ, Haggarty RJ (eds). *Reducing the Risks for Mental Disorder: Frontiers of Preventative Intervention Research*. Washington, DC: National Academy Press; 1994.
12. Miller TJ, McGlashan TH, Woods SW, et al. Symptom assessment in schizophrenic prodromal states. Psychiatr Q 1999; **70**(4):273–87.
13. Miller TJ, McGlashan TH, Rosen JL, et al. Prospective diagnosis of the initial prodrome for schizophrenia based on the Structured Interview for Prodromal Syndromes: preliminary evidence of

interrater reliability and predictive validity. Am J Psychiatry 2002; **159**(5):863–5.

14. Gross G, Huber G, Klosterkötter J, et al. *Bonner Skala für die Beurteilung von Basissymptomen.* Berlin: Springer; 1987.

15. Tsuang MT, Stone WS, Tarbox SI, Faraone SV. An integration of schizophrenia with schizotypy: identification of schizotaxia and implications for research on treatment and prevention. Schizophr Res 2002; **54**(1–2):169–75.

16. Cornblatt B, Lencz T, Obuchowski M. The schizophrenia prodrome: treatment and high-risk perspectives. Schizophr Res 2002; **54**(1–2):177–86.

17. Klosterkötter J, Hellmich M, Steinmeyer EM, Schultze-Lutter F. Diagnosing schizophrenia in the initial prodromal phase. Arch Gen Psychiatry 2001; **58**(2):158–64.

18. American Psychiatric Association. *Diagnostic and Statistical Manual of Mental Disorders* (4th edn). Washington, DC: American Psychiatric Association; 1994.

19. McGorry PD, Yung AR, Phillips LJ, et al. Randomized controlled trial of interventions designed to reduce the risk of progression to first-episode psychosis in a clinical sample with subthreshold symptoms. Arch Gen Psychiatry 2002; **59**(10):921–8.

20. Yung AR, Phillips LJ, Yuen HP, et al. Psychosis prediction: 12–month follow up of a high-risk ("prodromal") group. Schizophr Res 2003; **60**(1):21–32.

21. Phillips LJ, Velakoulis D, Pantelis C, et al. Nonreduction in hippocampal volume is associated with higher risk of psychosis. Schizophr Res 2002; **58**(2–3):145–58.

22. Pantelis C, Velakoulis D, McGorry PD, et al. Neuroanatomical abnormalities before and after onset of psychosis: a cross-sectional and longitudinal MRI comparison. Lancet 2003; **361**(9354):281–8.

23. Brewer WJ, Wood SJ, McGorry PD, et al. Impairment of olfactory identification ability in individuals at ultra-high risk for psychosis who later develop schizophrenia. Am J Psychiatry 2003; **160**(10):1790–4.

24. Carr V, Halpin S, Lau N, et al. A risk factor screening and assessment protocol for schizophrenia and related psychosis. Aust N Z J Psychiatry 2000; **34**(suppl): 170–80.

25. Amminger G, Leicester S, Yuen HP, McGorry PD. Age predicts transition to psychosis in prodromal

schizophrenia. Schizophr Res 2003; **60**(1, Suppl 1):32–3.

26. Räsänen S, Veijola J, Hakko H, et al. Gender differences in incidence and age at onset of DSM-III-R schizophrenia. Preliminary results of the Northern Finland 1966 birth cohort study. Schizophr Res 1999; **37**:197–8.

27. Falloon IR. Early intervention for first episodes of schizophrenia: a preliminary exploration. Psychiatry 1992; **55**(1):4–15.

28. Woods SW, Breier A, Zipursky RB, et al. Randomized trial of olanzapine versus placebo in the symptomatic acute treatment of the schizophrenic prodrome. Biol Psychiatry 2003; **54**(4):453–64.

29. Morrison AP, Bentall RP, French P, et al. Randomised controlled trial of early detection and cognitive therapy for preventing transition to psychosis in high-risk individuals. Study design and interim analysis of transition rate and psychological risk factors. Br J Psychiatry Suppl 2002; **43**:S78–84.

30. Meyer JM. A retrospective comparison of weight, lipid, and glucose changes between risperidone- and olanzapine-treated inpatients: metabolic outcomes after 1 year. J Clin Psychiatry 2002; **63**(5):425–33.

31. Goff DC, Coyle JT. The emerging role of glutamate in the pathophysiology and treatment of schizophrenia. Am J Psychiatry 2001; **158**(9): 1367–77.

32. Farber NB, Kim SH, Dikranian K, et al. Receptor mechanisms and circuitry underlying NMDA antagonist neurotoxicity. Mol Psychiatry 2002; **7**(1):32–43.

33. Fenton WS, Hibbeln J, Knable M. Essential fatty acids, lipid membrane abnormalities, and the diagnosis and treatment of schizophrenia. Biol Psychiatry 2000; **47**:8–21.

34. Khan M, Evans D, Gunna V, et al. Reduced erythrocyte membrane essential fatty acids and increased lipid peroxides in schizophrenia at the never-medicated first-episode of psychosis and after years of treatment with antipsychotics. Schizophr Res 2002; **58**(1):1–10.

35. Horrobin DF, Jenkins K, Bennett CN, Christie WW. Eicosapentaenoic acid and arachidonic acid: collaboration and not antagonism is the key to biological understanding. Prostaglandins Leukot Essent Fatty Acids 2002; **66**(1):83–90.

36. Peet M, Brind J, Ramchand CN, et al. Two double-blind placebo-controlled pilot studies of eicosapentaenoic acid in the treatment of schizophrenia. Schizophr Res 2001; **49**(3):243–51.

37. Emsley R, Myburgh C, Oosthuizen P, van Rensburg SJ. Randomized, placebo-controlled study of ethyl-eicosapentaenoic acid as supplemental treatment in schizophrenia. Am J Psychiatry 2002; **159**(9):1596–8.

38. Peet M, Horrobin DF. A dose-ranging exploratory study of the effects of ethyl-eicosapentaenoate in patients with persistent schizophrenic symptoms. J Psychiatr Res 2002; **36**(1):7–18.

39. Fenton WS, Dickerson F, Boronow J, et al. A placebo-controlled trial of omega-3 fatty acid (ethyl eicosapentaenoic acid) supplementation for residual symptoms and cognitive impairment in schizophrenia. Am J Psychiatry 2001; **158**(12):2071–4.

40. Lewis S. Is treatment research in people at high risk of psychosis ethical? J Ment Health 2003; **12**(4):359–62.

41. Edwards J, McGorry PD. *Implementing Early Intervention in Psychosis: A Guide to Establishing Early Psychosis Services.* London: Martin Dunitz; 2002.

42. McGorry PD, Yung A, Phillips L. Ethics and early intervention in psychosis: keeping up the pace and staying in step. Schizophr Res 2001; **51**(1):17–29.

43 Hashimoto R, Hough C, Nakazawa T, et al. Lithium protection against glutamate excitotoxicity in rat cerebral cortical neurons: involvement of NMDA receptor inhibition possibly by decreasing NR2B tyrosine phosphorylation. J Neurochem 2002; **80**(4):589–97.

22

The Significance of Cognitive Functioning in First Episode Psychosis

Ross Norman and Laurel Townsend

Introduction

There is a large body of research demonstrating that individuals with schizophrenia spectrum disorders, such as schizophrenia, schizophreniform, and schizoaffective disorders, often demonstrate performance below normal controls on a variety of cognitive tasks.[1] Many issues related to the significance of such deficits for understanding the nature of these disorders await final resolution. For instance, there has long been an interest in the extent to which the cognitive dysfunctions observed in schizophrenia spectrum disorders reflect relatively static neurodevelopmental anomalies, an ongoing process of cognitive deterioration, or a state-specific disruption of cognition that improves with reduction in primary clinical symptoms. While comparisons of cognitive deficits in first episode and more longstanding patients sometimes suggest greater cognitive deficits in the latter, this could reflect more profound dysfunctions being a risk factor for chronicity instead of a progressive worsening. The strongest evidence regarding the course of cognitive dysfunction associated with schizophrenia would come from studies in which first episode patients are followed over time. Reviews of these latter studies in general provide little evidence of ongoing deterioration in cognitive functioning.[2,3]

Similarly, the evidence regarding the relationship between duration of untreated psychosis and cognitive functioning certainly does not provide consistent support for the experience of untreated psychosis being associated with increased deficits.[4–8]

Most research on cognitive functioning in schizophrenia patients focuses on average performance for a sample of patients. While attending to averages can be informative for many purposes, it is important to recognize that there is considerable variation between patients in their level of cognitive performance. Within a single patient there can also be considerable variation in performance across different cognitive domains. Examination of this variation may have important implications for our understanding of the heterogeneity of these disorders.[9] Such variation may also have important clinical implications. There is evidence that formal cognitive assessments sometimes predict aspects of community adjustment and functioning,[10] and the implications of such deficits are likely to be particularly prominent for first episode patients who are generally young and at a transitional period in their lives with respect to education and employment.

Clinical implications of cognitive assessments in first episode patients

Over the past seven years, one of the authors (LT), a clinical psychologist with a particular interest in cognitive functioning, has become particularly aware of the clinical value of cognitive assessment of first episode patients while working in the Prevention and Early Intervention Program for Psychoses (PEPP) in London, Ontario. This program is dedicated to providing early detection and treatment services to those with psychotic disorders, primarily within the schizophrenia spectrum, who have not previously been treated. Details of the services provided by PEPP are available elsewhere.[11]

For several years assessment of a variety of areas of cognitive functioning has been part of the assessment protocol used in PEPP. These assessments include the Wechsler Adult Intelligence Scale-third edition (WAIS III), the Wechsler Memory Scale-third edition (WMS III), as well as measures of speed of processing (Paced Auditory Serial Addition Test, PASAT), selective attention and mental flexibility (Stroop Test), concept formation and ability to shift and maintain a mental set (Wisconsin Card Sorting Test, WCST), visuomotor sequencing (Trail Making Test), sustained attention (CPT numerical identical pairs version), and word fluency (Thurstone Word Fluency Test). This battery is typically completed soon after entry into the program when the client is considered likely to tolerate and attend to up to two hours of activity without interference from active psychotic symptoms. The battery is repeated after one year of treatment. It is worth noting that each of the instruments is likely to include multiple aspects of cognitive functioning, although each is designed to be particularly sensitive to one or two processes, such as memory, planning, selective attention, etc. While it can be a disadvantage for some research purposes that performance on any one test is likely to be determined by multiple aspects of functioning,[12] such complexity can provide parallels to tasks encountered in everyday life.

This cognitive assessment protocol in PEPP has been used to address research issues related to cognitive functioning,[13,14] but at least equal importance, the results of such assessments have also been found useful clinically. A previous report by several of our colleagues described the value of neuropsychological assessment in the rehabilitation of clients with longstanding psychotic disorders, particularly in setting and achieving realistic vocational and educational goals.[15] Here, we wish to highlight the potential value of such information in several aspects of clinical care for first episode patients.

Clarifying contributors to clinical presentation

It is well recognized that psychotic disorders are often accompanied by other psychiatric conditions or psychological states, such as anxiety, depression, obsessionality, and learning disabilities. The presence of such phenomena, even when they do not warrant a formal diagnosis, can have a substantial influence on the presentation and course of the individual's symptoms, as well as their recovery and functioning.

Both the results of formal cognitive assessments and observations made by an examiner during assessment can suggest important hypotheses about prominent emotional states, cognitive styles or difficulties in types of information processing or performance—particularly under challenging circumstances. For instance, significant discrepancies between performance on timed and untimed tests may reflect anxiety or susceptibility to stress. Prolonged delay in initiating responses can suggest depression. Difficulties in processing verbal as opposed to visual material may be reflected in differential performance on tasks as a function of the modalities in which material is presented.

While results on a single task or test cannot generally be interpreted as providing definitive evidence for the presence of a learning disability or prominent emotional state, consistent patterns of results across a range of tasks can, when interpreted by a skilled examiner, provide evidence that could then be cross-validated by additional psychometric methods and clinical observations.

Measuring change

Routine assessment of cognitive functioning can provide a broader perspective on change over time and response to treatment than outcome indices focused entirely on symptoms. Our experience has been that many clients do improve in cognitive functioning over the first year or two of treatment.[14] We sometimes find that changes in cognitive functioning are in many ways more compelling evidence of improvement than reduction in symptoms. The validity of these assessments can be more apparent to clients because they are often quite aware in their daily lives of the change in cognitive functioning that has occurred and its possible implications for their goals. For example, many clients describe increased endurance for reading following a period of recovery and this is often reflected in improved scores on concentration tasks.

Because changes in cognitive functioning are sometimes clearly perceived by the client and examiner as corresponding to changes in symptoms or degree of adherence to treatment, these changes can also be a ready source of feedback and reinforcement of progress being made in the treatment program. Many clients have reported that seeing improvement over time in their cognitive functioning has provided great encouragement to them in their efforts to get on with their lives after experiencing psychotic illness. Similarly, a worsening of attention or memory following a period of substance use or non-compliance with medication can also reinforce the importance of risk reduction.

Evaluating personal strengths and challenges

Providing careful and thoughtful feedback to clients about their performance on cognitive testing can help them develop an accurate perception of their areas of comparative strength and weakness. It must be emphasized that the interpretation of test results for this purpose and the provision of feedback requires considerable training, expertise, and experience and cannot by reduced to a simple formulaic procedure! An appreciation of the need to triangulate different sources of information, including test results, in identifying relative level of performance on underlying domains of cognition is essential, as are good therapeutic skills in providing constructive and encouraging yet realistic feedback in terms that clients can relate to their own lives.

In general, there are three comparisons that are critical in providing such comparative evaluations. One is the comparison of the individual's current performance to relevant population norms. This is intended to provide information by which the clients can assess his or her likelihood of meeting or exceeding typical expectations of performance in various areas. For instance, it may be helpful for an individual to have their impression that they are 'better with words', but 'not as good with their hands' than most of their peers confirmed through a comparison of their performance with the level typical for someone of comparable age and the same gender. One particularly interesting aspect of this type of feedback is when an individual comes to adjust his or her self-evaluation of an ability because it had been formulated on the basis of very limited or misleading personal comparisons. For instance, some individuals have come to suppose that because working with mathematics is not as easy for them as for a particularly gifted friend or family member that they have poor ability in this area whereas it may turn out that they actually have average or above average ability in this domain. Less enjoyable, but equally useful, can be feedback indicating that their perception of themselves as being exceptionally gifted in a particular area may not be justified by objective indices of their performance in comparison to others. Finally, comparison of the individual's perceived strengths and weaknesses to those supported by psychometric test results can also provide information regarding the degree of insight they have regarding their own level of cognitive functioning or actual capabilities.

A second important comparison is of an individual's own performance across domains. This personal profile of performance strengths and weaknesses can under some circumstances be used to help the individual develop more effective strategies for approaching tasks or processing information – for instance using visual schematics as opposed to verbal propositions in summarizing or remembering material. Such information can also provide the individual with a better basis for making important life decisions, such as those discussed in the next section, as well as adding credibility to other aspects of the assessment.

Finally, skilled interpretation of cognitive assessments may help the individual to appreciate the likelihood of change in their performance over time. As noted above, there is little evidence that the course of cognitive functioning for first episode patients is an inevitable decline and some improve during treatment.[14] In general, there is no way of predicting with certainty the likelihood of future improvement. Nevertheless, to the extent that the pattern of results suggests that current performance is at least partially a reflection of negative emotional states or the distraction of residual psychotic symptoms then further improvement appears possible. Again, offering hope and encouragement while maintaining realistic expectations requires well informed and skilled clinical judgment.

Academic and vocational planning

The onset of psychotic disorders most often occurs in late adolescence or early adulthood, which are critical time periods for many challenging transitions in people's lives including planning and undertaking initiatives in the areas of employment and education. These are areas in which level and profile of cognitive functioning can have important implications. Decisions made at this point in a young person's life can be difficult and have far reaching consequences even without the additional complications and challenges of dealing with a psychotic disorder.

For many first episode patients, the onset of psychosis is associated with a disruption in education at the high school, community college or university level. The occurrence of psychosis typically results in many challenges with respect to continuing education. It has been our experience that many young people hesitate to return to their education because of issues related to embarrassment and stigma, and it is important to help them cope with such social challenges. The occurrence of psychosis represents a form of trauma for many which reduces their self-confidence. It is, therefore, important that their return to school be under circumstances that are likely to prove rewarding.

We are aware of many instances in which young people with psychotic disorders and their families have been explicitly told by clinicians and educators, without relevant experience, that the occurrence of a psychotic disorder inevitably rules out any possibility of further educational achievement and likely means, at best, vocational stagnation. Our experience has been that many first episode patients are able to return to school, college or university and complete diplomas and degrees that can help assure them of good jobs and a better quality of life than might otherwise be possible. The results of cognitive assessments can be of considerable value with respect to advising on whether, when and how to return to school. Level of functioning, especially in such critical areas as sustained attention, speed of information processing and memory can be very useful in helping clients decide when they are sufficiently recovered to return, the level of coursework to take, the type of courses that are most likely to be appropriate and any modifications or accommodations that should be sought from the educational institution.

Clients can be helped in making prudent decisions by consideration of current level of cognitive functioning in combination with emotional states, any residual symptoms of psychotic illness and level of skills for coping with the demands of studying. Again, no one test result is likely to be sufficient in this respect, but rather skilled interpretation of a pattern of results is vital. A combination of circumstances often results in the recommendation being made for a gradual return to school, for instance, taking less than a full course load at the beginning and gradually increasing it as confidence is restored, social stress reduced and academic skills established or re-established. Cognitive assessments can provide evidence by which to guide the establishment of compensatory strategies for any areas of comparative weakness such as adaptation of note taking strategies, making memory friendly summaries of readings, scheduling breaks, and tape recording lectures. Schools and universities have considerable experience in adapting classroom procedures and examination circumstance to the needs of the physically disabled and the adaptations for the needs of our clients are typically relatively minor. Request for such adaptations being supported by reports from an appropriate assessment by a licensed psychologist can be of considerable assistance in this respect.

Similar considerations are relevant when individuals are addressing vocational issues. Formally assessed cognitive functioning considered in combination with the individual's interests and educational background can help identify the most viable employment options. For many clients, such assessments can help better inform not just the most appropriate types of jobs for the person, but also help identify the types of employment support interventions that may be most critical for them to receive.

Informing treatment decisions

Many decisions made in the course of treating a first episode client can be better informed by consideration of the results of formal cognitive assessments. Group interventions often require the ability to maintain selective and sustained attention and concentration over time. The ability to manage medication independently can be compromised by difficulties in memory—particularly prospective memory. A relative weakness in this area may point to the need for use of a dosette in a visible place to aid recall for medication intake. Decisions about level of support required in community living can also benefit from information with respect to functioning in such areas as working and prospective memory, concentration, planning and, other areas of executive functioning. In addition, information concerning the most effective ways of an individual being able to comprehend and retain material can be useful in helping clinicians determine the best way of presenting information. For example, clients with a relative weakness in auditory verbal learning may benefit from key points of treatment sessions being written down for them to review later. Assessment results of this nature may also aid the clinician in determining the appropriate amount of information to present in any one session and the frequency with which this should be reviewed.

Conclusions

Although the use of formal cognitive assessments has most often been associated with addressing research issues in first episode psychosis or early intervention, experience suggests that such assessments can be of considerable assistance in making clinical decisions. Carrying out careful assessments of cognitive functioning and meaningful and valid interpretation of the results requires very specific and specialized training and experience. Unfortunately, psychologists with the requisite skills are not always readily available in first episode and early intervention programs.

Our experience of the Prevention and Early Intervention Program for Psychosis (PEPP) was one in which a cognitive assessment protocol was initially introduced and funded for research purposes. Over time, the clinical value of the assessments has become so apparent that we hope to be able to maintain many aspects of these assessments in order to meet patient care needs.

References

1. Heinrichs RW, Zakzanis KK. Neurocognitive deficit in schizophrenia: A quantitative review of the evidence. Neuropsychology 1998; **12:**426–45.
2. Rund BR. A review of longitudinal studies of cognitive functioning in schizophrenia patients. Schizophr Bull 1998; **24:**425–35.
3. Townsend LA, Norman RMG. The course of cognitive functioning in first episode schizophrenia spectrum disorders. Exp Rev Neurotherapeutics 2004; **4:**89–96.
4. Amminger GP, Edwards J, Brewer WJ, et al. Duration of untreated psychosis and cognitive deterioration in first-episode schizophrenia. Schizophr Research 2002; **54:**223–30.
5. Barnes TRE, Hutton SB, Chapman MJ. West London first-episode study of schizophrenia: Clinical correlates of duration of untreated psychosis. Br J Psychiatry 2000; **177:**207–11.
6. Hoff AL, Sakuma M, Razi BK, et al. Lack of association between duration of untreated illness and severity of cognitive and structural brain deficits at the first episode of schizophrenia. Am J Psychiatry, 2000; **157:**1824–8.
7. Joyce E, Hutton S, Mutsatsa S, et al. Executive dysfunction in first-episode schizophrenia and relationship to duration of untreated psychosis: The West London Study. Br J Psychiatry 2002; **43**(Suppl): 538–44.
8. Norman RMG, Townsend LA, Malla AK. Duration of untreated psychosis and cognitive functioning in first episode patients. Br J Psychiatry 2002; **179:** 340–5.
9. Heinrichs RW. Schizophrenia and the brain. Am Psychol 1993; **48:**221–33.
10. Green MF. What are the functional consequences of neurocognitive deficits in schizophrenia? Am J Psychiatry 1996; **153:**321–30.
11. Malla AK, Norman RM, Manchanda R, et al. Status of patients with first-episode psychosis after one year of phase-specific community-oriented treatment. Psychiatr Serv 2002; **53:**458–63.
12. Kolb B, Wishaw IQ. *Fundamentals of Human Neuropsychology.* New York: WH Freeman; 1990.
13. Townsend LA, Malla AK, Norman RMG. Cognitive functioning in stabilized first episode patients. Psychiatry Res 2001; **104:**119–31.
14. Townsend LA, Norman RMG, Malla AK, et al. Changes in cognitive functioning following comprehensive treatment for first episode patients with schizophrenia spectrum disorders. Psychiatry Res 2002; **113:**69–81.
15. Malla AK, Lazosky A, McLean T, et al. Neuropsychological assessment as an aid to psychosocial rehabilitation in severe mental disorders. Psychiatr Rehab J 1997; **21:**169–73.

23

Family Intervention in First Episode Psychosis

William R McFarlane

Introduction

Among all medical disorders, schizophrenia is one of the most costly and most severe, creating nearly continuous disability for a lifetime in the great majority of cases. It is a devastating disorder for families, who often assume major care-taking and psychological burdens secondary to the functional deficits that this and other psychotic disorders impose. The functional disability that is particularly devastating in schizophrenia appears to be secondary to the negative symptoms that usually begin prior to the psychotic symptoms, often persist despite treatment and usually get worse with time and with each subsequent episode. These deficit symptoms are often the most burdensome for family members, because they usually do not identify them as part of the disorder but they nevertheless find themselves supporting the affected member to compensate for those deficits. The reactions many family members have to the emerging symptoms often become one of the stressors that have a negative influence on those symptoms, longer-term outcomes and degree of disability. This chapter describes the interaction of family and biological processes and a powerful treatment method that has been shown to reverse these negative processes and help family members become irreplaceable and remarkably effective contributors to the treatment and rehabilitation process.

Mutually reinforcing biological and social processes

The prodromal and early psychosis phases

Studies of first episode psychosis document that the average time between onset of psychotic symptoms and the initiation of treatment is one to two years, depending on the study.[1] Frequency and severity of recurrence may be increased by exposure to periods of untreated psychosis and decreased by effective treatment.[2,3] The earlier one provides treatment, the more effective is that treatment, the better the prognosis, and the less the functional deficit, perhaps preventing the persistent residual deficits common in these disorders. Early identification of those with active symptoms allows initiation of state-of-the-art treatment that can continue for as long as the person remains vulnerable.

While the scientific evidence is increasingly showing that the major psychotic disorders are based in genetic or developmental defects involving brain function, there is also abundant evidence that the final development of psychotic symptoms is the result of psychosocial stress. The stress-diathesis or stress-vulnerability model provides a widely accepted, empirically supported and useful framework for describing the relationships among provoking agents (stressors), vulnerability, symptom formation (diathesis), and outcome.[4] Thus, a genetically or developmentally vulnerable person with a low tolerance for stress may experience a first episode of psychotic illness following exposure to excessive internally or externally generated stimulation. This principle underlies the biosocial hypothesis (see box).

> Major psychotic disorders are the result of the continual interaction of specific biologic disorders of the brain with specific psychosocial and other environmental factors.

Psychosocial factors are usually the proximal causes of relapse in established cases and the initial psychotic episode. The treatment described here is based on a simple and now plausible theory: the first episode occurs in a biologically vulnerable individual in an already evolving disorder in which the types of proximal causes of the first episode are the same as those of later relapses. Those include major stresses imposed by role transitions and other life events, social isolation, family expressed emotion, family conflict and exasperation, separation from family of origin, and stigma. A review of pertinent literature supports this biosocial causal theory, yielding an interactive, feedback-based model for the final stages of onset, as compared to a simpler linear-causal model. Therefore, treatments that prevent relapse by counteracting those proximal causes can ameliorate the first episode, prevent subsequent relapse, and reduce the vulnerability to developing deficit symptoms.

Expressed emotion (EE)

High levels of criticism and emotional over-involvement are strongly predictive of exacerbation or relapse of symptoms.[5] In an extensive meta-analysis, Bebbington and Kuipers cite the overwhelming evidence from 25 studies representing 1346 patients in 12 different countries for a predictive relationship between high levels of expressed emotion and relapse of schizophrenia and bipolar disorder.[6] Inclusive reciprocal models have been proposed to increase the accuracy of the construct.[7] For example, Strachan et al.[8] and Goldstein et al.[9] found that expressed emotion among key relatives is a reflection of transactional processes between the patient and family, supporting the conclusion that family functioning is affected by aspects of the illness, as well as the converse.

Attribution—relatives' beliefs about the causes of illness-related behavior—is also associated with expressed emotion. Relatives described as critical or hostile misperceive the patient as somehow responsible for unpleasant, symptomatic behavior, whereas more accepting relatives see identical behaviors as characteristic of the illness itself.[10] This is an especially acute risk in the prodromal phase and in the first episode, during which symptoms and deficits often develop slowly, appearing to reflect personality or behavioral faults. An individual who is cognitively impaired, denying illness, paranoid, angry, hostile, affectively labile, socially withdrawn or anhedonic will be much less available to receive the support needed to function at an optimal level.[11] If family members confronted by such symptoms in a loved one have little formal knowledge of the illness, they are likely to respond with increased involvement, emotional intensity or criticism. One of the few prospectively validated predictors of the onset of schizophrenic psychosis in vulnerable adolescents is negative affective style, an analog of EE.[12]

Stigma

Stigma is often associated with withdrawal of social support, demoralization, and loss of self-esteem, and can have far-reaching effects on daily functioning, particularly at work or school. Link and colleagues observed that stigma had a strong continuing negative impact on well-being, even though proper diagnoses and treatment improved symptoms and levels of functioning over time.[13] Stigma affects the family as well. Effects include withdrawal and isolation on the part of family members, which in turn are associated with a decrease in social network size and emotional support, increased burden, diminished quality of life, and exacerbations of medical disorders.[14] Self-imposed stigma tends to reduce the likelihood that early signs will be addressed and treatment sought and accepted, especially during the first episode.[15]

Communication deviance

Communication deviance, a measure of distracted or vague conversational style, has been consistently associated with schizophrenia. This, and family negative affective style, are the two predictive factors in the onset of schizophrenic psychosis in disturbed, but non-psychotic, adolescents.[12] Studies have demonstrated that communication deviance is correlated with cognitive dysfunction in relatives, which is of the same type as in patients with schizophrenia, but of lower severity.[16] This suggests that some family members have difficulty holding a focus of attention, with important implications for treatment design. A child with subtle cognitive deficiencies may learn to converse in a communication milieu that is less able to compensate and correct. These difficulties are not personality defects; rather they are manifestations of the schizophrenic diathesis playing itself out in the interpersonal as well as in the neurological and genetic domains.

Social isolation

Research on several severe and chronic illnesses indicates that access to social contact and support prevents the deterioration of patients and improves the course of their illnesses.[17] Family members of the most severely ill patients are isolated, preoccupied with, and burdened by, the patient. Social support buffers the impact of adverse life events,[18] and is one of the key factors predicting medication compliance,[19] behavior

toward treatment in general, schizophrenic relapse, and quality of life.[20] Availability of social support to the family is associated with subjective burden experienced by relatives.[21] Brown et al. showed that 90% of the families with high expressed emotion were small in size and socially isolated.[5] Social network size decreases with number of episodes, is lower than normal prior to onset and decreases during the first episode.[22]

Life events prior to onset

Disruption of social networks leads to destabilization and relapse. Steinberg and Durrell found that the vast majority (nearly 80%) of first episodes in an Australian sample occurred after separation from home and family—on entering college or the military.[23] Life events have been shown to be associated with, or predictive of, relapse in schizophrenia.[24] For young adults and adolescents the most potent events tend to be those that involve loss of supportive social ties, especially separation from, or death of, family members, romantic/marital losses for women, and occupational disruptions for men.

Effects of psychosis on the family

Because there is so much evidence that some family members of patients with established psychotic disorders share subclinical forms of similar deficits and abnormalities, treatment for early stages of psychosis must be designed to compensate for some of those difficulties. Those deficits lead to diminished coping ability, which is required in abundance in order to provide a therapeutic influence on the affected family member. Psychotic disorders exact an enormous toll on family members, in anxiety, anger, confusion, stigma, rejection, and exacerbation of medical disorders.[14] Most families undergo organizational changes, including alienation of siblings, exacerbation or initiation of marital conflict, severe disagreement regarding support versus behavior control, even divorce. Almost every family undergoes a degree of demoralization and self-blame, which may be inadvertently reinforced by some clinicians. During the prodromal phase, family members are mystified by the often dramatic emotional, cognitive, and behavior changes that they are seeing, and react in a wide variety of ways, from anger to denial to profound anxiety and worry. The result is a slow-moving crisis that cannot be guided or resolved from within the family.

A model of reciprocal causation

For the genetically or developmentally vulnerable person, subclinical cognitive deficits, effects of the psychosis on the family, family expressed emotion and exasperation, and characteristic coping styles combine to contribute to illness-generated stresses that induce a spiraling and deteriorating process that ends in a major psychosis. The proximal causes described above are potential targets for psychosocial treatment. The psychoeducational multifamily group model assumes that these stress factors can be countered or ameliorated by family and social-network intervention.

Outcomes of family intervention

Established and first episode cases

The family psychoeducational model defines schizophrenia as a brain disorder sensitive to the social environment. Thus, this form of treatment is bimodal, influencing both the disease, through medication, and the social environment, through techniques that deliberately reduce stimulation, rate of change, and complexity to tolerable levels. The approach achieves these goals by providing education, training, and support to family members and others, who in turn provide support, protection, and guidance to the patient.

The efficacy of family intervention, variously termed family 'psychoeducation', 'family behavioral management', or 'family work' (but not family therapy) is remarkable. Outcome studies by Goldstein, Leff, Falloon, Hogarty, Tarrier, Schooler, and Randolph report a reduction in

annual relapse rates for medicated, non-institutionalized patients of as much as 40%, using a variety of educational, supportive, and behavioral techniques.[25,26] The average relapse rates in these studies are 40% for individual treatment without family involvement, and under 15% for family approaches. This effect equals the reduction in relapse in medicated versus unmedicated patients in most drug maintenance studies. In over 20 controlled clinical trials, the track record for symptomatic, relapse, and functional superiority of family over non-family based routine treatment is clear: it is effective, in nearly any country, population, socioeconomic environment, class, gender or ethnic group, when applied in schizophrenia.[27] Psychoeducational multiple family groups (PMFGs) reduce relapse to even lower frequencies and enhance vocational and social rehabilitation outcomes, especially regarding competitive employment.[28,29]

In a study in which 69% of the cases were having their first episode, there were no relapses among the first episode group in the cohort that received family crisis therapy during the six months of the trial, significantly lower than in the cohort without family involvement.[30] A long-term follow-up disclosed remarkably good outcomes in the period from three to six years after intervention. In two studies of differential effects in schizophrenia of single- (SFT) and multi-family group (MFG) forms of the same psychoeducational treatment method, better outcomes were observed for multifamily groups among those having their first hospitalization.[28,31]

Psychoeducational multi-family group treatment

First episode psychosis

The psychoeducation multi-family group treatment model described here is designed to assist families directly in coping with major burdens and reducing stresses during the prodromal and psychotic phases of these disorders. This approach:

1. Allays anxiety and exasperation;
2. Replaces confusion with knowledge, direct guidance, problem solving and coping skill training;
3. Reverses social withdrawal and rejection by participation in a multi-family group that counteracts stigma and demoralization; and
4. Reduces anger by providing a more scientific and socially acceptable explanation for symptoms and functional disability.

In short, it relieves the burdens of coping while more fully engaging the family in the treatment and rehabilitation process, and compensating—non-pejoratively—for the expected subclinical symptoms that many relatives can be expected to manifest. The goal of intervention is to provide optimal treatment as early as possible for those who are experiencing a first episode of psychosis.

These groups address expressed emotion, social isolation, stigmatization, and burden directly by education, training, and modeling. Much of the effectiveness of the groups results from increasing the size and density of the social network, by reducing the experience of being stigmatized, by providing a forum for mutual aid, and by providing an opportunity to hear similar experiences and find workable solutions.

Five to seven families meet with two clinicians on a biweekly basis for one to three years. Unless psychotic, the patients also attend the group, although the decision to attend is based upon the patient's mental status and susceptibility to stimulation. Each session lasts for 1.5 to 2 hours. The multi-family group intervention is described briefly here and in detail elsewhere.[32]

The intervention model consists of four treatment stages roughly corresponding to the phases of an episode of schizophrenia, from the acute phase through the recuperative and rehabilitation phases. These stages are:

1. Engagement
2. Education
3. Re-entry
4. Social and vocational rehabilitation.[33]

Engagement

Contact with the family and with the newly admitted individual is initiated within 48 hours of hospital admission or the onset of psychosis. The aim is to establish rapport and to gain consent to include the family in the ongoing treatment process. The clinician emphasizes that the goal is to collaborate with the family in helping their relative recover and avoid further deterioration or relapse. The family is asked to join with the clinician in establishing a working alliance or partnership, the purpose of which is to provide the best post-hospital environment for recovery. Initial contacts with the patient are deliberately brief and non-stressful. The young person is included in at least one of the joining sessions and is excluded from at least one. If the patient is actively psychotic, they are not included in these sessions, but only engaged in a patient-clinician format. This phase is typically three to seven single-family sessions for the multiple family group version, but more may be required until a sufficient number of families is engaged.

Education

Once the family is engaged and while the patient is still being stabilized, the family is invited to a workshop conducted by the clinicians who will lead the group. These six hour sessions are conducted in a formal, classroom-like atmosphere, involving five or six cases. Biological, psychological, and social information about psychotic disorders and their management is presented with videotapes, slide presentations, lectures, discussion, and question-and-answer periods. Information about how clinicians, patient, and family will work together is presented. The families are introduced to guidelines for management of the disorder and the underlying vulnerability to stress and information overload. Patients attend these workshops if clinically stable, willing, interested, and seemingly able to tolerate the social and informational stress.

The clinicians tailor education and information-sharing to each patient and family's unique and evolving experience, as assessed during the engagement process. Psychosis is defined as a reversible, treatable condition, like diabetes. The genetic or developmental vulnerability is presented as an unusual sensitivity to sensory stimulation, prolonged stress and strenuous demands, rapid change, complexity, social disruption, illicit drugs and alcohol, and negative emotional experience. As for blame and assigning fault, the clinicians take an important position: neither the patient nor the family caused the sensitivity. Whatever the underlying biological cause might be, it is part of the person's physical personhood, with both advantages and disadvantages. Families are explicitly urged not to blame themselves for this vulnerability.

Families receive rather specific guidelines to use in relating to, and attempting to help, their relative with the illness. Table 23.1 presents the guidelines that are specific to the early phases of psychosis.

Re-entry

Following the workshop, the families and patients meet with the clinicians every two weeks in the

---

Table 23.1 Guidelines for families: ways to hasten recovery and to prevent a recurrence

Believe in your power to affect the outcome: you can

Make forward steps cautiously, one step at a time
Go slowly. Allow time for recovery. Recovery takes time. Rest is important. Things will get better in their own time. Build yourself up for the next life steps. Anticipate life stresses.

Consider using medication to protect your future
A little goes a long way. The medication is working and is necessary even if you feel fine. Work with your doctor to find the right medication and the right dose. Have patience, it takes time. Take medications as they are prescribed. Take only medications that are prescribed.

Try to reduce your responsibilities and stresses, at least for the next six months or so
Take it easy. Use a personal yardstick. Compare this month to last month rather than last year or next year.

Use the symptoms as indicators
If they reappear, slow down, simplify and look for support and help, quickly. Learn and use your early warning signs and changes in symptoms. Consult with your family clinician or psychiatrist.

Create a protective environment

Keep it cool
Enthusiasm is normal. Tone it down. Disagreement is normal. Tone it down too.

Give each other space
Time out is important for everyone. It's okay to reach out. It's okay to say 'no'.

Set limits
Everyone needs to know what the rules are. A few good rules keep things clear.

Ignore what you can't change
Let some things slide. Don't ignore violence or concerns about suicide.

Keep it simple
Say what you have to say clearly, calmly, and positively.

Carry on business as usual
Re-establish family routines as quickly as possible. Stay in touch with family and friends.

Solve problems step-by-step

multiple family group format. The goal of this stage of treatment is to develop and implement strategies to cope with the vicissitudes of a person recovering from acute psychosis. Treatment compliance, stress reduction, buffering and avoiding life events, avoiding street drugs and/or alcohol, lowering of expectations during the period of negative symptoms, and a temporary increase in tolerance for these symptoms are major topics. Two special techniques are introduced to support the families' efforts to follow the guidelines introduced in the earlier workshop: formal problem solving and communications skills training.[34]

Social and vocational rehabilitation

Approximately one year following initiation of treatment most patients begin to show signs of returning to spontaneity and active engagement with those around them. Negative symptoms are diminishing and the patient can now be challenged more intensively. The focus of this phase deals with his/her relationship to the wider world, addressing specifically three areas of functioning in which there are commonly deficits: social skills, academic challenges, and the ability to get and maintain employment.

Each family receives education that takes into account the specific features of the symptom constellation of their ill family member during the initial engagement process; this continues during the multi-family group process as well. The pace of reentry is guided by clinical status, the subsidence of negative symptoms, and the continued remission of positive symptoms. Careful, forward progress is the key. In particular, full use is made of precipitants as a guide to situations and factors that may be destabilizing for the specific individual with a psychosis or prodromal symptoms and signs. Temporarily reducing expectations might be suggested around those specific areas. The approach emphasizes fostering patient-to-patient relationships and friendships.

Conclusions

Family psychoeducation and multi-family groups have shown remarkable outcomes in first episode cases in several studies and multi-family groups appear to have a specific efficacy in earlier phases. Empirical evidence and our experience suggests strongly that family-oriented, supportive, psychoeducational treatment is acceptable to families and in clinical trials appears to meet many of their needs. There is theoretical support for the likely efficacy of these methods, with their strategy of stress-avoidance, protection, and buffering, while the multi-family group format adds an inherent element of social support and network expansion.

References

1. Loebel AD, Lieberman JA, Alvir MJ, et al. Duration of psychosis and outcome in first-episode schizophrenia. Am J Psychiatry 1992; **149**:1183–8.
2. Lieberman JA, Koreen AR, Chakos M, et al. Factors influencing treatment response and outcome of first-episode schizophrenia: Implications for understanding the pathophysiology of schizophrenia. J Clin Psychiatry 1996; **57**:5–9.
3. Haas GL, Garratt LS, Sweeney JA. Delay to first antipsychotic medication in schizophrenia: Impact on symptomatology and clinical course of illness. J Psychiatr Res 1998; **32**:151–9.
4. Zubin J, Steinhauer SR, Condray R. Vulnerability to relapse in schizophrenia. Br J Psychiatry 1992; **161**(suppl 18):13–18.
5. Brown GW, Birley JLT, Wing JK. Influence of family life on the course of schizophrenic disorders: A replication. Br J Psychiatry 1972; **121**:241–58.
6. Bebbington P, Kuipers L. The predictive utility of expressed emotion in schizophrenia: An aggregate analysis. Psychol Med 1994; **24**:707–18.
7. Kuipers L, Bebbington P. Expressed emotion research in schizophrenia: Theoretical and clinical implications. Psychol Med 1988; **18**:893–909.
8. Strachan A, Feingold D, Goldstein M, et al. Is expressed emotion an index of a transactional process? II. Patient's coping style. Fam Process 1989; **28**:169–81.

9. Goldstein M, Rosenfarb I, Woo S, Nuechterlein K. Intrafamilial relationships and the course of schizophrenia. Acta Psychiatr Scand Suppl 1994; **384**:60–6.

10. Brewin C, MacCarthy B, Duda R, Vaughn C. Attribution and expressed emotion in the relatives of patients with schizophrenia. J Abnorm Psychol 1991; **100**:546–55.

11. McFarlane WR, Lukens EP. Insight, families, and education: An exploration of the role of attribution in clinical outcome. In: Amador XF, David AS (eds). *Insight and Psychosis.* Oxford University Press; 1998: 317–31.

12. Goldstein M. Family factors that antedate the onset of schizophrenia and related disorders: The results of a fifteen year prospective longitudinal study. Acta Psychiatr Scand 1985; **71**:7–18.

13. Link BG, Mirotznik J, Cullen FT. The effectiveness of stigma coping orientations: Can negative consequences of mental illness labeling be avoided? J Health Soc Behav 1991; **32**:302–20.

14. Johnson D. The family's experience of living with mental illness. In: Lefley HP, Johnson DL (eds). *Families as Allies in Treatment of the Mentally Ill: New Directions for Mental Health Professionals.* Washington, DC: American Psychiatric Press; 1990: 31–65.

15. Phelan JC, Bromet EJ, Link BG. Psychiatric illness and family stigma. Schizophr Bull 1998; **24**:115–26.

16. Wagener DK, Hogarty GE, Goldstein MJ, et al. Information processing and communication deviance in schizophrenic patients and their mothers. Psychiatr Res 1986; **18**:365–77.

17. Penninx BWJH, Kriegsman DMW, van Eijk JTM, et al. Differential effect of social support on the course of chronic disease: A criterion-based literature review. Fam, Syst Health 1996; **14**:223–44.

18. Lin N, Ensel W. Depression-mobility and its social etiology: The role of life events and social support. J Health Soc Behav 1984; **25**:176–88.

19. Fenton WS, Blyler CR, Heinssen RK. Determinants of medication compliance in schizophrenia: Empirical and clinical findings. Schizophr Bull 1997; **23**:637–51.

20. Becker T, Leese M, Clarkson P, et al. Links between social network and quality of life: An epidemiologically representative study of psychotic patients in south London. Soc Psychiatry Psychiatr Epidemiol 1998; **33**:229–304.

21. Solomon P, Draine J. Subjective burden among family members of mentally ill adults: Relation to stress, coping, and adaptation. Am J Orthopsychiatry 1995; **65**:419–27.

22. Anderson C, Hogarty G, Bayer T, Needleman R. Expressed emotion and social networks of parents of schizophrenic patients. Br J Psychiatry 1984; **144**:247–55.

23. Steinberg H, Durell J. A stressful social situation as a precipitant of schizophrenia. Br J Psychiatry 1968; **114**:1097–105.

24. van Os J, Fahy TA, Bebbington P, et al. The influence of life events on the subsequent course of psychotic illness. A prospective follow-up of the Camberwell Collaborative Psychosis Study. Psychol Med 1994; **24**:503–13.

25. Penn DL, Mueser KT. Research update on the psychosocial treatment of schizophrenia. Am J Psychiatry 1996; **153**:607–17.

26. Dixon L, Adams C, Lucksted A. Update on family psychoeducation for schizophrenia. Schizophr Bull 2000; **26**:5–20.

27. McFarlane WR, Dixon L, Lukens E, Lucksted A. Family psychoeducation and schizophrenia: A review of the literature. J Marital Fam Ther 2003; **29**:223–45.

28. McFarlane WR, Lukens E, Link B, et al. Multiple-family groups and psychoeducation in the treatment of schizophrenia. Arch Gen Psychiatry 1995; **52**:679–87.

29. McFarlane WR, Dushay RA, Stastny P, et al. A comparison of two levels of Family-aided Assertive Community Treatment. Psychiatr Serv 1996; **47**:744–50.

30. Goldstein M, Rodnick E, Evans J, et al. Drug and family therapy in the aftercare treatment of acute schizophrenia. Arch Gen Psychiatry 1978; **35**:1169–77.

31. McFarlane WR, Link B, Dushay R, et al. Psychoeducational multiple family groups: Four-year relapse outcome in schizophrenia. Fam Process 1995; **34**:127–44.

32. McFarlane WR. *Multifamily Groups in the Treatment of Severe Psychiatric Disorders.* New York: Guilford Press; 2002.

33. Anderson C, Hogarty G, Reiss D. *Schizophrenia and the Family: A Practitioner's Guide to Psychoeducation and Management.* New York: Guilford Press; 1986.

34. Falloon I, Boyd J, McGill C. *Family Care of Schizophrenia.* New York: Guilford Press; 1984.

24

Cognitive Therapies

Tania Lecomte and Richard P Bentall

Origins/history

Of the existing psychosocial interventions, cognitive behavioral therapy (CBT) is recognized by many researchers and clinicians as an effective treatment of choice for people struggling with psychotic symptoms, particularly when offered as an adjunct to pharmacotherapy.[1–3] CBT was originally developed by AT Beck as a treatment for depression,[4] but has since been used to treat many other difficulties, such as anxiety, personality disorders or substance abuse. CBT, adapted to individuals with psychosis, aims at diminishing psychological distress, which is often linked to dysfunctional beliefs and behaviors. It also attempts to address cognitive and reasoning biases thought to underlie symptoms, such as hallucinations and delusions. Although most studies investigating the effects of CBT with patients with psychotic disorders have reported significant decreases in symptoms, the goal of the therapy is to help patients with a multitude of difficulties they might experience, such as stress, anxiety, depression or low self-esteem. CBT works by teaching the link between perceptions, beliefs, and emotional or behavioral reactions; by questioning the apparent evidence supporting abnormal beliefs; by encouraging self-monitoring of thoughts; and also by teaching effective coping strategies for dealing with distressing experiences, such as hallucinatory voices.

Numerous studies investigating the effects of CBT on psychotic symptoms have been published, mostly in Britain, including more than 13 randomized controlled trials and three meta-analyses.[3,5–22] (See Table 24.1.) Although results vary and more studies are warranted in order to understand how and for whom CBT works best,[7,23] CBT is, to date, the most efficacious psychosocial individually targeted intervention for patients with psychosis. No negative effects from CBT have ever been reported and most studies show significant improvements in clinical and psychosocial measures, such as self-esteem and positive symptoms.[2,24–26]

Although interest in using CBT with first episode patients is recent, many arguments support the need for CBT with this patient group. First, optimal antipsychotic treatment for young people presenting with a first episode is very difficult to achieve because more than 50% abandon their medication in the first year of treatment,[27] and those who continue take, on average, 58% of the prescribed dose.[28] This is often because of distressing side effects or because the treatment is not perceived as effective.[29] Second, further episodes may lead to increasing treatment resistance. Birchwood and Spencer describe two

Table 24.1 Summary of trials of cognitive behavioral therapy CBT for psychosis

Authors	Groups	Follow-ups	Outcomes	Comments
Tarrier et al. (1993)[6]	CBT vs PST vs WL ($n = 27$)	Post treatment, 6 mths	Both treatment groups improved, CBT greater improvements on delusions and anxiety.	No random allocation.
Garety et al. (1994)[9]	CBT vs WL ($n = 20$)	Post treatment	Improvements in total symptoms, delusions, and depression for CBT.	No random allocation.
Drury et al. (1994; 2000)[10,11]	CBT vs RT ($n = 40$)	Baseline – wkly for 9 mths, + 5 yrs	Superior decline in positive symptoms for CBT. No difference at follow-up on symptoms, or relapse rates. Perceived control over illness greater for CBT.	Assessment carried out by therapist; non-engaged patients excluded from analysis. Acute phase inpatients.
Kuipers et al. (1997)[12]	CBT vs TAU ($n = 60$)	Baseline + 9 mths, 18 mths	Improvements in total symptoms only for CBT (25% reduction), continued improvements for CBT at 18 mths.	
Tarrier et al. (1998)[13]	CBT vs SC vs TAU ($n = 87$)	Post treatment, 12 mths	CBT significantly superior to SC and TAU on positive symptoms, at 12 mths only superior to TAU.	
Pinto et al. (1999)[19]	CBT + SST vs SC ($n = 41$)	Baseline + 6 mths	Both groups improved at post-treatment, CBT significantly superior to SC for positive symptoms and total symptoms at 6 mths.	Combination clozapine + CBT.
Sensky et al. (2001)[14]	CBT vs BF; 9 mth treatment period ($n = 90$)	Post treatment and + 9 mths	Both groups improved post-treatment; gains maintained in CBT but not BF group.	

Table 24.1 continued

Authors	Groups	Follow-ups	Outcomes	Comments
Turkington et al. (2002)[5]	CBT targeted at improving insight vs TAU; CBT was 6 sessions + 3 sessions for carers (n = 422)	Post treatment	Post treatment CBT superior on insight, depression and overall symptoms.	Therapy delivered by nurses in receipt of 10 day training program.
Morrison et al. (2002; in press)[21,22]	CBT vs M (n = 31)	Baseline, 6–12 mths of monitoring	Significantly less transition to psychosis with CBT.	Individuals at risk for psychosis, in prodromal phase.
Lewis et al. (2002)[17] Tarrier et al. (2004)[18]	CBT vs SC vs TAU (n = 315) 5 wk therapy window plus 2 booster sessions	Post treatment, baseline + 9 mths, and baseline + 18 mths	No effects post treatment; modest effects for CBT (best outcome) and SC at final follow-up.	About 80% of first episode patients. Acutely ill recently admitted patient.
Durham et al. (2003)[15]	CBT vs SC vs TAU; 9 mth treatment period (n = 66)	Post treatment and + 3 mths	Modest improvements in total symptoms found for CBT at follow-up but not post treatment. About 1/3 CBT-treated patients showed a 25% reduction in total symptoms.	Therapy delivered by nurses.
Rector et al. (2003)[16]	CBT + ETAU vs ETAU (n = 42)	Post treatment and + 6 mths	No differences post-treatment (both groups improved on positive, negative and total symptoms). At follow-up CBT superior for negative symptoms.	
Granholm et al. (in press)[20]	CBT + SST vs TAU (n = 76)	Baseline, post treatment, and 18 mths	No effects on symptoms. CBT superior for psychosocial functioning and cognitive insight. No differences on symptoms.	Group therapy. Older patients (M = 55).

Treatments are: BF, befriending; CBT, cognitive behavior therapy; ETAU, enriched treatment as usual; RT, recreational therapy and support; PST, problem solving therapy; SST, social skills training; SC, supportive counseling; TAU, treatment as usual; WL, waiting list; M, monitoring.

studies where patients' symptoms become less responsive to medication following successive relapses; in some cases, symptoms appeared that were not present prior to relapse.[30] Third, a first episode typically occurs during adolescence or early adulthood, a period during which the person's sense of identity and belonging can be shattered by psychotic experiences, leading to social withdrawal or substance abuse.[31–34] Treatment by medication alone does not address these difficulties whereas CBT can.

Fundamental assumptions

The development of cognitive behavioral interventions for psychotic patients has occurred alongside a reappraisal of several fundamental assumptions about the nature of symptoms, such as hallucinations and delusions.[35] Whereas it has often been assumed that these kinds of experiences must be understood exclusively in biomedical terms so that, for example, delusions are 'empty speech acts, whose informational content refers to neither world or self',[36] cognitive behavioral researchers have argued that they can often be explained in terms of psychological processes that are amenable to psychotherapeutic intervention. Moreover, in contrast to medically orientated clinicians, who have often assumed that lack of insight is a cardinal feature of disorders such as 'schizophrenia' and 'bipolar disorder', cognitive behavioral therapists start from the assumption that patients are inherently rational and, with appropriate support, are capable of considering evidence that either supports or counts against their unusual beliefs and experiences.

These assumptions made by cognitive behavioral therapists have received some support from empirical research. For example, a number of investigators have suggested that the auditory hallucinations of psychotic patients may be a consequence of patients misattributing their inner speech to sources that are external or alien to the self.[37,38] In this context 'inner speech' refers to the internal dialogue or verbal thought that occurs throughout periods of wakefulness, and which is thought to have a self-regulatory function.[39] When adults engage in inner speech, covert activations of the speech muscles can be detected by means of electromyography,[40] and similar 'subvocalizations' can be detected when psychotic patients experience auditory hallucinations.[41–43] These observations suggest that people who experience hallucinations may be suffering a deficit in 'source monitoring', the process involved in distinguishing between self-generated cognitive events and events in the real world, and a number of experimental studies support this conclusion.[44–46] Importantly, a number of studies also show that the source monitoring judgments of psychotic patients can be influenced by patients' beliefs.[47,48] Consistent with this observation, it has been observed that patients who cope poorly with their voices and seek treatment, compared with those who do not, tend to regard themselves as weak in comparison with their voices,[49] and that challenging patients' beliefs about the omniscience and omnipotence of their voices can lead to therapeutic gains.[50]

Research on delusions has similarly emphasized the modifiability of the responsible psychological processes. In fact, patients' conviction in their delusional beliefs often fluctuates over time, so that beliefs that are held as self-evidently true one day may be questioned on the next.[51] The fact that most delusional systems concern core existential themes,[52] or the individual's position in the social universe,[53] suggests that they might result from biases in social reasoning. In fact, a number of reasoning biases have been demonstrated in patients suffering from abnormal beliefs. Patients with delusions, in general, have a tendency to jump to conclusions on the basis of limited data when trying to evaluate evidence relevant to their hypotheses.[54] Patients with persecutory or grandiose delusions also seem to have an abnormal style of reasoning about the causes of events, so that negative events are excessively attributed to causes other than the self.[55] It has been argued that this bias represents a dysfunctional method of regulating self-esteem, but this account remains controversial.[56] Whatever the truth, it is clear that delusions arise, at least in part, from processes that should be amenable to psychological intervention.

Cognitive behavioral therapy (CBT) for individual patients

The earliest published research on CBT for psychosis consisted of single case studies or multiple baseline investigations with small numbers of patients suffering from positive symptoms. These reported the effects of specific, usually very time-limited interventions, such as systematic desensitization or thought stopping, for patients suffering from auditory hallucinations,[56] or various ways of challenging the beliefs of patients suffering from delusions.[57,58] Gradually, however, researchers investigated more integrated styles of delivering CBT which were designed to address a wide range of problems, and which were more consonant with the broad cognitive behavioral approach developed for depressed and anxious patients by Beck and others. These approaches have recently been tested in large-scale clinical trials.

A number of good manuals designed to educate therapists in the use of CBT with psychotic patients are now available.[59–61] When working with individuals, cognitive behavioral interventions should be formulation-based, rather than prescriptively targeted at specific symptoms. In practice, this involves the patient and therapist agreeing on a problem list, which is then prioritized so that there is a shared understanding about which problems will be addressed first. Although symptoms, such as hallucinations and delusions, may appear as high priorities on this list, this is not always the case. Given that patients sometimes find their psychotic experiences, especially hallucinations, to be pleasant or even helpful,[62] and given that psychotic patients often experience problems of mood,[63,64] anxiety, depression or even relationship difficulties may be addressed first. Once the therapeutic goals

have been established, the patient and therapist work together in a spirit of collaborative empiricism to identify and assess factors that influence the difficulties, to construct a shared formulation about their origins and any processes that may be maintaining them, and to devise interventions that may help to bring about change. It is usually helpful if the therapist adopts an 'it just might be true' attitude towards patients' unusual experiences and beliefs. Delusional beliefs may then be questioned by means of a Socratic dialogue, or an agreement may be reached to carry out suitable behavioral experiments that will enable core beliefs to be tested (e.g. testing the belief that 'the newsreader is reading out my thoughts' by writing down thoughts while video-recording news bulletins and then watching them later). In the case of auditory hallucinations, it may be particularly important to address patients' beliefs about the malevolence and omnipotence of their voices,[50] and also their meta-cognitive beliefs about their own thought processes, which may be responsible for dysfunctional thought-control strategies.[65] Cognitive behavioral therapists also typically address issues of self-esteem, as negative beliefs about the self may exacerbate psychotic symptoms.[66] Attention may be paid to patients' coping strategies, and also strategies for avoiding relapse.

Most clinical trials of CBT for psychosis have focused on chronically ill patients who have failed to respond adequately to antipsychotic medication. The quality of trials has varied but most must be considered good by the standards used to evaluate pharmacological interventions. Only two studies (see Table 24.1) have specifically addressed the effects of CBT with acutely ill patients, including first episode patients, who had recently been admitted to hospital. Although Drury and colleagues reported excellent results from an intensive intervention with recently admitted patients, this trial was compromised by the fact that outcomes were assessed by the therapist, and by the exclusion of patients who failed to engage with treatment from the analysis of the results.[10] A five year follow-up of the patients found little evidence that the earlier reported gains had been sustained.[25] The recent SoCRATES (Study of Cognitive Re-Alignment Therapy in Early Schizophrenia) trial is the only study to examine the effects of this kind of CBT specifically in early schizophrenia. Over 300 first episode and second episode patients were randomly assigned to three conditions: treatment as usual (typically, admission to a ward and medication); treatment as usual plus supportive counseling; and treatment as usual plus cognitive behavioral therapy. An important limitation of this study is that the therapy, delivered within two weeks of admission, was limited to a five week therapy window plus a small number of booster sessions. However, outcomes were assessed by blinded psychiatrists up to 18 months after inception to the study, and approximately 75% of patients remained in the study at this point. Outcome following the treatment phase showed no advantage to psychological therapy, almost certainly because any treatment effects were overshadowed by the first-time use of antipsychotic drugs.[17] However, at 18 month follow-up modest advantages were observed for psychological therapy, especially cognitive behavioral therapy, in terms of symptom improvements, although not in terms of relapse rates.[18] Experience during the trial indicated that delivering psychological therapy immediately after admission, when patients were often highly emotional and confused, may have impeded engagement. Furthermore, the short therapy window meant that therapists often found that they were just beginning to make progress when therapy was terminated. It seems likely, therefore, that cognitive behavioral interventions for first episode patients will be more effective if introduced some weeks after initial pharmacotherapy, and if treatment is sustained for the kind of period (typically six months) normally allocated for the treatment of other disorders.

CBT as a group intervention

Studies by Wykes et al.,[67] Levine et al.,[68] and Granholm et al.[69] all showed significant decreases in positive symptoms following CBT in group format. Though none of the group studies involved individuals with a first psychotic episode, these significant results nonetheless support the use of CBT group interventions for treating psychotic symptoms. A randomized controlled trial still underway is comparing group CBT for first episode patients to a skills training approach and to a waiting list. Preliminary results suggest that the group approach helps patients decrease positive symptoms, increase self-esteem, and manage stress in their lives.[70] Other arguments coming from the group's participants further support the use of a group format for first episode patients: group interventions foster social support between patients and therefore increase feelings of normalcy through their sharing of common experiences and coping strategies. The study is also demonstrating that group CBT can reliably be offered by mental health staff after receiving a few days of training, instead of the many years necessary in individual therapy. A structured and manualized group format also entails treating more people while necessitating fewer therapists than an individual format.[71]

The structured group approach was developed in a manual,[71] which had to be adapted for people in their late teens and early adult years who had no prior experience in psychosocial interventions for psychosis. The manual consists of 24 activities, equally divided in four parts:

1. Stress: how it affects me
2. Testing hypotheses and looking for alternatives
3. Drugs, alcohol, and how I feel
4. Coping and competence.

In the group approach, the first few sessions aim at building the group cohesion and alliance by first introducing non-threatening concepts, such as stress and its impact on physical and mental health, as well as the vulnerability-stress model as a potential explanatory framework. The second part aims at exploring concepts such as normalization (i.e. others, including those in the group, can experience delusions and hallucinations); perceptions (there is often more than meets the eye); the ABCs of CBT, that is, for a given situation or antecedent (A), people can hold different beliefs (B), which will lead to different emotional and behavioral consequences (C); alternative explanations can explain a situation; seeking facts instead of jumping to conclusions; and how attributions influence our outlook on life. The third section aims at gaining insight into using drugs and alcohol, as well as exploring coping skills and enhancing self-esteem in order to deal better with difficult emotions, such as depression, suicidality, and aggression. Although the CBT group is not meant as a treatment for substance abuse, a few relevant activities are included because of the high prevalence of substance abuse in first episode patients.[72] The last section focuses on coping strategies that are best suited for each individual participant according to different levels of distress. A relaxation technique is practiced. Participants exchange and try out new coping strategies to control voices (e.g. focusing, distraction, humming) or to improve their mood. A relapse-prevention plan (called 'Coping my own way') is also developed for each participant, where resources and coping strategies (either behavioral or cognitive) are chosen by participants according to level of stress and distress anticipated.

In a group setting, concepts are typically introduced with neutral examples ('What are all the possible explanations for a traffic jam?') to more personal examples ('What other alternative explanation could you find for your belief that others want to harm you?'). One of the advantages of working in a group context is that much of the therapeutic work is distributed among members; normalization, Socratic questioning, alternative seeking, as well as checking the facts, can all be used and/or suggested by the clinicians and the participants. However, one of the challenges in conducting group CBT with first episode patients is initially to get them to attend a group, especially when the person no longer experiences vivid psychotic symptoms and wishes to forget ever having experienced a psychotic episode. A good relationship with a therapist, who believes in the benefits of the group, and ideally support from the patient's family, are essential in order to bring a first episode patient to engage in any intervention, including CBT.

Process issues

CBT brings something of a paradigm shift to the treatment of psychosis by changing the way clinicians interact with their patients. Whereas before (and unfortunately in many places still) the clinician was considered the keeper of knowledge, who decided what the patient needed, and would not listen to the patient if his or her speech content was considered 'delusional', CBT proposes the opposite. In fact, the patient is the expert on his or her own experience and decides what is central for him or her to work on. As can be observed in Table 24.2, the role of the CBT clinician is of a facilitator in a collaborative relationship who tries to understand the patient's distress and underlying beliefs regardless of whether they are based in reality or not. Although CBT techniques play an important role in the treatment, they are used as tools and would be inefficient, or even harmful, if used by themselves without the appropriate context and relationship.[23] Above and beyond the strict use of CBT techniques, process variables such as the therapeutic alliance come into play.

Though the therapeutic alliance is rarely measured in most trials, psychotherapy studies estimate the quality of the relationship, or the alliance, as explaining as much as 45% of the outcome.[73] Svensson and Hansson found a positive relationship between initial therapist alliance and treatment outcome in CBT for individuals with severe mental illness.[74] Similarly, in a study in

Table 24.2 Role of the cognitive behavioral therapist	
Do	**Do not**
Establish a good alliance and collaborative working relationship.	Impose your view or your formulation of the patient's issues.
Set treatment goals with patient.	Try to convince the patient to see things differently.
Offer a stable and consistent structure for the therapy.	Aim at modifying the psychotic symptoms at all costs.
Try to understand the patient's beliefs.	Act as an expert.
Work on the most distressing beliefs first.	Demean a patient's belief as 'only a symptom of your illness'.
Protect and enhance self-esteem.	Be inconsistent or interpretative.
Help the patient to discover his or her best ways of coping.	Apply CBT techniques at random.
Promote the use of homework between sessions.	Use CBT for psychosis without appropriate training and supervision.

which schizophrenia patients treated with psychodynamic therapy were found to do no better than patients receiving a control therapy, Frank and Gunderson found that patients who had formed good alliances with their therapist or caregiver had fewer relapses, responded better to treatment, and had better outcomes at two year follow-up than those who did not form such alliances.[75] Similarly, in the SoCRATES cognitive behavioral therapy study with first episode patients,[76] the therapeutic alliance, as rated by the patient (but not as rated by the therapist) predicted the long-term (18 month) improvements in positive symptoms and in general psychopathology.[77] These studies not only stress the importance of the alliance as a major variable related to outcome, but as an active ingredient in therapeutic changes. The alliance is influenced by many other variables, such as the patient's and therapist's personality traits, attachment styles, cognitive schemas, etc. Further investigations of the interaction between patient and therapist variables, and the techniques used, will undoubtly

uncover the most active therapeutic ingredients involved in CBT.

Further likely developments

CBT is already going through multiple changes, some of which will be quite relevant for first episode patients. For one, more and more mental health staff, including nurses, occupational therapists, psychologists, psychiatrists, and social workers, are becoming sensitized to the approach and are receiving some basic training in CBT for psychosis. This suggests openness in certain settings, such as in Canada and the UK,[15,70] to following a philosophy of care that is patient-based, respectful, and collaborative. Other current initiatives include the integration of CBT and vocational rehabilitation,[78] CBT with skills training for patients with more enduring cognitive deficits,[79] CBT for post-traumatic stress disorder in patients with psychosis,[80] CBT for individuals in the prodromal phase to prevent or delay transition to psychosis,[21] and CBT integrated dual disorder treatment programs for substance abuse and psychosis.[81] Other avenues, such as teaching CBT principles to family members or assertive community treatment workers (ACT), could also bring important benefits to patients, families, and ACT teams. Regarding CBT and first episode patients, multiple studies are currently underway by various investigators. For instance, in Canada, Lecomte and colleagues are conducting studies looking into the impact of personality traits on the working alliance and on CBT treatment outcomes, the combination of motivational interviewing and CBT for improving treatment adherence, and integrated dual disorder treatment for first episode patients with methamphetamine abuse. Also in Canada, Addington and colleagues are investigating CBT for first episode patients which addresses adaptation, functional recovery and symptomatic recovery with a focus on affect, early development, attachment, and interpersonal processes.

More studies are, of course, warranted to improve our understanding of how a psychological treatment, such as CBT, can help individuals in the long term and whether this kind of intervention can contribute to maintaining a higher quality of life with less distress linked to symptoms and relapses. It is not clear, for instance, if the treatment effects observed in current studies are a result of patient empowerment or if they are dependent on the presence of specific social or environmental contingencies. Other research questions are more systemic: Can a change in treatment philosophy, such as CBT, decrease perceived stigma towards individuals with psychosis?

References

1. Chadwick PD, Birchwood M. Challenging the omnipotence of voices : A cognitive approach to auditory hallucinations. Br J Psychiatry 1994; **164:**190–201.
2. Garety P, Fowler D, Kuipers E. Cognitive-behavioral therapy for medication-resistant symptoms. Schizophr Bull 2000; **26:**73–86.
3. Gould RA, Mueser KT. Cognitive therapy for psychosis in schizophrenia: An effect size analysis. Schizophr Res 2001; **48:**335–42.
4. Beck AT, Rush AJ, Shaw BF, Emery G. *Cognitive Therapy of Depression.* New York: Guilford Press; 1979.
5. Turkington D, Kingdon D, Turner T, Group IiSR. Effectiveness of a brief cognitive-behavioural therapy intervention in the treatment of schizophrenia. Br J Psychiatry 2002; **180:**523–7.
6. Tarrier N, Beckett R, Harwood S, et al. A trial of two cognitive-behavioural methods of treating drug-resistant residual psychotic symptoms in schizophrenic patients. I: Outcome. Br J Psychiatry 1993; **162:**524–32.
7. Cormac I, Jones C, Campbell C. Cognitive behaviour therapy for schizophrenia (Cochrane review). Cochrane Database Syst Rev 2002; 1.
8. Pilling S, Bebbington P, Kuipers E, et al. Psychological treatments in schizophrenia: I. Meta-analysis of family intervention and cognitive behaviour therapy. Psychol Med 2002; **32:**763–82.
9. Garety PA, Kuipers E, Fowler D, et al. Cognitive behavioural therapy for drug-resistant psychosis. Br J Med Psychology 1994; **67:**259–71.
10. Drury V, Birchwood M, Cochrane R, MacMillan F. Cognitive therapy and recovery from acute psychosis: I. Impact on psychotic symptoms. Br J Psychiatry 1996; **169:**593–601.
11. Drury V, Birchwood M, Cochrane R. Cognitive therapy and recovery from acute psychosis: a controlled trial. 3. Five-year follow-up. Br J Psychiatry 2000; **177:**8–14.
12. Kuipers E, Garety P, Fowler D, et al. The London-East Anglia randomised controlled trial of cognitive-behaviour therapy for psychosis I: Effects of the treatment phase. Br J Psychiatry 1997; **171:**319–27.
13. Tarrier N, Yusupoff L, Kinney C, et al. Randomised controlled trial of intensive cognitive behaviour therapy for chronic schizophrenia. BMJ 1998; **317:**303–7.
14. Sensky T, Turkington D, Kingdon D, et al. A randomized controlled trial of cognitive-behaviour therapy for persistent symptoms in schizophrenia resistant to medication. Arch Gen Psychiatry 2000; **57:**165–72.
15. Durham RC, Guthrie M, Morton RV, et al. Tayside-Fife clinical trial of cognitive-behavioural therapy

for medication-resistant psychotic symptoms. Br J Psychiatry 2003; **182**:303–11.

16. Rector NA, Seeman MV, Segal ZV. Cognitive therapy for schizophrenia: A preliminary randomized controlled trial. Schizophr Res 2003; **63**:1–11.

17. Lewis S, Tarrier N, Haddock G, et al. A randomised, controlled trial of cognitive-behaviour therapy in early schizophrenia: Acute phase outcomes in the SoCRATES trial. Br J Psychiatry 2002; **43**(Suppl): 591–7.

18. Tarrier N, Lewis SW, Haddock G, et al. 18 month follow-up of a randomised, controlled trial of cognitive-behaviour therapy in first episode and early schizophrenia. Br J Psychiatry 2004; **184**:231–9.

19. Pinto A, La Pia S, Mennella R, et al. Cognitive-behavioral therapy and clozapine for clients with treatment-refractory schizophrenia. Psychiatr Serv 1999; **50**:901–4.

20. Granholm E, McQuaid JR, McClure F, et al. A randomized controlled trial of cognitive behavioral social skills training for middle-aged and older outpatients with very chronic schizophrenia. Am J Psychiatry (in press).

21. Morrison AP, Bentall RP, French P, et al. Randomised controlled trial of early detection and cognitive therapy for preventing transition to psychosis in high-risk individuals. Study design and interim analysis of transition rate and psychological risk factors. Br J Psychiatry 2002; **43**(Suppl): S78–S84.

22. Morrison AP, French P, Walford L, et al. A randomised controlled trial of cognitive therapy for the prevention of psychosis in people at ultra-high risk. Br J Psychiatry (in press).

23. Lecomte T, Lecomte C. Toward uncovering robust principles of change inherent to Cognitive-Behavioral therapy for psychosis. Am J Orthopsychiatry 2002; **72**:50–7.

24. Barrowclough C, Haddock G, Tarrier N, et al. Randomized controlled trial of motivational interviewing, cognitive behavior therapy, and family intervention for patients with comorbid schizophrenia and substance use disorders. Am J Psychiatry 2001; **158**:1706–13.

25. Drury V, Birchwood M, Cochrane R. Cognitive therapy and recovery from acute psychosis: A controlled trial: 3. Five-year follow-up. Br J Psychiatry 2000; **177**:8–14.

26. Sensky T, Turkington D, Kingdon D, et al. A randomised controlled trial of cognitive-behavioral therapy for persistent symptoms in schizophrenia resistant to medication. Arch Gen Psychiatry 2000; **57**:165–72.

27. Kasper S. First-episode schizophrenia: The importance of early intervention and subjective tolerability. J Clin Psychiatry 1999; **60**:5–9.

28. Cramer J, Rosenheck R. Compliance with medication regimens for mental and physical disorders. Psychiatr Serv 1998; **49**:196–201.

29. Sheitman BB, Lee H, Strauss R, Lieberman JA. The evaluation and treatment of first-episode psychosis. Schizophr Bull 1997; **23**:653–61.

30. Birchwood M, Spencer E. Early intervention in psychotic relapse. Clin Psychol Rev 2001; **21**:1211–26.

31. Linszen DH, Dingemans PMAJ, Nugter MA, et al. Patient attributes and expressed emotion as risk factors for psychosis relapse. Schizophr Bull 1997; **23**:119–30.

32. Morrison AP, Bowe S, Larkin W, Nothard S. The psychological impact of psychiatric admission: Some preliminary findings. J Nerv Ment Dis 1999; **187**:250–3.

33. Mueser KT, Rosenberg SD, Goodman LA, Trumbetta SL. Trauma, PTSD, and the course of severe mental illness: An interactive model. Schizophr Res 2002; **53**:123–43.

34. Aguilar EJ, Haas G, Manzanera FJ, et al. Hopelessness and first-episode psychosis: A longitudinal study. Acta Psychiatr Scand 1997; **96**:25–30.

35. Bentall RP. *Madness Explained: Psychosis and Human Nature*. London: Penguin; 2003.

36. Berrios G. Delusions as 'wrong beliefs': A conceptual history. Br J Psychiatry 1991; **159**:6–13.

37. Bentall RP. The illusion of reality: A review and integration of psychological research on hallucinations. Psychol Bull 1990; **107**:82–95.

38. Hoffman RE. Verbal hallucinations and language production processes in schizophrenia. Behav Brain Sci 1986; **9**:503–48.

39. Vygotsky LSV. *Thought and Language*. Cambridge, MA: MIT Press; 1962.

40. McGuigan FJ. *Cognitive Psychophysiology: Principles of Covert Behavior*. Englewood Cliffs, NJ: Prentice Hall; 1978.

41. Gould LN. Auditory hallucinations and subvocal speech. J Nerv Ment Dis 1949; **109**:418–27.

42. Inouye T, Shimizu A. The electromyographic study of verbal hallucination. J Nerv Ment Dis 1970; **151**:415–22.

43. McGuigan FJ. Covert oral behavior and auditory hallucinations. Psychophysiology 1966; **3**:73–80.

44. Bentall RP, Slade PD. Reality testing and auditory hallucinations: A signal-detection analysis. Br J Clin Psychology 1985; **24**:159–69.

45. Morrison AP, Haddock G. Cognitive factors in source monitoring and auditory hallucinations. Psychol Med 1997; **27**:669–79.

46. Brebion G, Amador X, David A, et al. Positive symptomatology and source monitoring failure in schizophrenia: An analysis of symptom-specific effects. Psychiatry Res 2000; **95**:119–31.

47. Haddock G, Slade PD, Bentall RP. Auditory hallucinations and the verbal transformation effect: The role of suggestions. Personality Indiv Diff 1995; **19**:301–6.

48. Young HF, Bentall RP, Slade PD, Dewey ME. The role of brief instructions and suggestibility in the elicitation of hallucinations in normal and psychiatric subjects. J Nerv Ment Dis 1987; **175**: 41–8.

49. Honig A, Romme MAJ, Ensink BJ, et al. Auditory hallucinations: A comparison between patients and nonpatients. J Nerv Ment Dis 1998; **186**:646–51.

50. Chadwick P, Birchwood M. The omnipotence of voices: A cognitive approach to auditory hallucinations. Br J Psychiatry 1994; **164**:190–201.

51. Brett-Jones J, Garety P, Hemsley D. Measuring delusional experiences: A method and its application. Br J Clin Psychol 1987; **26**:257–65.

52. Musalek M, Berner P, Katschnig H. Delusional theme, sex and age. Psychopathology 1989; **22**:260–7.

53. Bentall RP. Cognitive biases and abnormal beliefs: Towards a model of persecutory delusions. In: Cutting J (ed). *The Neuropsychology of Schizophrenia.* London: Erlbaum; 1994:337–60.

54. Garety P, Freeman D. Cognitive approaches to delusions: A critical review of theories and evidence. Br J Clin Psychol 1999; **38**:113–54.

55. Bentall RP, Corcoran R, Howard R, et al. Persecutory delusions: A review and theoretical integration. Clin Psychol Rev 2001; **21**:1143–92.

56. Slade PD, Bentall RP. *Sensory Deception: A Scientific Analysis of Hallucination.* London: Croom-Helm; 1988.

57. Chadwick P, Lowe CF. The measurement and modification of delusional beliefs. J Consult Clin Psychol 1990; **58**:225–32.

58. Watts FN, Powell EG, Austin SV. The modification of abnormal beliefs. Br J Med Psychol 1973; **46**:359–63.

59. Kingdon DG, Turkington D. *Cognitive-behavioural Therapy of Schizophrenia.* Hove, UK: Erlbaum; 1994.

60. Fowler D, Garety P, Kuipers E. *Cognitive-behaviour Therapy for Psychosis: Theory and Practice.* Chichester: Wiley; 1995.

61. Morrison AP, Renton JC, Dunn H, et al. *Cognitive Therapy for Psychosis: A Formulation-based Approach.* New York: Brunner-Routledge; 2003.

62. Miller LJ, O'Connor E, DePasquale T. Patients' attitudes to hallucinations. Am J Psychiatry 1993; **150**:584–8.

63. Norman RMG, Malla AK. Dysphoric mood and symptomatology in schizophrenia. Psychol Med 1991; **21**:897–903.

64. Siris SG. Depression and schizophrenia. In: Weinberger DR (ed). *Schizophrenia.* Oxford: Blackwell; 1995:128–45.

65. Morrison AP. The interpretation of intrusions in psychosis: An integrative cognitive approach to hallucinations and delusions. Behav Cogn Psychother 2001; **29**:257–76.

66. Barrowclough C, Tarrier N, Humphreys L, et al. Self-esteem in schizophrenia: The relationship between self-evaluation, family attitudes and symptomatology. J Abnorm Psychol 2003; **112**:92–9.

67. Wykes T, Parr A-M, Landau S. Group treatment of auditory hallucinations. Br J Psychiatry 1999; **175**:180–5.

68. Levine J, Barak Y, Granek I. Cognitive group therapy for paranoid schizophrenics: Applying cognitive dissonance. J Cogn Psychother 1998; **12**:3–12.

69. Granholm E, McQuaid J, McClure F, et al. A randomized controlled pilot study of cognitive behavioral social skills training for older patients with schizophrenia. Schizophr Res 2002; **53**:167–9.

70. Lecomte T, Leclerc C, Wykes T, Lecomte J. Group CBT for clients with a first episode of psychosis. J Cogn Psychother 2003; **17**:375–83.

71. Lecomte T, Leclerc C, Wykes T. CBT—Participant's workbook and clinician's supplement; 2001.

72. Addington J, Addington D. Effect of substance misuse in early psychosis. Br J Psychiatry Suppl 1998; **172**:134–6.

73. Gaston L, Marmar CR, Callaghes D, Thompson LW. Alliance prediction of outcome beyond in-

treatment symptomatic change as psychotherapy processes. Psychother Res 1991; **1**:104–13.

74. Svensson B, Hansson L. Therapeutic alliance in cognitive therapy for schizophrenic and other long-term mentally ill patients: Development and relationship to outcome in an in-patient treatment programme. Acta Psychiatr Scand 1999; **99**:281–7.

75. Frank AF, Gunderson JG. The role of the therapeutic alliance in the treatment of schizophrenia: Relationship to course and outcome. Arch Gen Psychiatry 1990; **47**:228–35.

76. Lewis S, Tarrier N, Haddock G, et al. Randomised controlled trial of cognitive-behavioural therapy in early schizophrenia: Acute-phase outcomes. Br J Psychiatry 2002; **181**:S91–S97.

77. Bentall RP, Lewis S, Tarrier N, et al. Relationships matter: The impact of the therapeutic alliance on outcome in schizophrenia. Schizophr Res 2003; **60**:319.

78. Davis LW, Lysaker PH, Lancaster RS, et al. The Indianapolis Vocational Intervention Program: A cognitive behavioral approach to addressing rehabilitation issues in schizophrenia. J Rehab Res Dev (in press).

79. McQuaid J, Granholm E, McClure F, et al. Development of an integrated cognitive-behavioral, social skills training intervention for older patients with schizophrenia. J Psychother Pract Res 2000; **9**:149–56.

80. Rosenberg SD, Mueser KT, Friedman MJ, et al. Developing effective treatments for posttraumatic disorders among people with severe mental illness. Psychiatr Serv 2001; **52**:1453–61.

81. Mueser KT, Noordsy DL, Drake RE, Fox LB. *Integrated Treatment for Dual Disorders—A Guide to Effective Practice*. New York: Guilford Press; 2003.

25

Psychosocial Interventions in Early Psychosis

Jean Addington and Donald Addington

Introduction

This chapter focuses on the importance of psychosocial interventions for individuals who are recovering from a first episode of psychosis. Progress in the research and development of such interventions can easily be overshadowed by progress in psychopharmacology. For psychosocial interventions there are no glossy inserts of new advances. Empirical testing takes time and money; is labor-intensive and does not lead to a highly profitable product. There are fewer data available to assess efficacy and the interventions are rarely widely tested beyond development settings. The questions this chapter will address are: Why these young people need psychosocial interventions? What psychosocial interventions are available and are they effective?

Why is there a need for early intervention?

The need to recover

First, the overarching goal is to support the concept of recovery from psychosis. The formal definition of the word recovery means 'to get back: regain' or 'to restore (oneself) to a normal state' (*Webster's Dictionary*, 1984). The term 'recovery' is used to include concepts such as awareness

of the toll of the illness, recognition of the need to change, insight as to how this change can begin, and the determination it takes to recover. Ralph identifies four dimensions of recovery.[1] These include internal factors, self-managed care, external factors, and empowerment. Internal factors are those within the individual, such as awareness of the toll the illness has taken, recognition of the need to change, insight as to how this change can begin, and the determination it takes to recover. Self-managed care is an extension of the internal factors in which individuals describe how they manage their own mental health and how they cope with the difficulties and barriers they face. External factors include interconnectedness with others, the supports provided by family, friends, and professionals, and having people who believe that they can cope with, and recover from, their mental illness. Finally, empowerment is a combination of internal and external factors where internal strengths are combined with interconnectedness to provide self-help, advocacy, and caring about what happens to us and to others.[1]

Developmental issues and collateral damage

Young people with psychosis face several developmental issues and subsequent interpersonal and social problems. The onset of psychosis may complicate or interfere with many of the developmental tasks that the young adult is attempting to accomplish at this time.[2,3] These include individuating from the family, developing interests, hobbies and skills, discovering and experimenting with sexuality, forming and maintaining relationships, and engaging in further and/or higher education and vocational activities. Identity formation is one of the first major tasks of young adults.[2] Developing social interactions with others is an important component of this process in terms of the development of a good sense of self-esteem and self-worth.[3] As the young person approaches adulthood he or she becomes dependent on peers more than on family members for these interactions. Clearly, for people experiencing a first episode of psychosis, these important social interactions are often missed if, because of psychosis, the individual begins to withdraw from friends and peers.

When these young individuals develop a psychosis they often fall out of step with their peers, become socially isolated, have an altered self-perception, and are unable to complete their education or training. They experience changes in their sense of self and maturation of the personality. The potential for achievement is reduced and, as the gap between themselves and their peers widens, catching up becomes more difficult. The potential for achievement is further reduced if these individuals delay completion of education or vocational training because of difficulties resulting from their illness. Thus, failure or difficulty in accomplishing these developmental tasks, along with any experiences of stigma, has a major impact on the young person over and above the psychotic illness itself.

Functional vs symptomatic recovery

Recovery from psychotic symptoms is common after the first episode with 75% to 90% achieving remission from positive symptoms one year after treatment.[4–6] However, even in the case of best practice there are limitations to biological treatments. Despite modern pharmacotherapy, there is a limited impact on negative symptoms.[4] Adherence rates to medication are low in first episode patients.[7] Some patients are characterized as 'slow-responders', others are at risk of treatment resistance even when adherence is addressed. Even with ideal biological interventions, relapse rates are very high after the first year of follow-up.[6,8,9] However, functional recovery (e.g. social, vocational, interpersonal) remains a major challenge. The illness remains disabling and problematic for patients and their families since symptom improvement is not always matched with functional improvement.[10,11] Thus, it is critical that we develop treatment approaches to complement pharmacotherapy to help achieve improved outcome. Furthermore, such treatment needs to focus on limiting psychosocial damage by offering sustained treatment during this critical early period when the vulnerability is at its peak and 'we have the best opportunity to provide a degree of damage control' (McGorry: 156).[12]

Goals of psychosocial interventions

There are several goals for psychosocial interventions (Box 25.1). In order to achieve the goals of a psychosocial treatment program it is necessary to take into account not only the symptoms of the illness, but also the impact of the illness on an individual. This includes isolation from families and friends, damage to social and working relationships, depression and demoralization, and an increased risk of self-harm, aggression, and

---

Box 25.1 Goals of psychosocial interventions

- Increase the understanding of psychotic disorders
- Promote adaptation to the disorder
- Increase self-esteem, coping, and adaptive functioning
- Reduce emotional disturbance
- Prevent relapse.

substance abuse. Persistent symptoms that remain after the early recovery phase are an additional problem and add to the already disrupted developmental trajectory. Since the overall goal is to enhance both symptomatic and functional recovery these interventions should be available to everyone within an early psychosis program.

What psychosocial interventions are available?

There is a range of psychosocial interventions available to help recovery from a first episode. They include psychoeducation, individual cognitive behavioral therapy, phase-specific groups, and interventions for substance misuse. Family work is a valuable component of any psychosocial intervention program,[13] but is addressed elsewhere in this text.

Psychoeducation

Through psychoeducation we can give information about symptoms, etiology, and treatment of psychosis. This is a technique used in clinical practice that has the goals of increasing understanding and changing behavior. Individuals have the right to be fully informed about the nature of their illness. In this way they can gain knowledge that helps them understand and integrate their experiences of themselves and their world. This understanding is empowering as it helps clients to take an active role in the management of their illness. Thus, as an integral part of the overall therapeutic process psychoeducation can be delivered individually or in a group format.

Psychoeducation is particularly important in early psychosis since individuals and their families probably have little experience with or knowledge about psychosis. Topics include symptoms and diagnoses, models and theories of psychoses, impact of substance use, medications, warning signs, avoiding relapse, and agencies and personnel involved in treatment. The origins of the illness and factors influencing it are presented in terms of a stress-vulnerability model. Psychosis-

education should be provided for all clients and their families. In addition to the information given by the therapist or group leader, we need to include the client's own explanation of illness and recovery style. A comprehensible, explanatory model for understanding psychosis involving both the individual's and therapist's accounts should be developed since it helps the young person to have some understanding of the concept of psychosis and what it means for them, rather than just providing facts and information. It is important that psychoeducation is sensitive to cultural diversity and the individual's life circumstances and offers a positive outlook. It should always be considered as part of a broader therapeutic approach.

Cognitive behavioral therapy (CBT)

We propose a modular approach to CBT for first episode psychosis. This approach, which has been described elsewhere,[14] parallels the theoretical shift in CBT over the last decade in its consideration of affect, early development, attachment, interpersonal processes, and the therapeutic relationship. The modules include: engagement, education, addressing adaptation, treating coexisting anxiety or depression, coping strategies, relapse prevention, and treating positive and negative symptoms. The development of the modules has been guided by a wide range of texts and manuals of empirically supported treatment models that offer both unique and complementary perspectives of CBT for psychosis.

One of the advantages of offering a modular approach is that there is a range of interventions to meet many of the needs of first episode clients and thus there is less need for 'exclusion criteria'. It is recommended that CBT be introduced to first episode patients once medication, stabilization, and symptom remission has begun, in order to enhance the goal and expectation of optimum recovery. Typically, the length of treatment is approximately 20 sessions over six months. This allows strategies to be offered to those who may be experiencing a prolonged symptomatic

Table 25.1 Modular approach to cognitive behavior therapy

1. Engagement, assessment, and formulation phase
- Formation and development of the therapeutic alliance
- Use of instruments assessing functioning and symptoms
- Use of instruments specifically relevant to the focus of the therapy
- Development of an individualized formulation begins at the first session and continues through several sessions
- Identification of problem areas
- Development of understanding of the key elements leading to the psychotic disorder and of the factors that maintain the problem areas
- Assessment of the background to psychosis for biological, psychological, and social context presentation to client with therapist's understanding of the etiology, development, and maintenance of the problem
- Presentation of a rationale for the intervention and length and frequency of sessions
- Development of a consensus about treatment goals
- Continued elaboration and refinement of the formulation

2. Psychoeducation
- Offered in an individual or group format

3. Adaptation to psychosis
- Individual's understanding of the disorder
- Impact of psychosis on the self
- Adaptation to the psychosis

4. Treatment of secondary morbidity
- Depression, anxiety, and substance abuse
- Challenging underlying beliefs and assumptions

5. Coping strategies
- Strategies for positive and negative symptoms
- Strategies for functional and emotional problems that arise from the symptoms
- Use of distraction and focusing techniques for voices
- Use of behavioral self-monitoring, paced activity scheduling, assertiveness training, and diary recording of mastery and pleasure for negative symptoms

6. Relapse prevention
- Monitoring for early warning signs of relapse
- Cognitive restructuring of enduring self-schema associated with elevated risk of relapse

7. Techniques to address delusions and beliefs about voices
- *For auditory hallucinations*: collaborative critical analysis of beliefs about the origin and nature of the voice(s), use of voice diaries, reattribution of the cause of the voices, and generation of possible coping strategies
- *For delusions*: identifying precipitating and maintenance factors, modifying distressing appraisal of the symptoms and generating alternative hypotheses for abnormal beliefs.

recovery. A brief description of the modules is presented in Table 25.1.

Phase-specific group treatment

Participating in groups encourages the development of a positive social role. Groups promote self-awareness and identify skills and abilities to enhance the development of identity, especially when self-esteem is low.[15,16] Communicating with peers who are having similar experiences of psychosis, in combination with opportunities to explore alternative explanatory models of illness, can assist with the development of a personal model of psychosis that enhances, rather than hinders, a positive self-esteem. The group provides the opportunity to develop and maintain social skills, improve social relationships, and develop an understanding of the illness. Additionally, participation in groups can provide support and encouragement to take an active role in personal and group decision-making and thus help with the establishment of realistic and practical life goals. It is valuable to have contacts with others who may be at different points in the recovery process. Support and hope can be offered to those who are feeling stuck, lost, or demoralized that recovery is taking too long.[15,16] Groups should be designed to help the individual to manage different phases of illness and recovery following the first episode. As the group addresses later stages of recovery the focus moves from being educational to more cognitive behavioral and eventually encompasses some aspects of interpersonal therapy.[17]

A range of groups can be offered as presented and may be specific to the phase of recovery as in Figure 25.1. These may include psychosis education, recovery, interpersonal skills, and substance abuse. The content of these groups is presented in Tables 25.2–25.4, and have been described in more detail elsewhere.[7] A substance group can be part of a more comprehensive approach to address substance use.[18,19]

Do psychosocial interventions help?

One of the concerns about psychosocial interventions is the lack of quality outcome studies. Out of 2000 published randomized controlled trials (RCTs) for schizophrenia only 8% involved psychological interventions compared with 86% examining medication.[20] Very little information is available about outcome of groups for individuals with psychosis, let alone for those who are presenting with a first episode. There are some preliminary reports in uncontrolled trials of success

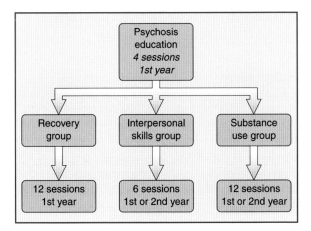

Figure 25.1 Phase-specific group treatment

> **Table 25.2 Psychosis education group**
>
> - Four one-hour sessions
> - Offers information and education
> - Goal is to facilitate acceptance of treatments
> - Educates about:
>   - symptoms
>   - diagnoses
>   - theories and models of psychosis
>   - individual explanatory models
>   - impact of substance use
>   - use of medications
>   - identification of warning signs
>   - avoidance of relapse
>   - introduction to the program.

<table>
<tr><td>Table 25.3 Recovery group</td></tr>
<tr><td>

- 12 weekly sessions
- Includes psychoeducation
- Uses CBT strategies
- Clients:
  - are 3–4 months into recovery
  - have completed psychosis education group
  - are experiencing some symptom remission
- Six sessions focus on understanding impact of illness
- Six session focus on recovery strategies
- Recovery group goals are to:
  - reinforce education on psychosis
  - promote sharing of ideas and experiences
  - increase communication about psychosis
  - promote recovery
  - improve coping
  - decrease isolation and facilitate social reintegration
  - decrease shame
  - improve coping with psychosis
  - help prevent relapse.

</td></tr>
</table>

<table>
<tr><td>Table 25.4 Interpersonal skills group</td></tr>
<tr><td>

- Six sessions
- Specifically for symptoms of social anxiety
- Offers CBT strategies
- Interpersonal skills group goals, to:
  - increase understanding of social anxiety
  - learn strategies for coping with social anxiety
  - decrease level of anxiety in social situations
  - increase confidence in social interactions
  - improve level of social skills and confidence in social situations
  - reduce social alienation and isolation.

</td></tr>
</table>

<table>
<tr><td>Table 25.5 Substance use group</td></tr>
<tr><td>

- Serious implications for psychosis
- Address through all aspects of treatment
- Offer a specialty group
- Specialty group sessions include:
  - education of effects of substances
  - relationship between substances and psychosis
  - goal-setting
  - barriers to quitting
  - learning problem-solving skills
  - relapse prevention.

</td></tr>
</table>

in addressing substance abuse.[18] Cognitive behavioral therapy (CBT) is gaining recognition as a potentially effective treatment for improving outcome among patients with schizophrenia.[21] Four separate RCTs have demonstrated effectiveness of CBT.[22–27] However, only one trial has addressed the use of CBT at the first episode. Results of this trial suggested that at 70 days there were trends towards faster improvement of positive symptoms in the CBT group and at 18 months follow-up, CBT demonstrated significant advantages in outcome over routine care and some advantages over supportive therapy.[28–29]

A major effort is needed to demonstrate the effectiveness of a range of psychosocial interventions at the first episode. Such studies need to examine which treatments are most effective for which individuals and at which stage of recovery.

Summary

We have suggested a range of options for interventions to meet psychosocial needs and to aid recovery from a first episode. It is possible that psychosocial interventions have the potential for improved recovery after the first episode that would render them more than a 'useful adjunct to medication'. There is some preliminary evidence that these interventions make a difference but there is a need for more sophisticated outcome trials. Thus, a major goal for the use of psychosocial treatment is to demonstrate the effectiveness of these interventions at the first episode.

References

1. Ralph RO. *Review of Recovery Literature: A Synthesis of a Sample of Recovery Literature.* Alexandria, VA: National Technical Assistance Center for State Mental Health Planning (NTAC); 2000.
2. Erikson EH. *Childhood and Society.* New York: Norton; 1950.
3. Muuss RE. *Theories of Adolescence.* New York: McGraw-Hill; 1988.
4. Addington J, Leriger E, Addington D. Symptom outcome one year after admission to an early psychosis program. Can J Psychiatry 2003; **48:**204–7.
5. Edwards J, Maude D, McGorry PD, et al. Prolonged recovery in first-episode psychosis. Br J Psychiatry 1998; **172**(Suppl 33):107–16.
6. Lieberman J, Jody D, Geisler S, et al. Time course and biologic correlates of treatment response in first-episode schizophrenia. Arch Gen Psychiat 1993; **50:**369–76.
7. Coldham EL, Addington J, Addington D. Medication adherence of individuals with a first episode of psychosis. Acta Psychiatr Scand 2002; **106:** 286–90.
8. Edwards J, Maude D, Herrmann-Doig T, et al. A service response to prolonged recovery in psychosis. Psychiatr Serv 2002; **50:**1067–9.
9. Robinson D, Woerner MG, Alvir J, et al. Predictors of relapse following response from a first episode of schizophrenia or schizoaffective disorder. Arch Gen Psychiatry 1999; **56:**241–7.
10. Addington J, Young J, Addington D. Social outcome in early psychosis. Psychol Med 2003; **33:**1119–24.
11. Tohen M, Strakowski SM, Zarate CA, et al. The McLean-Harvard first-episode project: 6-month symptomatic and functional outcome in affective and nonaffective psychosis. Biol Psychiatry 2000; **48:**467–76.
12. McGorry PD. The detection and optimal management of early psychosis. In: Lieberman J, Murray RM (eds). *Comprehensive Care of Schizophrenia.* London: Martin Dunitz; 2002:153–66.
13. Addington J, Burnett P. Working with families in the early stages of psychosis. In McGorry PD, Gleeson JF (eds). *Psychological Interventions in Early Psychosis: A Treatment Book.* Chichester: Wiley.
14. Addington J, Gleeson J. Implementing cognitive behavior therapy for first episode psychosis (submitted).
15. Albiston DJ, Francey SM, Harrigan SM. Group programmes for recovery from early psychosis. Br J Psychiatry 1998; **172**(suppl 33):117–21.
16. Early Psychosis Prevention and Intervention Centre (EPPIC). *Working with Groups in Early Psychosis.* [No. 3 in a series of early psychosis manuals]. Victoria, Australia: Psychiatric Services Branch, Human Services; 2000.
17. Addington J, Addington D. Phase specific group treatment for recovery in an early psychosis program (in press).
18. Addington J, Addington D. Impact of an early psychosis program on substance use. J Psychiatr Rehab 2001; **25:**60–7.
19. Addington J. An integrated treatment approach to substance abuse in an early psychosis program. In: Graham H, Mueser K, Birchwood M, Copello A (eds). *Substance Misuse in Psychosis: Approaches to Treatment and Service Delivery.* Chichester: Wiley.
20. Thornley B, Adams C. Content and quality of 2000 controlled trials in schizophrenia over 50 years. BMJ 1998; **317:**1181–4.
21. Cormac I, Jones C, Campbell C. Cognitive behavior therapy for schizophrenia. The Cochrane Database Syst Rev 2002; **2:**1–46.
22. Garety P, Fowler D, Kuipers E, et al. London-East Anglia randomised controlled trial of cognitive-behavioural therapy for psychosis: II. Predictors of outcome. Br J Psychiatry 1997; **171:**319–27.
23. Kuipers E, Garety P, Fowler D, et al. London-East Anglia randomised controlled trial of cognitive-behavioural therapy for psychosis: I. Effects of the treatment phase. Br J Psychiatry 1997; **171:**319–27.
24. Sensky T, Turkington D, Kingdon D, et al. A randomized controlled trial of cognitive-behavioral therapy for persistent symptoms in schizophrenia resistant to medication. Arch Gen Psychiatry 2000; **57:**165–72.
25. Tarrier N, Yusopoff L, Kinney C, et al. Randomized controlled trial of intensive cognitive behavior therapy for patients with chronic schizophrenia. BMJ 1998; **317:**303–7.

26. Tarrier N, Wittkowski A, Kinney C, et al. Durability of the effects of cognitive-behavioural therapy in the treatment of chronic schizophrenia: 12 month follow-up. Br J Psychiatry 1999; **174**:500–4.

27. Tarrier N, Kinney C, McCarthy E, et al. Brief reports: Two-year follow-up of cognitive-behavioral therapy and supportive counseling in the treatment of persistent symptoms in chronic schizophrenia. J Consult Clin Psychol 2000; **68**:917–22.

28. Lewis S, Tarrier N, Haddock G, et al. Randomised controlled trial of cognitive-behavioral therapy in early schizophrenia: Acute-phase outcomes. Br J Psychiatry 2002; **181**:S91–S97.

29. Lewis S, Tarrier N, Haddock G, et al. Cognitive therapy improves 18–month outcomes but not time to relapse in first episode schizophrenia. Schizophr Res 2002; **53**:14.

26

Pharmacological Management

Diana O Perkins and Jeffrey A Lieberman

Introduction

Pharmacological management is the cornerstone of schizophrenia treatment, improving or relieving symptoms and so maximizing patients' ability to benefit from other interventions. The target symptoms and optimal management strategies change as patients move through the acute, recovery, and maintenance treatment phases.

First treatment contact and initiation of antipsychotic medication marks the beginning of the acute phase, targeting positive and acute mood symptoms. The risk of distressing side effects should be minimized at this stage in order to avoid adding to the trauma of a first episode.

In the recovery phase, the patient and their family are coming to terms with the diagnosis, and thus the potential for a disabling, chronic, stigmatizing disorder. Target symptoms include residual positive symptoms, as well as negative and cognitive symptoms. Comorbid disorders, including substance use and major depression, are actively addressed.

Pharmacological management in the maintenance phase targets relapse prevention and functional recovery. Although most individuals recover from a first episode with minimal to no residual psychotic symptoms, relapse risk is high. Acceptance of the high relapse risk may be diffi-cult for recovered patients and their significant others, understandably influencing adherence behavior. Many patients will opt for trials off antipsychotic medication. Despite the fact that most patients will experience positive symptoms remission, most do not achieve functional recovery. Minimizing relapse risk and achieving functional recovery is the challenge of first episode treatment.

Acute phase

The problem of treatment delay

While subclinical 'prodromal' symptoms commonly precede psychosis schizophrenia (and the related schizophreniform and schizoaffective disorders) disorder onset occurs with the onset of psychotic symptoms. Pharmacological treatment should be initiated as close to illness onset as possible for a number of reasons. First, the emerging psychotic and other symptoms of schizophrenia impair social and occupational or school function, with significant functional decline occurring in the first few years of illness. The onset of illness is in late teens to early twenties for about 70% of affected individuals:[1,2] a crucial time for psychosocial development. Emerging psychosis often derails normal development, and early intervention may minimize functional losses. Second, psychosis is associated with behavioral disturbances that later may be viewed as embarrassing or that are criminal and have legal consequences. Third, the onset of psychosis is a period when individuals are at increased risk of aggressive behaviors towards others, property, or themselves.[3] While there is little systematic study of this issue, it stands to reason that the sooner psychosis is appropriately treated, the less the opportunity and thus the risk for aggressive behaviors. Finally, there is emerging evidence that delay in medication treatment may influence likelihood and level of recovery.[4] In most communities on average a year or more elapses from the time psychosis first occurs to first treatment, with the median time to treatment about 3–4 months.[5] The reasons for the treatment delays are not well understood. However, it appears that despite the presence of frank psychotic symptoms the illness may not be recognized by the patient, family, and healthcare provider as a psychosis.[6] While not systematically investigated, it follows that early intervention may improve prognosis. Recent specialized programs directed at community and healthcare provider education and outreach have proven successful in dramatically reducing treatment delays.[7,8]

Antipsychotic choice and dosing

There has been little empiric data to guide optimal pharmacological management of a first episode. There is a general consensus, however, that one of the second generation antipsychotics should be first choice.[9] This consensus is based on the decreased risk of neurological side effects, especially tardive dyskinisia, and the better subjective tolerability of the second generation antipsychotics. With the exception of clozapine, which is reserved for treatment-resistant patients due to its side effect profile, there is no evidence of clinically meaningful differences in efficacy among the second generation antipsychotics.[9] The second generation antipsychotics vary in risk for side effects, including metabolic, endocrine, cardiovascular, weight gain, and sedation.[9] In addition, adolescents and young adults may have greater sensitivity to antipsychotic side effects than patients in later stages of the illness.[10]

The dose of antipsychotic needed to achieve positive symptom remission is typically lower than the dose needed in chronically ill patients and use of lower doses often minimizes side effect risk.[11,12] For example, in a dose-finding study with first generation antipsychotics, first episode patients developed parkinsonian symptoms at much lower doses than chronic patients.[13] In another study, a post-hoc analysis found that low dose risperidone (maximum of equal to or less than 6 mg/day) was more effective and better tolerated than high dose risperidone (greater than 6 mg/day) in first episode subjects.[14] A recent study of 49 acutely psychotic, neuroleptic-naïve patients with schizophrenia, schizophreniform disorder, or schizoaffective disorder found 2 mg or 4 mg daily of risperidone equally efficacious with an advantage for the lower dose in fine motor functioning.[15] Younger patients are also more susceptible to other side effects, such as weight gain.[16,17] Consistent with these studies, the American Psychiatric Association's Guideline for the Treatment of Schizophrenia and the Schizophrenia Patient Outcomes Research Team recommended that patients in a first psychotic episode should be treated with doses that are about half of the dose used in chronic populations.[9,18]

The median time to positive symptom remission is about three months, but many patients will take six months to a year to realize the maximal benefit of the antipsychotic.[19] Clinicians need to avoid pressures to rapidly escalate dose past reasonable target doses, especially in the first few weeks of treatment. Early dose escalation increases the risk of poorly tolerated side effects without the likelihood of more rapid or better symptom response. Furthermore, since the first episode is a time when patients form their attitudes about treatment, efforts that minimize unpleasant side effects may influence patients' willingness to take medications long term. In a study of first episode patients, the only variable that predicted whether patients would attend a follow-up assessment was antipsychotic dose, with those on higher doses less likely to comply.[20]

Treatment of positive symptoms

Studies consistently find positive symptom remission or near remission with both first and second generation antipsychotics. For example, in 70 first episode patients treated with first generation antipsychotics 83% remitted by one year, with mean and median time to remission of 35.7 and 11 weeks, respectively.[21] A more recent randomized double blind clinical trial in 160 first episode patients found that most patients achieved positive symptom remission by one year, whether treated with clozapine (81%) or chlorpromazine (79%).[22] Subjects randomized to clozapine responded more quickly and remained in remission longer than those receiving chlorpromazine, however, suggesting some advantage for the second generation antipsychotic. The positive symptom responsivity of first episode patients is also found in community treatment programs; in one clinical program 37/53 (70%) treated primarily with second generation antipsychotics achieved complete positive symptom remission by one year.[23]

Recovery phase

Treatment of negative and cognitive symptoms

While positive symptoms in first episode patients tend to respond well to antipsychotic drug treatment, negative and cognitive symptoms of schizophrenia generally take longer to respond and are less responsive to antipsychotic medications.[17,24,25] This indicates that negative and cognitive symptoms may have a different time course for response than positive symptoms and/or that the relative refractoriness of negative and cognitive symptoms may contribute to the less than optimal functional recovery that is often observed in first episode patients. Improving treatments for negative and cognitive symptoms in the first episode of

schizophrenia is an area of major importance in future research and drug development efforts, especially since these symptoms probably affect these patients' functional abilities.

Treatment of residual symptoms

Severity of residual positive, and to a greater extent negative and cognitive symptoms, is correlated with level of functional recovery.[26] Residual positive symptoms are often addressed by sequential trials of different antipsychotics, since there may be profound individual differences in response to any given antipsychotic. If residual positive symptoms persist a trial of clozapine or the addition of adjunctive treatments (e.g. valproate[27]) should be considered.[9] Non-pharmacological strategies, specifically cognitive behavioral therapy, have demonstrated efficacy for residual positive symptoms in clinical trial.[28]

There is little systematic study to guide clinicians when confronted with residual mood lability, dysphoria, or anxiety in first episode patients. Benzodiazepines are effective in treating anxiety, but their use is limited if a comorbid substance abuse disorder is present.[29] Mood stabilizers, including anticonvulsants and lithium, are widely used in patients with schizophrenia and there is some evidence that they may also have a role in reducing impulsivity and aggression.[9]

On presentation with an acute psychotic episode, first episode patients often have mood symptoms.[30] Depressive symptoms will often resolve as psychotic symptoms remit,[31] however, in some cases these symptoms may persist or occur in the episode's aftermath ('post-psychotic depression'). The sparse available clinical trial data give mixed results for the value of antidepressants in patients with schizophrenia, even those who meet full major depression syndrome criteria.[32,33] Most clinicians will opt for an antidepressant trial, however, when presented with a depressed patient.[9]

Residual negative symptoms that are primary to schizophrenia (the deficit syndrome) are uncommon in first episode schizophrenia.[34] For most patients, negative symptoms are either secondary to antipsychotic sides effects (e.g. parkinsonian related akinesia or apathy), depression (e.g. social withdrawal, anhedonia), or the effects of illness on self-esteem (e.g. poor motivation due to concerns about failure). Here, treatment should address the underlying cause. Residual primary negative symptoms are difficult to treat, with no proven treatment options. Medications under study include those that effect the N-methyl-D-aspartic acid (NMDA) receptor, such as glycine,[35] d-cycloserine,[36] and also neuro-steroids.[37]

Neurocognitive function is typically impaired in first episode patients, and with antipsychotic treatment neurocognitive function usually stabilizes or improves.[38,39] Similar to negative symptoms, there are few proven treatments to address residual cognitive symptoms. The second generation antipsychotics improve neurocognitive function in first episode patients compared to first generation antipsychotics, with the impact likely to be clinically meaningful.[14,40]

Suicidal risk

A suicide attempt is made by a significant minority (~15–25%) of first episode patients prior to treatment.[41–43] While depression in the presenting psychotic episode or in the post-psychotic period is an important risk factor for suicide, patients with schizophrenia may attempt suicide in the absence of prominent depressive symptoms as a result of hallucinations, paranoia, disorganization, or other symptoms considered more primary to psychosis or other factors. Mounting literature supports the use of clozapine in patients with psychotic disorder and suicidal behaviors.[44] Though its use in first episode schizophrenia has been studied recently,[22] clozapine is not considered at this time a first line drug for first episode schizophrenia. It should be considered early in the course of treatment only in patients who are unresponsive to other second generation antipsychotic drugs or in whom suicidality remains a prominent residual symptom.

Substance use disorders

Substance use and substance use disorders are common in first episode patients. Use of certain substances, in particular marijuana and psychostimulants, may be environmental factors that affect vulnerability to psychosis and impair recovery.[45–47] Illicit substance use is also associated with poor adherence to treatment and thus is associated with increased relapse risk.[48] In addition, the proportion of patients with schizophrenia who are addicted to tobacco is very high, increasing risk of various medical disorders. Thorough evaluation and targeted treatment of substance use is thus a critical component of first episode treatment. The use of pharmacological strategies is not well researched, and clinicians often turn to strategies proven to be useful in substance-dependent patient populations.[49]

Maintenance phase

Relapse prevention

The risk of eventual relapse after recovery from a first psychotic episode is very high and is greatly diminished by maintenance antipsychotic treatment. However, the majority of patients proceed to have one or more psychotic relapses from which some proportion fail to recover, at least to the same degree as from their first episode.[50] This process of psychotic relapse, treatment failure, and incomplete recovery, leads many patients to a chronic course of illness.[51] The deterioration process predominantly occurs in the early phases of the illness, during the first five to 10 years after the initial episode.

However, even with strong evidence of the risk of relapse without antipsychotic medication, there is still no clear consensus on the recommended duration of treatment for patients who have recovered from a first episode of schizophrenia. The recently published American Psychiatric Association's Practice Guideline for the Treatment of Schizophrenia (p. 26) recommends:[9]

In arriving at a plan of treatment with remitted first-episode patients, clinicians should engage patients in discussion of the long-term potential risks of maintenance treatment with the prescribed antipsychotic versus risk of relapse (e.g. effect of relapse on social and vocational function, risk of dangerous behaviors with relapse, and risk of developing chronic treatment-resistant symptoms). Prudent treatment options that clinicians may discuss with remitted patients include either 1) indefinite antipsychotic maintenance medication or 2) medication discontinuation with close follow-up and a plan of antipsychotic reinstitution with symptom recurrence.

During both the acute phase and, more importantly, the maintenance phase of treatment close monitoring for medication side effects is necessary. This should include regular monitoring for abnormal involuntary movements and parkinsonian symptoms, sexual side effects, weight gain, metabolic status (e.g. glucose, cholesterol, triglycerides), and sedation.[9]

Functional recovery

First episode patients treated in routine clinical settings typically have a deteriorating illness course despite good initial symptomatic response. For example, in a study of 349 patients followed up to 15 years after their first onset of schizophrenia, 17% had no disability at follow-up, while 24% still suffered from severe disability, and the remaining 69% had varying degrees of disability.[52] Specialized first episode treatment programs may improve functional outcomes.[8,25,53] While functional recovery is probably maximized with long-term maintenance antipsychotic treatment and the use of adjunctive pharmacological treatments for any residual symptoms, for most patients, optimal pharmacological treatment will not be sufficient. The best psychosocial interventions for first episode patients are still not known, although specialized first episode treatment programs may employ a combination of strategies with some indication of success.

Conclusions

The treatment goal for first episode patients is positive symptom remission, amelioration of negative and cognitive symptoms, and functional recovery. Sequential trials of adequate dose and duration of antipsychotics and adjunctive treatments should be employed to help patients achieve their optimal response and so set the stage for benefiting from available psychosocial therapies. Once remission from the first episode is reached the clinician and patient face the difficult issue of maintenance treatment duration. Despite remission, relapse risk is very high. Clinically useful predictors of the small minority who maintain remission without pharmacotherapy have not yet been identified, and the optimal length of maintenance treatment for recovered patients is not known.

Atypical antipsychotics represent an advance in the treatment of first episode schizophrenia with strong evidence for greater tolerability with equal or better therapeutic efficacy. While future research will help to characterize their efficacy relative to one another and define the effect of their use on the long-term outcomes of schizophrenia, available evidence and consensus expert opinion support their use as first line treatment in first episode schizophrenia.

References

1. Alda M, Ahrens B, Lit W, et al. Age of onset in familial and sporadic schizophrenia. Acta Psychiatr Scand 1996; **93:**447–50.
2. Hafner H, Nowotny B, Loffler W, Maurer K. When and how does schizophrenia produce social deficits? Eur Arch Psychiatry Clin Neurosci 1995; **246:**17–28.
3. Milton J, Amin S, Singh SP, et al. Aggressive incidents in first-episode psychosis. Br J Psychiatry 2001; **178:**433–40.
4. Norman RM, Malla AK. Duration of untreated psychosis: a critical examination of the concept and its importance. Psychol Med 2001; **31:**381–400.
5. Larsen TK, Friis S, Haahr U, et al. Early detection

and intervention in first-episode schizophrenia: a critical review. Acta Psychiatr Scand 2001; **103**:323–34.

6. Addington J, van Mastrigt S, Hutchinson J, Addington D. Pathways to care: help seeking behaviour in first episode psychosis. Acta Psychiatr Scand 2002; **106**:358–64.

7. Johannessen JO, McGlashan TH, Larsen TK, et al. Early detection strategies for untreated first-episode psychosis. Schizophr Res 2001; **51**:39–46.

8. Malla A, Norman R, McLean T, et al. A Canadian programme for early intervention in non-affective psychotic disorders. Aust N Z J Psychiatry 2003; **37**:407–13.

9. Practice guideline for the treatment of patients with schizophrenia (2nd edn). Am J Psychiatry 2004; **161**:1–56.

10. Walter G, Wiltshire C, Anderson J, Storm V. The pharmacologic treatment of the early phase of first-episode psychosis in youths. Can J Psychiatry 2001; **46**:803–9.

11. Cullberg J. Integrating intensive psychosocial therapy and low dose medical treatment in a total material of first episode psychotic patients compared to 'treatment as usual': a 3 year follow-up. Med Arh 1999; **53**:167–70.

12. Chakos MH, Alvir JM, Woerner MG, et al. Incidence and correlates of tardive dyskinesia in first episode of schizophrenia. Arch Gen Psychiatry 1996; **53**:313–19.

13. McEvoy JP, Hogarty GE, Steingard S. Optimal dose of neuroleptic in acute schizophrenia. A controlled study of the neuroleptic threshold and higher haloperidol dose. Arch Gen Psychiatry 1991; **48**:739–45.

14. Emsley RA. Risperidone in the treatment of first-episode psychotic patients: a double-blind multicenter study. Risperidone Working Group. Schizophr Bull 1999; **25**:721–9.

15. Merlo MC, Hofer H, Gekle W, et al. Risperidone, 2 mg/day vs. 4 mg/day, in first-episode, acutely psychotic patients: treatment efficacy and effects on fine motor functioning. J Clin Psychiatry 2002; **63**:885–91.

16. Kumra S, Jacobsen LK, Lenane M, et al. Case series: spectrum of neuroleptic-induced movement disorders and extrapyramidal side effects in childhood-onset schizophrenia. J Am Acad Child Adolesc Psychiatry 1998; **37**:221–7.

17. Lieberman JA, Tollefson G, Tohen M, et al. Comparative efficacy and safety of atypical and conventional antipsychotic drugs in first-episode psychosis: a randomized, double-blind trial of olanzapine versus haloperidol. Am J Psychiatry 2003; **160**:1396–404.

18. Lehman AF, Steinwachs DM. Translating research into practice: the Schizophrenia Patient Outcomes Research Team (PORT) treatment recommendations. Schizophr Bull 1998; **24**:1–10.

19. Loebel AD, Lieberman JA, Alvir JM, et al. Duration of psychosis and outcome in first-episode schizophrenia. Am J Psychiatry 1992; **149**:1183–8.

20. Jackson H, McGorry P, Henry L, et al. Cognitively oriented psychotherapy for early psychosis (COPE): a 1-year follow-up. Br J Clin Psychol 2001; **40**(Pt 1):57–70.

21. Robinson DG, Woerner MG, Alvir JM, et al. Predictors of treatment response from a first episode of schizophrenia or schizoaffective disorder [see comments]. Am J Psychiatry 1999; **156**:544–9.

22. Lieberman JA, Phillips M, Gu H, et al. Atypical and conventional antipsychotic drugs in treatment-naïve first-episode schizophrenia: a 52–week randomized trial of clozapine vs chlorpromazine. Neuropsychopharmacology 2003; **28**:995–1003.

23. Malla AK, Norman RM, Manchanda R, et al. Status of patients with first-episode psychosis after one year of phase-specific community-oriented treatment. Psychiatr Serv 2002; **53**:458–63.

24. Kopala LC, Fredrikson D, Good KP, Honer WG. Symptoms in neuroleptic-naïve, first-episode schizophrenia: response to risperidone. Biol Psychiatry 1996; **39**:296–8.

25. Addington J, Leriger E, Addington D. Symptom outcome 1 year after admission to an early psychosis program. Can J Psychiatry 2003; **48**:204–7.

26. Malla AK, Norman RM, Manchanda R, Townsend L. Symptoms, cognition, treatment adherence and functional outcome in first-episode psychosis. Psychol Med 2002; **32**:1109–19.

27. Casey DE, Daniel DG, Wassef AA, et al. Effect of divalproex combined with olanzapine or risperidone in patients with an acute exacerbation of schizophrenia. Neuropsychopharmacology 2003; **28**:182–92.

28. Haddock G, Tarrier N, Spaulding W, et al. Individual cognitive-behavior therapy in the treatment of hallucinations and delusions: a review. Clin Psychol Rev 1998; **18**:821–38.

29. Wolkowitz OM, Pickar D. Benzodiazepines in the treatment of schizophrenia: a review and reappraisal. Am J Psychiatry 1991; **148:**714–26.

30. Addington D, Addington J, Patten S. Depression in people with first-episode schizophrenia. Br J Psychiatry Suppl 1998; **172:**90–2.

31. Koreen AR, Siris SG, Chakos M, et al. Depression in first-episode schizophrenia [see comments]. Am J Psychiatry 1993; **150:**1643–8.

32. Addington D, Addington J, Patten S, et al. Double-blind, placebo-controlled comparison of the efficacy of sertraline as treatment for a major depressive episode in patients with remitted schizophrenia. J Clin Psychopharmacol 2002; **22:**20–5.

33. Levinson DF, Umapathy C, Musthaq M. Treatment of schizoaffective disorder and schizophrenia with mood symptoms. Am J Psychiatry 1999; **156:**1138–48.

34. Mayerhoff DI, Loebel AD, Alvir JM, et al. The deficit state in first-episode schizophrenia. Am J Psychiatry 1994; **151:**1417–22.

35. Heresco-Levy U, Javitt DC, Ermilov M, et al. Efficacy of high-dose glycine in the treatment of enduring negative symptoms of schizophrenia. Arch Gen Psychiatry 1999; **56:**29–36.

36. Goff DC, Tsai G, Levitt J, et al. A placebo-controlled trial of D-cycloserine added to conventional neuroleptics in patients with schizophrenia. Arch Gen Psychiatry 1999; **56:**21–7.

37. Strous RD, Maayan R, Lapidus R, et al. Dehydroepiandrosterone augmentation in the management of negative, depressive, and anxiety symptoms in schizophrenia. Arch Gen Psychiatry 2003; **60:**133–41.

38. Townsend LA, Norman RM, Malla AK, et al. Changes in cognitive functioning following comprehensive treatment for first episode patients with schizophrenia spectrum disorders. Psychiatry Res 2002; **113:**69–81.

39. Hoff AL, Sakuma M, Wieneke M, et al. Longitudinal neuropsychological follow-up study of patients with first-episode schizophrenia. Am J Psychiatry 1999; **156:**1336–41.

40. Keefe RSE, Seidman LJ, Christensen BK, et al. and the HGDH Research Group. Comparative effect of atypical and conventional antipsychotic drugs on neurocognition in first-episode psychosis: a randomized double-blind trial of olanzapine versus haloperidol. Am J Psychiatry 2004 (in press).

41. Cohen S, Lavelle J, Rich CL, Bromet E. Rates and correlates of suicide attempts in first-admission psychotic patients. Acta Psychiatr Scand 1994; **90:**167–71.

42. Steinert T, Wiebe C, Gebhardt RP. Aggressive behavior against self and others among first-admission patients with schizophrenia. Psychiatr Serv 1999; **50:**85–90.

43. Addington J, Williams J, Young J, Addington D. Suicidal behaviour in early psychosis. Acta Psychiatr Scand 2004; **109:**116–20.

44. Meltzer HY, Alphs L, Green AI, et al. Clozapine treatment for suicidality in schizophrenia: International Suicide Prevention Trial (InterSePT). Arch Gen Psychiatry 2003; **60:**82–91.

45. Linszen DH, Dingemans PM, Lenior ME. Cannabis abuse and the course of recent-onset schizophrenic disorders. Arch Gen Psychiatry 1994; **51:**273–9.

46. Hambrecht M, Hafner H. Cannabis, vulnerability, and the onset of schizophrenia: an epidemiological perspective. Aust N Z J Psychiatry 2000; **34:**468–75.

47. Andreasson S, Allebeck P, Engstrom A, Rydberg U. Cannabis and schizophrenia. A longitudinal study of Swedish conscripts. Lancet 1987; **2:**1483–6.

48. Coldham EL, Addington J, Addington D. Medication adherence of individuals with a first episode of psychosis. Acta Psychiatr Scand 2002; **106:**286–90.

49. Noordsy DL, Green AI. Pharmacotherapy for schizophrenia and co-occurring substance use disorders. Curr Psychiatry Rep 2003; **5:**340–6.

50. Lieberman JA, Alvir JM, Koreen A, et al. Psychobiologic correlates of treatment response in schizophrenia. Neuropsychopharmacology 1996; **14:**13S–21S.

51. Lieberman JA. Is schizophrenia a neurodegenerative disorder? A clinical and neurobiological perspective. Biol Psychiatry 1999; **46:**729–39.

52. Wiersma D, Nienhuis FJ, Slooff CJ, Giel R. Natural course of schizophrenic disorders: a 15-year follow-up of a Dutch incidence cohort. Schizophr Bull 1998; **24:**75–85.

53. Carbone S, Harrigan S, McGorry PD, et al. Duration of untreated psychosis and 12–month outcome in first-episode psychosis: the impact of treatment approach [see comments]. Acta Psychiatr Scand 1999; **100:**96–104.

Index